OCULUS RES GESTAE
A Neophyte's Animative & Videographic Compendium

OCULUS RES GESTAE
A Neophyte's Animative & Videographic Compendium

Editors-in-Chief
Prasanna Venkatesh Ramesh
MS (Gold Medal) DNB MNAMS FICO (Glaucoma) FAICO (Glaucoma) FAICO (Cataract/Phaco)(Gold Medal)
Fellow in Glaucoma Surgery and Research (Dr Sathyan's)
DNB Coordinator, Medical Officer
Mahathma Eye Hospital Private Limited
Tiruchirappalli, Tamil Nadu, India

Shruthy Vaishali Ramesh
MS (Gold Medal) DNB MNAMS FICO (Cataract/Phaco) FAICO (Cataract/Phaco) FRCOphth
Fellowship in Comprehensive Ophthalmology and Phacoemulsification
Ophthalmic Specialty Doctor
Blackpool Victoria Hospital
England, UK

Forewords
Lalit Verma, S Natarajan, Shibal Bhartiya, Mohan Rajan,
VR Vijayaraghavan, P Sathyan, Diva Kant Misra

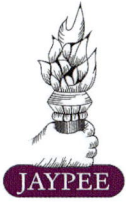

JAYPEE BROTHERS MEDICAL PUBLISHERS
The Health Sciences Publisher
New Delhi | London

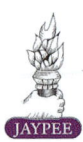 **Jaypee Brothers Medical Publishers (P) Ltd**

Headquarters
Jaypee Brothers Medical Publishers (P) Ltd
EMCA House, 23/23-B
Ansari Road, Daryaganj
New Delhi 110 002, India
Landline: +91-11-23272143, +91-11-23272703
+91-11-23282021, +91-11-23245672
Email: jaypee@jaypeebrothers.com

Corporate Office
Jaypee Brothers Medical Publishers (P) Ltd
4838/24, Ansari Road, Daryaganj
New Delhi 110 002, India
Phone: +91-11-43574357
Fax: +91-11-43574314
Email: jaypee@jaypeebrothers.com

Overseas Office
JP Medical Ltd
83 Victoria Street, London
SW1H 0HW (UK)
Phone: +44 20 3170 8910
Fax: +44 (0)20 3008 6180
Email: info@jpmedpub.com

Website: www.jaypeebrothers.com
Website: www.jaypeedigital.com

© 2025, Jaypee Brothers Medical Publishers

The views and opinions expressed in this book are solely those of the original contributor(s)/author(s) and do not necessarily represent those of editor(s) or publisher of the book.

All rights reserved. No part of this publication may be reproduced, stored or transmitted in any form or by any means, electronic, mechanical, photocopying, recording or otherwise, without the prior permission in writing of the publishers.

All brand names and product names used in this book are trade names, service marks, trademarks or registered trademarks of their respective owners. The publisher is not associated with any product or vendor mentioned in this book.

Medical knowledge and practice change constantly. This book is designed to provide accurate, authoritative information about the subject matter in question. However, readers are advised to check the most current information available on procedures included and check information from the manufacturer of each product to be administered, to verify the recommended dose, formula, method and duration of administration, adverse effects and contraindications. It is the responsibility of the practitioner to take all appropriate safety precautions. Neither the publisher nor the author(s)/editor(s) assume any liability for any injury and/or damage to persons or property arising from or related to use of material in this book.

This book is sold on the understanding that the publisher is not engaged in providing professional medical services. If such advice or services are required, the services of a competent medical professional should be sought.

Every effort has been made where necessary to contact holders of copyright to obtain permission to reproduce copyright material. If any have been inadvertently overlooked, the publisher will be pleased to make the necessary arrangements at the first opportunity.

Inquiries for bulk sales may be solicited at: jaypee@jaypeebrothers.com

Oculus Res Gestae: A Neophyte's Animative & Videographic Compendium
First Edition: **2025**

ISBN: 978-93-6616-348-2

Printed at: Samrat Offset Pvt. Ltd.

Dedication

To Amma and Appa, for shaping my journey; to my family, for their unwavering love and support; to my teachers, for lighting the path of knowledge; to God, for strength and guidance; and to Mahathma Eye Hospital Private Limited and the Mahathma Centre of Moving Images Pvt Ltd (MCMI) Team for making this journey possible.
With heartfelt gratitude, I dedicate this work to you all.

*Learning is the supreme light that removes the darkness of ignorance,
just as medicine cures disease.*

Contributors

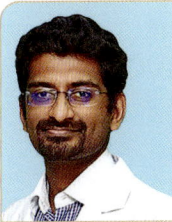

Prasanna Venkatesh Ramesh
MS (Gold Medal) DNB MNAMS FICO (Glaucoma) FAICO (Glaucoma) FAICO (Cataract/Phaco) (Gold Medal) Fellow in Glaucoma Surgery and Research (Dr Sathyan's)
DNB Coordinator, Medical Officer
Mahathma Eye Hospital Private Limited
Trichy, Tamil Nadu, India
email2prajanna@gmail.com

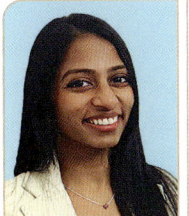

Shruthy Vaishali Ramesh
MS (Gold Medal) DNB MNAMS FICO (Cataract/Phaco) FAICO (Cataract/Phaco) FRCOphth
Fellowship in Comprehensive Ophthalmology and Phacoemulsification
Ophthalmic Specialty Doctor
Blackpool Victoria Hospital
England, UK
vaishusmail@gmail.com

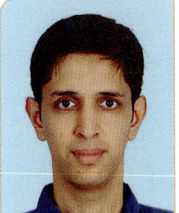

Aditya Maitray
MS FMRF
Senior Consultant
Vitreoretina Services and Ocular Oncology
Aravind Eye Hospital
Chennai, Tamil Nadu, India
aditya.maitray@gmail.com

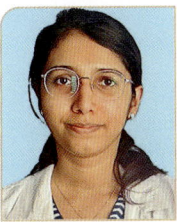

Ajanya K Aradhya
BSc Optometry (GMC Kozhikode)
Consultant Optometrist
Mahathma Eye Hospital Private Limited
Tiruchirappalli, Tamil Nadu, India
ajanyak777@gmail.com

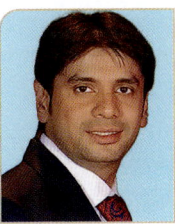

Aman Khanna
MBBS MS FVRS
Consultant (Vitreo-Retina, Uvea and Phaco)
Khanna Eye Centre
New Delhi, India
dramanrkhanna@gmail.com

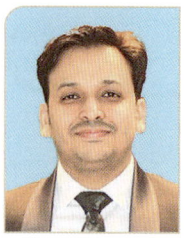

Ankit Agrawal
MD Pediatrics (Gold Medalist) DM Pediatric Gastroentrology
Assistant Professor
Department of Pediatric Gastroentrology
Post Graduate Institute of Child Health
Noida, Uttar Pradesh, India
ankitagrawal456798@gmail.com

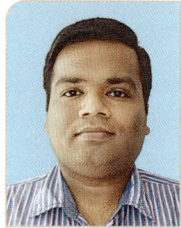

Ankit Agrawal
MBBS MS
Consultant and Phaco-Refractive Surgeon
Krishna Eye Foundation
Eye Clinic
Prayagraj, Uttar Pradesh, India
ankit1989@gmail.com

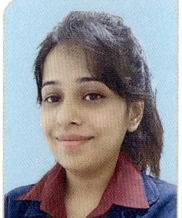

Ankita Aishwarya Agrawal
MS (Gold Medalist) FIOOP FICO MRCSEd (UK)
Senior Resident
Department of Ophthalmology
Post Graduate Institute of Child Health
Noida, Uttar Pradesh, India
anki.twinki@gmail.com

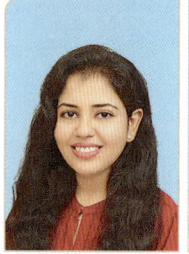

Ankita Mulchandani
MBBS MS DNB FPRS
Consultant
Ophthalmologist and Cataract and Refractive Surgeon
Mumbai Eye Care Cornea and LASIK Centre
An ASG Enterprise
Mumbai, Maharashtra, India
dr.ankita02@gmail.com

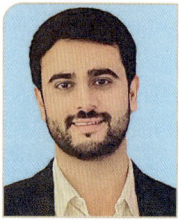

Anuj Kodnani
MS (Ophth) DNB FWCRS FTVPEI (Cornea & Refractive Surgery) (Moorfields - London, Bascom Palmer - USA, CFS, London Vision Clinic) AHA-CLS (Retina & Glaucoma, LVPEI) MNAMS FAGE
anuj_kodnani@yahoo.co.in

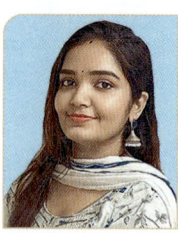

Anugraha Balamurugan
MBBS MS FVRS
Head (Vitreo Retinal Services)
Mahathma Eye Hospital Private Limited
Tiruchirappalli, Tamil Nadu, India
anuumoonn@gmail.com

Contributors

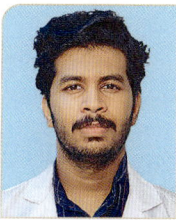

Ashik Azad
BSc Optometry JIPMER
Consultant Optometrist
Mahathma Eye Hospital Private Limited
Tiruchirappalli, Tamil Nadu, India
ashiqazad27@gmail.com

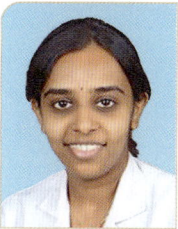

Bhavatharini M
FRCS (Gl)
Senior Consultant
Department of Ophthalmology
Pushpagiri Eye Institute
Hyderabad, Telangana, India
btharini@gmail.com

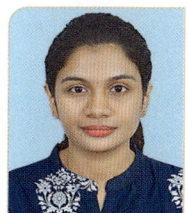

Deepika Beeraka
MS (Ophthalmology) FICO
Consultant
Aravind Eye Hospital and Postgraduate Institute of Ophthalmology
Madurai, Tamil Nadu, India
deepika.brk849@gmail.com

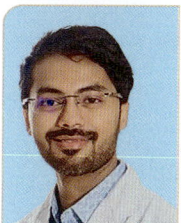

Dhaivat Shah
MBBS MS DNB FMRF (Sankara Nethralaya, Chennai)
Joint Medical Director and Head
Department of Vitreoretina, Research and Academics
Choithram Netralaya
Indore, Madhya Pradesh, India
dhaivatkshah@gmail.com

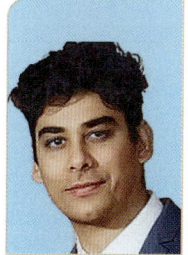

Gaurav M Kohli
MD DNB FVRS
Assistant Professor
Era's Medical College, Lucknow
Consultant (Vitreo-Retina, Uvea and ROP)
Era Group of Hospitals
Lucknow, Uttar Pradesh, India
Drkohligaurav@gmail.com

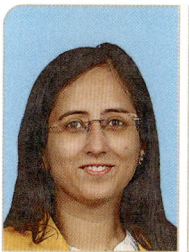

Gunjan Saluja
MD (AIIMS, New Delhi) DNB FICO FRCS FAICO (Pediatric Ophthalmology and Strabismus) Ex Senior Resident AIIMS, New Delhi
Director and Consultant
Strabismus and Oculoplasty Services
Bhatia Netralaya
Bhilai, Chhattisgarh, India
gunjansaluja2015@gmail.com

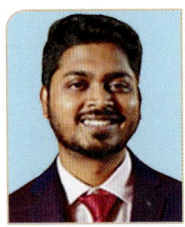

Himanshu Prakash
MBBS MS (Ophthalmology)
Lady Hardinge Medical College
New Delhi, India
himanshu.maurya1509@gmail.com

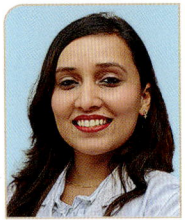

Isha Acharya
MBBS MS FVRS FAICO (Retina & Vitreous)
Vitreo-retina Consultant
Sharp Sight Eye Hospital
New Delhi, India
dr.acharyaisha@gmail.com

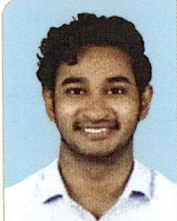

Kalyan Basa
MBBS MS (Ophthalmology) (2nd year)
Junior Resident
Department of Ophthalmology
Jawaharlal Institute of Postgraduate Medical Education and Research
Puducherry, India
kalyanbasa.kb@gmail.com

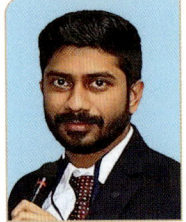

Karthikeyan Mahalingam
MBBS MD (Ophthalmology)
Assistant Professor
Department of Ophthalmology
Jawaharlal Institute of Postgraduate Medical Education and Research
Puducherry, India
kalingachit@gmail.com

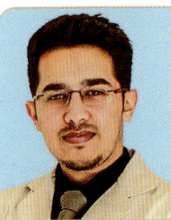

Kshitij Raizada
MBBS MS (Ophthalmology)
Vitreo-Retina, Uvea and ROP Specialist
Dr Raizaday Eye Centre
raizada.13@gmail.com

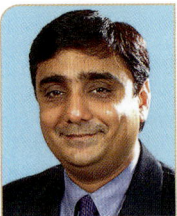

Kumar Doctor
MBBS MD DNB
Cataract and Refractive Surgeon
Doctor Eye Institute, Mumbai, India
kumarlaser@gmail.com

Contributors **xi**

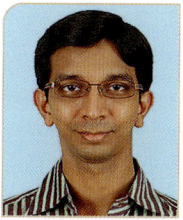

Kushal S Delhiwala
MBBS MS (Ophthalmology) FMRF FICO FAICO(VR)
Vitreoretina and Uvea Consultant
Netralaya Superspeciality Eye Hospital
Ahmedabad, Gujarat, India
kushal.delhiwala@yahoo.co.in

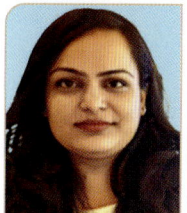

Lipi Mittal
MBBS MS FAICO (Refractive Surgery) FASGEH
Fellow (Cataract and Refractive Surgery)
ASG Eye Hospital
Jodhpur, Rajasthan, India
Lipi.26mittal@gmail.com

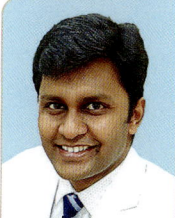

Madanagopalan VG
MS (Ophthalmology)
Consultant
Vitreoretinal Services
JB Eye Care and Retina Centre
Salem, Tamil Nadu, India
drmadanagopalan@gmail.com

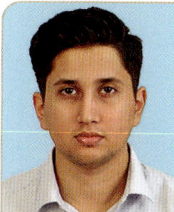

Manan Balvant Mistry
MBBS
Ophthalmology Resident
Aravind Eye Hospital
Chennai, Tamil Nadu, India
mistry.manan@outlook.com

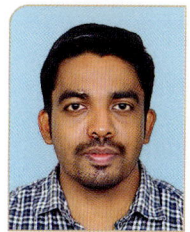

Mary Stephen
Academic Senior Resident (Glaucoma)
Department of Ophthalmology
Jawaharlal Institute of Postgraduate Medical Education and Research
Puducherry, India
stephen6752@gmail.com

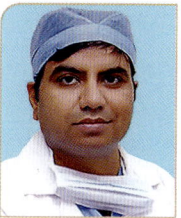

Mayank Sharma
MBBS MS FASGEH
Consultant and Head (Cataract and Refractive Surgery)
ASG Eye Hospital
Jodhpur, Rajasthan, India
drmayanksharma001@gmail.com

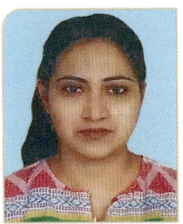

Mousumi Banerjee
MD (AIIMS, Delhi) FAICO (Retina)
Assistant Professor
Maharaja Agrasen Medical College
Agroha, Haryana, India
banerjeemou12@gmail.com

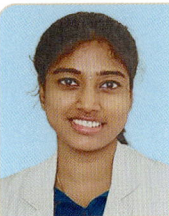

N Shastikaa
MS DNB
Fellow at Mahathma Eye Hospital Private Limited
Tiruchirappalli, Tamil Nadu, India
shastikaa.janani7@gmail.com

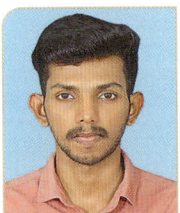

Navaneeth Krishna MP
BSc Optometry JIPMER
Consultant Optometrist
Mahathma Eye Hospital Private Limited
Tiruchirappalli, Tamil Nadu, India
nkmpchlr@gmail.com

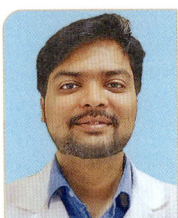

Nilesh Kumar
MBBS DOMS DNB
Consultant and Medical Director
Madhavi Netralaya
Arrah, Bihar, India
n.nilesh.kumar@gmail.com

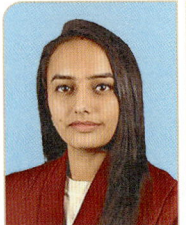

Nitika Beri
MS DNB FAICO (Glaucoma)
Assistant Professor
Department of Ophthalmology
University College of Medical Sciences and Guru Teg Bahadur Hospital
New Delhi, India
berinitika@gmail.com

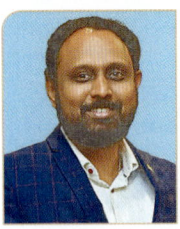

Nivean M
MS (Ophthalmology)
Vitreoretinal services
MN Eye Hospital
Chennai, Tamil Nadu, India
nivean69@gmail.com

Contributors xiii

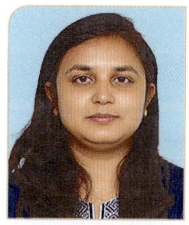

Pallavi Goel
MBBS DNB FVRS FICO
Vitreo Retina Fellow
Dr Shroff's Charity Eye Hospital
New Delhi, India
pg150393@gmail.com

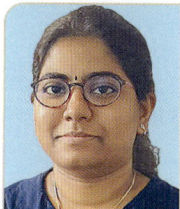

Pavithra P
MBBS DNB (Ophthalmology)
DNB Resident
Mahathma Eye Hospital, Pvt Ltd
Tiruchirappalli, Tamil Nadu, India
pavithrapannerselvam@gmail.com

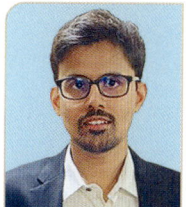

Pratik Shenoy
MBBS DNB FVRS FICO
Vitreo-Retina Consultant
Isha Netralaya
Thane, Maharashtra, India
drpratikshenoy@gmail.com

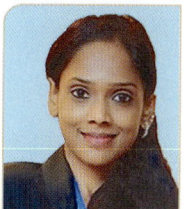

Puja Maitra
DNB FICO MRCS (Ed) FMRF
Consultant (Pediatric Retina and Ocular Oncology)
Aravind Eye Hospital
Chennai, Tamil Nadu, India
pujamaitra@gmail.com

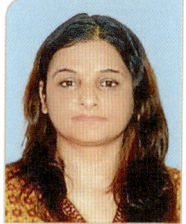

Rachna Agrawal
MS (Ophthalmology)
Additional Professor
Department of Ophthalmology
Sanjay Gandhi Postgraduate Institute of Medical Sciences
Lucknow, Uttar Pradesh, India
rachna7500@yahoo.co.in

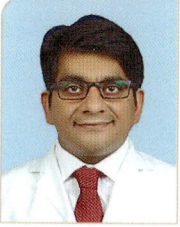

Rajat Kapoor
FRCS (Gl)
Senior Consultant
Department of Ophthalmology
Pushpagiri Eye Institute
Hyderabad, Telangana, India
drrajatkapoor86@gmail.com

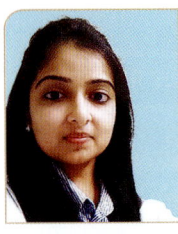

Rinal Pandit
MBBS MS (Gold Medalist) FMRF (Sankara Netralaya, Chennai) FAICO (Glaucoma)
Consultant (Glaucoma Services)
Choithram Netralaya
Indore, Madhya Pradesh, India
rinalpandit@gmail.com

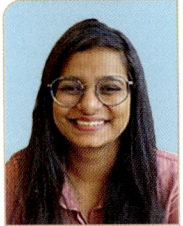

Ritu Singh
MS DNB MNAMS
Assistant Professor
All India Institute of Medical Sciences–Central Armed Police Forces Institute of Medical Sciences (CAPFIMS)
New Delhi, India
ritusingh.diya@gmail.com

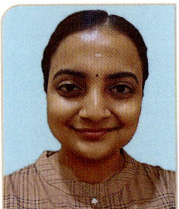

Sai Thaejesvi Gopalakrishnan
MBBS
Postgraduate Resident
Mahathma Eye Hospital Private Limited
Tiruchirappalli, Tamil Nadu, India
sai.thaejesvi@gmail.com

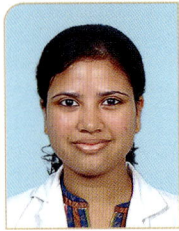

Sameeksha Agrawal
MBBS DNB MNAMS FVRS
Consultant and Vitreo-Retina Surgeon
Krishna Eye Foundation
Eye Clinic
Prayagraj, Uttar Pradesh, India
sameeksha.agrawal92@gmail.com

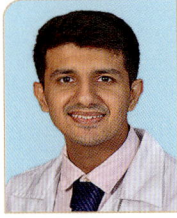

Sameer Chaudhary
MS (Ophthalmology)
Consultant
Aravind Eye Hospital and Postgraduate Institute of Ophthalmology
Madurai, Tamil Nadu, India
sameerchaudhary22@outlook.com

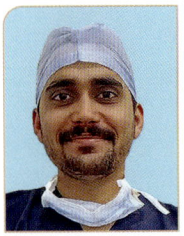

Sandeep Choudhary
MBBS MS
Consultant
Cataract, Refractive Surgery, Cornea and Glaucoma
ASG Eye Hospital
Jaipur, Rajasthan, India
drsandeep7001@gmail.com

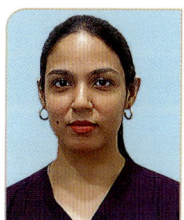

Shivani P Pattnaik
MBBS MS (Ophthalmology)
Cataract and Refractive Surgeon
Doctor Eye Institute
Mumbai, Maharashtra, India
drshivanipattnaik14@gmail.com

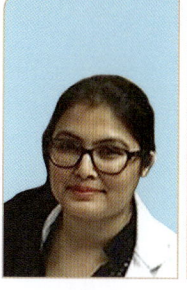

Sunandini Bose
MBBS MS (Ophthalmology) FSNC
Director
Dr Sunandini Eye Care and Cornea Clinic
Head
Department of Ophthalmology
Bhagat Hospitals Pvt Ltd
New Delhi, India
sunandini_bose@yahoo.in

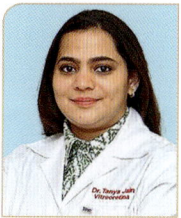

Tanya Jain
MBBS DNB FVRS FICO
Consultant
Dr Shroff's Charity Eye Hospital
New Delhi, India
tanyajain_t@yahoo.com

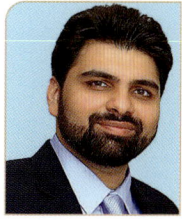

Zain Khatib
MBBS MS DNB FICO FAICO (Cataract) FAICO (Refractive Surgery)
Consultant Ophthalmologist
Khatib Eye Clinic
Mumbai, Maharashtra, India
zainkhatib89@gmail.com

Foreword

It is my proud privilege and honor to be writing a foreword for this beautiful masterpiece, *Oculus Res Gestae: A Neophyte's Animative & Videographic Compendium* by one of the finest innovators in ophthalmology Dr Prasanna Venkatesh Ramesh.

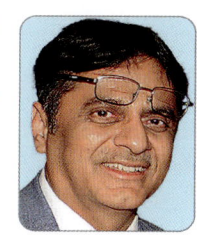

Oculus Res Gestae aspires to be a definitive resource for pedagogy, combining the expertise of distinguished professionals to offer invaluable insights to neophyte readers, particularly undergraduate (MBBS) and postgraduate (ophthalmology) students.

What sets Oculus Res Gestae apart is its emphasis on visual learning, incorporating multimedia elements such as images, videographic links, animative content, and equational explanations to enhance understanding—serving as essential tools for experiential learning. Each topic is thoroughly covered, from foundational concepts to advanced surgical procedures, with concise writeups designed to convey essential information clearly and effectively.

Besides being a Must for all budding ophthalmologists, it is also a useful read for seniors for a quick revision.

Congratulations to Dr Prasanna Venkatesh Ramesh, one of our very active members of Young Ophthalmologists Society of India (YOSI), and all the authors who have contributed to this wonderful, out-of-world masterpiece—I know it is not an easy task!

Lalit Verma
MD
Director (Vitreo-Retina Services)
Centre for Sight, New Delhi, India
Congress President, Asia-Pacific Academy of Ophthalmology
Past President, All India Ophthalmological Society
Secretary General, South Asian Academy of Ophthalmology

Foreword

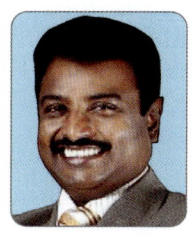

A landmark resource for aspiring ophthalmologists. In an era where the field of ophthalmology is rapidly advancing, it is essential that our methods of education evolve in tandem. *Oculus Res Gestae* stands as a landmark resource, thoughtfully crafted to meet the needs of future ophthalmologists. This book offers a harmonious blend of foundational principles and cutting-edge surgical insights, all presented through a modern multimedia framework that enhances the learning experience.

The thoughtfully organized chapters, authored by distinguished specialists in the field, exemplify the significance of clarity and precision in disseminating complex medical knowledge. Each contribution reflects a deep commitment to teaching, ensuring that readers not only grasp essential concepts but also cultivate the skills necessary for success in their careers.

Oculus Res Gestae is poised to become an indispensable companion for any student aspiring to excellence in ophthalmology. May it inspire and equip the next generation of eyecare professionals to navigate the challenges and opportunities that lie ahead.

With great anticipation,

S Natarajan
MBBS DO FRVS FICO (UK) FRCS FELAS
Principal Investigator
Aditya Jyot Eye Hospital, Mumbai, Maharashtra, India
Awarded the Padma Shri by the President of India
President, Tele Ophthalmology Society of India (TOSI)
Chief, Clinical Services, Aditya Jyot Eye Hospital (AJEH)
Chief, Vitreoretinal Services, Dr Agarwal's Group of Eye Hospitals World Wide
Trustee, International Council of Ophthalmology (ICO)
President, APOTS
Chief Patron, Sankara Nethralaya Alumni
Vice President, Global Eye Genetics Consortium
Board Member, RWC, ISOT
Chief Advisor, Ophthalmic Trauma Society of Africa
Managing Trustee, Kamala Sundaram Foundation
Founding Chairman & Director
Sundaram Natarajan Blind Free India Foundation

Foreword

It is with great honor and joy that I write the foreword for *Oculus Res Gestae: A Neophyte's Animative & Videographic Compendium*, a book that stands as a remarkable resource for both undergraduate and postgraduate students embarking on the journey of ophthalmology.

Ophthalmology is a dynamic and ever-evolving field, one that requires a profound understanding of both the foundational principles and the cutting-edge advancements that continually reshape patient care. This comprehensive work exemplifies the fusion of traditional knowledge and pedagogy with modern multimedia learning tools. Through a unique collaboration between editors and contributors, *Oculus Res Gestae* blends time-tested expertise with innovative technology. The inclusion of images, videos, animations, and interactive content provides an immersive experience—one that extends beyond the capabilities of traditional textbooks.

What truly sets *Oculus Res Gestae* apart is its multidisciplinary approach. Covering a vast array of topics—from the complexities of the cornea and lens to the intricacies of the retina and vitreous—each subject is explored with precision and clarity. The chapters span from basic anatomy to advanced surgical techniques, offering invaluable insight into the full scope of ophthalmic care. Specialized topics such as strabismus, ocular surface disorders, and vitreoretinal surgery further underscore the depth of knowledge contained within.

In an era where visual learning plays an essential role in medical education, this compendium sets a new standard by seamlessly integrating multimedia resources. This innovative approach not only reinforces theoretical knowledge but also provides students with a practical, hands-on understanding of procedures and conditions. Each chapter, contributed by renowned professionals in their respective fields, ensures that the content is both authoritative and approachable.

As the great Physician and Educator William Osler once said, "The good physician treats the disease; the great physician treats the patient who has the disease." *Oculus Res Gestae* is not just an educational tool but an invitation for students to engage deeply with the material, fostering a greater understanding and appreciation of the complexities of the human eye and the art of healing.

I am confident that this book will become an indispensable resource for aspiring ophthalmologists, equipping them with the knowledge, skills, and inspiration necessary to make meaningful contributions to the field. And on a personal note, I would like to congratulate Dr Prasanna Venkatesh Ramesh on his remarkable contribution to ophthalmic pedagogy: may this be the first of many!

Best wishes,

Shibal Bhartiya
MBBS MS (Ophthalmology)
Clinical Director
Department of Ophthalmology
Marengo Asia Hospitals, Gurugram
Program Director
Community Outreach and Wellness
Marengo Asia Hospitals
Gurugram and Faridabad, Haryana, India
Research Collaborator
Department of Ophthalmology
Mayo Clinic
Jacksonville, FL, USA

Foreword

Ophthalmology is a field where precision, clarity, and a deep understanding of anatomy and physiology are essential. Yet, for many students and practitioners, grasping the complexities of the eye through static images and dense text can be challenging. This book takes a different approach—bringing ophthalmology to life through the power of animation.

Visual learning has always been a cornerstone of medical education, but modern technology allows us to go beyond traditional diagrams. By using animations, this book transforms abstract concepts into dynamic, intuitive lessons. The movement of ocular structures, the pathophysiology of diseases, and even surgical techniques are easier to comprehend when seen in action. This method not only enhances retention but also makes learning engaging and efficient.

Whether you are a medical student, a resident, or a clinician looking for a fresh perspective, this book provides a visually rich and accessible foundation in ophthalmology. The animations, combined with clear explanations, ensure that even complex topics become approachable.

I am confident that this innovative approach will help bridge the gap between theory and practice, inspiring a deeper appreciation for the intricate world of ophthalmology. Enjoy the journey, and may this book illuminate your path to mastering the eye.

I compliment Dr Prasanna Venkatesh Ramesh on his innovative approach and lateral thinking in producing this masterpiece.

Mohan Rajan
MBBS DO FMRF MNAMS MCh FACS DNB DD FIAMS FRCS PhD DSc
Chairman and Medical Director
Rajan Eye Care Hospital
Chennai, Tamil Nadu, India
President SN Alumni Association
Past President, Tamil Nadu Ophthalmic Association
Past Secretary, Madras City Ophthalmic Association
Past President, Indian Intraocular Implant and Refractive Society of India

Foreword

It is a pleasure to write a foreword for the book edited by my dear student, Dr Prasanna Venkatesh Ramesh of Mahathma Eye Hospital Private Limited, Tiruchirappalli, Tamil Nadu, India. Dr Prasanna, a great hard-working ophthalmologist, who stood first in his postgraduate examination, has been doing a lot of work in innovative ophthalmology.

This book, *Oculus Res Gestae: A Neophyte's Animative & Videographic Compendium*, is a masterpiece. This book has topics which are very important for postgraduate students in ophthalmology. The topics are approached in a simple way that can be understood by all the students.

Understanding these topics will definitely help the students to appear for all the examinations including FRCS and others with great confidence. The topics in the book will have a lightbulb effect on students, helping them understand difficult concepts with ease. I am sure that Dr Prasanna, a gold medalist, will bring more innovative books in the future to help the student community. I wish him success.

I feel that he is an asset to the field of ophthalmology.

VR Vijayaraghavan
MBBS DO MS DNB FRCS
Academic Director
Arasan Eye Hospital
Erode, Tamil Nadu, India
Vice President, Tamil Nadu Ophthalmic Association

Foreword

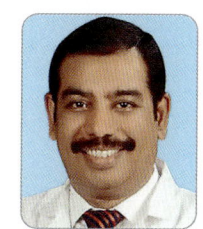

The field of ophthalmology continues to grow at an astonishing pace, fueled by advancements in technology and a deeper understanding of eye health and disease. Amid this dynamic landscape, the need for educational resources that engage and inspire learners has never been greater. *Oculus Res Gestae: A Neophyte's Animative & Videographic Compendium* arrives at just the right time to fill this vital role.

What makes this book particularly noteworthy is its commitment to clarity and accessibility. It combines well-structured concise explanations with carefully curated visual materials, including images, animations, and videographic contents to simplify complex concepts. This fresh perspective makes complex topics easier to understand and practical applications more accessible.

The book also excels in its comprehensiveness, addressing an array of subjects ranging from the basics of anatomy and physiology to the complexities of advanced surgical techniques. Its structure ensures that both budding learners and experienced practitioners will find immense value within its pages. Moreover, by focusing on clarity and precision, the compendium delivers knowledge in a way that respects the time and learning needs of its readers.

Behind this work is the collective expertise of contributors who are leaders in ophthalmology. The dedication of the authors and editors to crafting an effective, student-focused resource is evident in every chapter. By presenting content in a concise, well-organized format, they have ensured that this book will serve as a reliable reference for years to come.

It is a privilege to endorse *Oculus Res Gestae* as a meaningful contribution to ophthalmic education. I am confident that this work will inspire and guide the next generation of eye care professionals in their pursuit of excellence.

P Sathyan
MBBS DO DNB
Director Sathyan Eye Care Hospital and
Coimbatore Glaucoma Foundation (SEH and CGF)
President Glaucoma Society of India

Foreword

It is with great pleasure that I write the foreword for *Oculus Res Gestae: A Neophyte's Animative & Videographic Compendium*, an innovative and much-needed contribution to ophthalmic education. This book, curated under the able leadership of Dr Prasanna Venkatesh Ramesh, represents a paradigm shift in medical learning, catering to the evolving needs of young ophthalmologists in a visually immersive manner.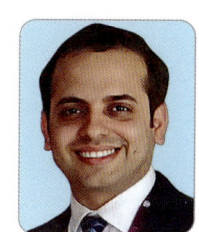

As we navigate the ever-expanding frontiers of ophthalmology, the integration of multimedia learning tools is becoming increasingly essential. This compendium, meticulously structured with animative content, videographic links, and equational explanations, provides an experiential learning approach that complements traditional pedagogical methods. The book effectively bridges the gap between theoretical knowledge and clinical practice, ensuring that both undergraduate and postgraduate students develop a nuanced understanding of key ophthalmic concepts and procedures.

One of the most compelling aspects of this work is its commitment to clarity and accessibility. The inclusion of fundamental topics, from ocular anatomy and physiology to intricate surgical techniques, makes it a comprehensive resource for students at different stages of their learning journey. Furthermore, the contributions from distinguished ophthalmologists lend the book a richness of perspective, offering readers insights from some of the finest minds in the field.

In today's dynamic educational landscape, where visual engagement enhances cognitive retention, *Oculus Res Gestae* stands out as a vital resource. It aligns perfectly with our collective goal of fostering a generation of well-trained, confident, and skillful ophthalmologists. I commend Dr Prasanna Venkatesh Ramesh and the esteemed contributors for their dedication in creating this masterpiece, which will undoubtedly leave a lasting impact on ophthalmic education.

I am honored to contribute this foreword and look forward to seeing this remarkable book benefit aspiring ophthalmologists worldwide.

Diva Kant Misra
MBBS DO DNB MNAMS FVRS
Director and Head (Retina Services)
Swarnjyoti Eye Hospital
Lucknow, Uttar Pradesh, India
President, Young Ophthalmologists Society of India

Preface

Ophthalmology is a field where visualizing concepts is as important as understanding them. Traditional textbooks often rely on extensive text to explain complex topics, but we believe that *a concise, multimedia-integrated approach* can significantly enhance learning. *Oculus Res Gestae: A Neophyte's Animative & Videographic Compendium* is designed to bridge this gap by combining precise textual content with videos, animations, and infographics, making learning more engaging and clinically relevant.

This book is tailored for *young ophthalmologists*, including those in training and early in their careers, as well as clinicians seeking a quick yet detailed reference. Each chapter is structured to prioritize clarity over verbosity, ensuring that essential concepts are easily grasped. The QR codes have been integrated throughout the book, linking to high-quality videos, animations, and surgical demonstrations, allowing readers to visualize procedures and techniques rather than relying solely on descriptions.

The content is based on up-to-date knowledge and clinical expertise, ensuring accuracy, credibility, and practical relevance. Additionally, we have collaborated with experts in the field to refine the material and ensure its clinical applicability. While we have aimed for brevity, important points have not been compromised, catering to those who prefer reading alongside visual learning.

We extend our gratitude to the contributors, mentors, and institutions that have supported this endeavor. This book is a product of extensive teamwork, innovation, and dedication. We hope it serves as a valuable resource, simplifying complex topics while enhancing understanding and clinical application.

Prasanna Venkatesh Ramesh
Shruthy Vaishali Ramesh

Acknowledgments

With utmost gratitude, I begin by expressing my deepest thanks to the Almighty, whose blessings have guided me through this journey.

I extend my heartfelt appreciation to my parents, Dr Ramesh Rajesekaran and Dr Meena Kumari, whose unwavering support and encouragement have been my greatest strength. Their dedication to medicine and education has been the foundation of my own journey. A special mention goes to my grandmother, Mrs Manonmani, whose blessings and wisdom continue to inspire me.

I am thankful to my wife, Dr B Anugraha Prasanna, and my wonderful daughters, Pranu and Hasanna, whose love, patience, and sacrifices have been my constant source of inspiration. Their unwavering belief in me has been the driving force behind my endeavors.

I am deeply grateful to my sister, Dr Shruthy Vaishali Ramesh, who has played a pivotal role in shaping this book as the Co-Chief Editor. Her dedication, expertise, and meticulous contributions have been instrumental in bringing this project to life.

A special note of appreciation extends to my father-in-law, Dr R Balamurugan, and my mother-in-law, Mrs B Vijayalakshmi, for their constant encouragement and support throughout my professional journey.

I am forever grateful to my mentor, Dr P Sathyan, whose guidance, wisdom, and encouragement have been instrumental in shaping my professional journey. His unwavering support has inspired me to strive for excellence in both clinical practice and academics.

I take immense pride in Mahathma Eye Hospital Private Limited, Tiruchirappalli, Tamil Nadu, India, which has been the foundation of my clinical and academic growth. The institution's commitment to excellence in ophthalmic care and education has provided me with invaluable opportunities to innovate and advance in the field. I extend my sincere gratitude to the staff and patients of Mahathma Eye Hospital, whose trust and experiences have shaped my perspective as a Clinician and Educator.

My heartfelt appreciation extends to my research team at the Mahathma Centre of Moving Images Pvt Ltd (MCMI) for their dedication to enhancing visual learning in this book. Mr Navaneeth Krishna MP, Mr Ashik Azad, Mr Pragash Raj, Mr Tensing Joshua, Mr Sheik Mohammed, Mrs Prajnya, Mr Aji K, and Ms Ajanya K Aradhya have contributed immensely through their expertise in high-quality imaging and content development, helping bridge the gap between theory and clinical practice.

A special acknowledgment goes to my alma maters, PSG Institute of Medical Sciences and Research, Coimbatore, Tamil Nadu and Mahatma Gandhi Medical College and Research Institute, Puducherry, for laying the strong academic foundation that has guided me throughout my career.

I am deeply thankful to all the authors who contributed their expertise and knowledge to each chapter, ensuring the book's comprehensive and insightful content. Their valuable contributions have helped shape *Oculus Res Gestae: A Neophyte's Animative & Videographic Compendium* into a resource that benefits both undergraduate and postgraduate students.

Finally, I extend my gratitude to M/s Jaypee Brothers Medical Publishers (P) Ltd, New Delhi, India, for believing in this vision and ensuring its wide distribution, making it accessible to students and professionals across the globe.

This book is a culmination of shared efforts, and I am forever grateful to each person who played a role in making *Oculus Res Gestae: A Neophyte's Animative & Videographic Compendium* a reality.

Prasanna Venkatesh Ramesh

Acknowledgments

As I pen this note of gratitude, I extend my deepest gratitude to my father, Dr Ramesh Rajesekaran, and my mother, Dr Meena Kumari, whose unwavering support and encouragement have shaped my academic and professional pursuits. Their dedication to the field of ophthalmology has been an enduring source of inspiration.

I extend my heartfelt appreciation to my brother, Dr Prasanna Venkatesh Ramesh, the Editor-in-Chief of Oculus Res Gestae. Collaborating on this book has been an incredible journey, and I am honored to have contributed as the Co-Chief Editor. His passion for innovation and knowledge has set a high benchmark, and his commitment to advancing ophthalmology is truly commendable.

I am deeply grateful to my husband, for his unwavering support, patience, and encouragement throughout this endeavor. His belief in my work and constant motivation have been invaluable in balancing my professional and personal aspirations.

A special note of thanks goes to Mahathma Eye Hospital Private Limited, Tiruchirappalli, Tamil Nadu, India, for being a pillar of excellence in ophthalmology and for fostering an environment that nurtures clinical and academic brilliance. The institution has played a crucial role in our professional journeys, providing a platform for research, learning, and innovation.

I am deeply appreciative of the research team at the Mahathma Centre of Moving Images Pvt Ltd (MCMI) for their dedication to creating high-quality visual content that enhances the learning experience. Mr Navaneeth Krishna MP, Mr Ashik Azad, Mr Pragash Raj, Mr Tensing Joshua, Mr Sheik Mohammed, Mrs Prajnya, Mr Aji K, and Ms Ajanya K Aradhya have been instrumental in integrating advanced imaging techniques that bridge the gap between theoretical knowledge and clinical practice.

My sincere gratitude extends to all the contributing authors whose expertise and knowledge have shaped each chapter of this book. Their valuable insights have ensured that *Oculus Res Gestae: A Neophyte's Animative & Videographic Compendium* serves as a comprehensive and insightful resource for both undergraduate and postgraduate students.

Lastly, I thank M/s Jaypee Brothers Medical Publishers (P) Ltd, New Delhi, India, for their support and belief in this project, enabling its reach to students and professionals worldwide.

This book is a testament to shared efforts, dedication, and a passion for knowledge. I am truly grateful to everyone who has played a role in bringing *Oculus Res Gestae* to life.

Shruthy Vaishali Ramesh

Contents

1. **Anatomy of Limbus** 1
   Zain Khatib

2. **Lens Embryology and Growth** 2
   Nilesh Kumar

3. **Physiology of Eye and Vision** 20
   Mary Stephen, Kalyan Basa, Karthikeyan Mahalingam

4. **Refraction Part 1** 30
   Zain Khatib

5. **Refraction Part 2** 31
   Zain Khatib

6. **Basic Concepts Related to Strabismus** 32
   Zain Khatib

7. **Evaluation of a Case of Squint** 33
   Zain Khatib

8. **Strabismus** 34
   Gunjan Saluja

9. **Ocular Surface Disorders** 54
   Ritu Singh

10. **Corneal Lacerations and Management Protocols** 58
    Sunandini Bose

11. **Keratoconus** 70
    Sai Thaejesvi, Prasanna Venkatesh Ramesh, Shruthy Vaishali Ramesh, Navaneeth Krishna MP, Ashik Azad, Pavithra P

12. **Posterior Polar Cataract** 74
    Lipi Mittal, Sandeep Choudhary, Mayank Sharma

13. **Pediatric Cataract** 79
    Rajat Kapoor, Bhavatharini M

14. **Mastering the Art of Capsulorhexis: A Transition to Forceps Continuous Curvilinear Capsulorhexis** 88
    Shivani P Pattnaik, Kumar Doctor

15. **Tips and Tricks in Phacoemulsification** 93
    Ankita Mulchandani

16. **Argentinian Flag Sign Management** 101
    Anuj Kodnani

17. 2.5-mm Blunt Tip Chopper to the Rescue 102
    Anuj Kodnani

18. CM-T Flex IOL and XNIT 103
    Madanagopalan VG, Nivean M

19. Decoding Secondary Glaucomas... 104
    Rinal Pandit

20. Secondary Angle-closure Glaucomas 107
    Rinal Pandit

21. Insights into Intraocular Pressure and Glaucoma Dynamics 109
    Nitika Beri

22. Recent Advances in Medical Management 111
    Rinal Pandit

23. Disorders of Vitreous 113
    Kushal S Delhiwala

24. Retinopathy of Prematurity 118
    Puja Maitra, Aditya Maitray, Manan Balvant Mistry

25. Diabetic Eye Disease 125
    Aman Khanna, Gaurav M Kohli, Tanya Jain, Pratik Shenoy, Pallavi Goel

26. Current Approaches in the Diagnosis and Management of
    Sub-internal Limiting Membrane Hemorrhage 144
    Dhaivat Shah

27. Optical Coherence Tomography Biomarkers in Diabetic Macular Edema 149
    Isha Acharya, Himanshu Prakash

28. Ocular Ultrasonography in Retinal Disorders 160
    Mousumi Banerjee

29. Vitrectomy 168
    *N Shastikaa, Prasanna Venkatesh Ramesh, Shruthy Vaishali Ramesh,
    Anugraha Balamurugan, Ashik Azad, Navaneeth Krishna MP, Ajanya K Aradhya*

30. Vogt–Koyanagi–Harada Disease 171
    Sameeksha Agrawal, Ankit Agrawal

31. Optic Neuritis 174
    Sameer Chaudhary, Deepika Beeraka

32. Thyroid Eye Disease 184
    Ankita Aishwarya Agrawal, Rachna Agrawal, Ankit Agrawal

33. Laser-induced Ocular Injuries 188
    Kshitij Raizada

Index *193*

Video Contents

Chapter 1: Anatomy of Limbus

Video 1: Anatomy of Limbus.

Chapter 3: Physiology of Eye and Vision

Video 1: Video demonstrating the parts of the eye.

Video 2: Video explaining the mechanism for aqueous humor formation.

Video 3: Video explaining the aqueous humor outflow. The aqueous humor is produced from nonpigmented epithelium of ciliary body and pass through posterior chamber into anterior chamber via pupil. With aqueous convection current, the aqueous humor produced pass to the angle and involves in two drainage pathways. Conventional trabecular pathway, where via trabecular meshwork pass through Schlemm's canal and drains to venous circulation. Uveoscleral outflow passes along the surface of iris and uveal tissue to pass through suprachoroidal space and drains to venous circulation.

Video 4: Self-explanatory video explaining the major factors which play a crucial role in maintaining corneal transparency and metabolism. The individual layers are explained in detail.

Video 5: Self-explanatory video of the lens metabolism and the various pathways which provides nutrient support to the lens.

Video 6: Video explaining the break of rhodopsin with light into opsin and retinal which then joins to form rhodopsin after passing through a cyclical change.

Video 7: Video demonstration of the three components of binocular single vision. Simultaneous binocular perception is represented by two dissimilar objects (cage in one eye and bird in one eye) seen by individual eyes which appear as single image (bird inside the cage). Fusion is represented by ability of human eyes to fuse two similar images (one image with hat and other image with shoe) with minor difference to form a single composite image (image with both hat and shoe). Stereopsis is the ability to obtain depth by superimposition of two pictures of same objects taken at slightly different angle (bucket handle orientation).

Video 8: Videographic representation of visual pathway starting from the light rays falling in retina till visual cortex. Retinal fibers are divided into nasal (decussate to opposite side) and temporal (passes in same side) go through optic nerve to reach optic chiasma and optic tract. From lateral geniculate body via optic radiations, the fibers will reach the occipital lobe. The various levels of damage in visual pathway are represented in the video. Damage of same side optic nerve results in total blindness of that side, lesion at optic chiasma leads to bitemporal hemianopia, with homonymous hemianopia in lesion posterior to optic chiasma.

Video 9: Videographic representation of the pupillary pathway where in light falls on the photoreceptors, the impulse passes through optic nerve, optic tract to reach pretectal nucleus from there both sides of Edinger–Westphal nucleus gets stimulated which via ciliary ganglion tends to cause pupillary constriction in both eyes resulting in both direct and consensual light reflex.

Chapter 4: Refraction Part 1

Video 1: Refraction Part 1.

Chapter 5: Refraction Part 2

Video 1: Refraction Part 2.

Chapter 6: Basic Concepts Related to Strabismus

Video 1: Basic concepts related to strabismus.

Chapter 7: Evaluation of a Case of Squint

Video 1: Evaluation of a case of squint.

Chapter 8: Strabismus

Video 1: Demonstration of extraocular movements.

Video 2: Cover test [performed for tropia (manifest squint). On occluding the normal eye of patient, the squinting eye takes up fixation].

Video 3: Uncover test (performed for latent squint. On uncovering, the eye under cover moves to take up fixation).

Video 4: Krimsky test and prism bar cover test. The apex of prism is kept toward the direction of deviation. The test is done for both distance and near fixation. Cover test is performed gradually with increasing strength of prism till no refixation movement is obtained.

Video 5: Measurement of near point convergence and near point accommodation using RAF rule. (measured with the help of RAF rule) Near point of convergence is the nearest point at which the target appears double. Normal NPC is 8–10 cm. Near point of accommodation is the nearest point at which target appears blurred.

Video 6: Synaptophore.

Video 7: Four prism base-out test for microtropia.

Video 8: V-pattern.

Video 9: Diplopia charting and Hess chart.

Video 10: Forced duction test.

Video 11: Active force generation test.

Video 12: Superior oblique palsy and head tilt test.

Video 13: Torsion evaluation.

Video 14: Sixth nerve palsy.

Video 15: Duane's retraction syndrome.

Video 16: Brown's syndrome.

Chapter 10: Corneal Lacerations and Management Protocols

Video 1: Siedel test-graft dehiscence.

Video 2: Subtenon block.

Video 3: Partial corneal tear with foreign body removal.

Chapter 13: Pediatric Cataract

Video 1: Demonstrating steps of pediatric lens aspiration, IOL implantation, primary posterior capsulotomy, and anterior vitrectomy.

Chapter 14: Mastering the Art of Capsulorhexis: A Transition to Forceps Continuous Curvilinear Capsulorhexis

Video 1: Creating a perfect continuous curvilinear capsulorhexis (CCC) with cystitome.

Video 2: Forceps continuous curvilinear capsulorhexis (CCC).

Video 3: Physics of continuous curvilinear capsulorhexis (CCC).

Video 4: How to enter the eye like a Pro?

Video 5: Grasping correctly.

Video 6: *Hybrid approach:* Needle initiation, forceps completion of continuous curvilinear capsulorhexis (CCC).

Chapter 15: Tips and Tricks in Phacoemulsification

Video 1: How to make a cystitome.

Video 2: Tips and tricks in phacoemulsification.

Chapter 16: Argentinian Flag Sign Management

Video 1: Argentinian flag sign management.

Chapter 17: 2.5-mm Blunt Tip Chopper to the Rescue

Video 1: 2.5-mm blunt tip chopper to the rescue.

Chapter 18: CM-T Flex IOL and XNIT

Video 1: CM-T Flex IOL.

Video 2: XNIT.

Chapter 23: Disorders of Vitreous

Video 1: Mittendorf dot with cloquet canal remnant.

Video 2: Vitreous degeneration.

Video 3: Vitreous hemorrhage.

Video 4: Intravitreal triamcinolone acetonide (IVTA).

Video 5: Vitritis.

Chapter 28: Ocular Ultrasonography in Retinal Disorders

Video 1: Retinal detachment.

Video 2: Giant retinal tear.

Video 3: Vitreous hemorrhage.

Video 4: Tractional retinal detachment.

Chapter 31: Optic Neuritis

Video 1: Animation showing a case scenario of a typical case of optic neuritis—its presentation, clinical features, and management.

Chapter 33: Laser-induced Ocular Injuries

Video 1: Large retinal hole following injury by Q-Switched Nd:YAG laser.

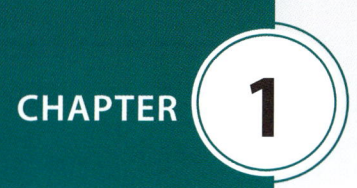

Anatomy of Limbus

Zain Khatib

The limbus, a transitional zone located at the junction between the cornea and the sclera, holds significant importance in both anatomical studies and surgical practices. Understanding its structural and functional characteristics requires consideration from two viewpoints: The anatomical limbus and the surgical limbus. Everything an ophthalmologist needs to know about the limbus and its clinical applications have been explained in detail in this chapter.

a. Understanding anatomical and surgical limbus
b. Concept of blue zone and white zone
c. Limbus with respect to angle and gonioscopy
d. Palisades of Vogt
e. Clinical application of limbus anatomy to surgery

Kindly scan the QR code below to access the online Videos.

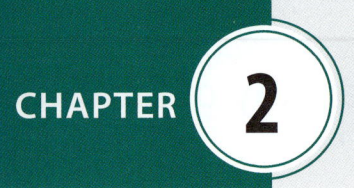

CHAPTER 2

Lens Embryology and Growth

Nilesh Kumar

INTRODUCTION

The lens develops from surface ectoderm beginning around day 22 of embryonic development. Key stages include:
- *Lens placode formation:* Thickening of surface ectoderm adjacent to optic vesicle
- *Lens pit formation:* Lens placode invaginates, forming a depression or pit
- *Lens vesicle formation:* Detachment of invaginated lens pit from surface ectoderm
- *Primary fiber cell formation:* Elongation of posterior lens vesicle cells
- *Secondary fiber cell formation:* Differentiation of equatorial epithelial cells

The lens expands continuously throughout life. New fiber cells are continually added at the lens's equator and resulting in a layered configuration with oldest cells at the core (nucleus) and youthful cells at the periphery (cortex).

Lens growth involves several key processes:[1]
- Proliferation of lens epithelial cells at the equatorial germinative zone
- Migration of epithelial cells posteriorly
- Differentiation into fiber cells, involving cell elongation and organelle loss
- Synthesis of crystallin proteins and other lens-specific proteins
- Formation of specialized membrane junctions between fiber cells

The rate of lens growth declines with age but continues throughout life. In humans, lens weight increases from approximately 65 mg at birth to 250 mg by age 80 years. This persistent growth contributes to age-related changes in lens morphology and function. A comprehensive understanding of lens embryology and growth patterns is essential for elucidating the pathogenesis of congenital cataracts and age-related lens alterations. It also informs surgical techniques, as different lens layers have distinct properties that impact cataract extraction.

ANATOMY OF THE LENS

The natural crystalline lens is positioned behind the iris diaphragm within the patellar fossa of the anterior vitreous face. It is held in place by the zonules, which attach it circumferentially to the ciliary body. The lens continues to grow throughout life, transitioning from a slightly rounded ovoid shape in childhood to a more flattened ovoid shape in old age. The lens always contains several key anatomical components:
- *Capsule:* The lens capsule originates as the basement membrane of the epithelial cells of the embryonic lens vesicle. As development progresses, the capsule differentiates into distinct anterior and posterior regions. The anterior capsule remains a basement membrane for the epithelial cells, while the posterior capsule becomes a thin membrane adherent to the fiber cells. With age, the capsule becomes thicker, particularly anteriorly, although it remains thinnest posteriorly. The elasticity of the capsule enables it to transmit forces from the ciliary body during accommodation, though it does

not significantly alter the lens shape. This elasticity also facilitates the expansion of openings created during Nd:YAG laser capsulotomy. Posterior capsule opacification (PCO) following cataract surgery occurs due to the proliferation and migration of epithelial cells along the intact capsule, a process that may reflect the natural movement of epithelial cells from the midperiphery to the equator. Understanding PCO formation has been an area of intense research, as its treatment is second only to cataract surgery itself in ophthalmic healthcare costs.

- *Epithelium:* The lens epithelium is composed of a single layer of cuboidal cells on the anterior surface, which extends to the lens bow, where new fiber cells are generated. As the individual ages, the epithelial cells become shorter in height and wider in width. The epithelium is metabolically active and vulnerable to injury. Recent studies have highlighted significant age-related changes in the lens epithelium, such as regions of markedly flattened cells and areas where epithelial coverage is entirely absent. However, these changes appear to be more related to aging than cataract formation specifically.
- *Cortex:* The lens cortex comprises the outer layers of lens fibers. Key regions include:
  - *Peripheral cortex:* Just beneath the anterior epithelium or posterior capsule
  - *Supranuclear cortex:* Adjacent to the adult nucleus
  - *Epinucleus:* Equivalent to the supranuclear region
  - *Sutures:* Lines formed by abutting ends of lens fibers
    The cortex continuously adds new fiber layers throughout life, with the posterior cortex remaining thinner than the anterior. An interesting difference exists between the anterior and posterior—posterior fibers peel off easily from the capsule during surgery, while anterior epithelial cells remain adherent.
- *Nucleus:* The lens nucleus consists of several concentric layers:
  - *Epinucleus:* Outermost nucleus/innermost cortex
  - *Adult nucleus:* Next innermost layer
  - *Fetal nucleus:* Corresponds to cotyledonous areas in clear adult lens
  - *Embryonal nucleus:* Innermost core

Surgically, the nucleus is characterized by a densely sclerotic posterior third, slightly less sclerotic central core, and softer peripheral shell. Nuclear sclerosis refers to the increasing rigidity with age, while nuclear opalescence describes the opacification. Brunescence refers to the yellowing/darkening of the nucleus color with age. Understanding of the lens's detailed surgical anatomy and its age-related changes is crucial for cataract surgeons to plan and execute successful procedures across patients of all ages. The increasing fragility of the capsule, syneretic vitreous, and hardening of the nucleus in older patients presents unique surgical challenges compared to pediatric or young adult cataracts.

OPTICAL BASIS OF TRANSPARENCY AND LIGHT SCATTERING

The transparency of the normal lens derives from its regular fiber arrangement and minimal spatial variation in refractive index relative to the wavelength of incident light. In cataractous lenses, more abrupt changes occur in the refractive index due to:

- Accumulation of low refractive index fluid between fiber cells in cortical and subcapsular cataracts

- Formation of very high molecular weight cytoplasmic protein aggregates in nuclear cataracts
- Binding of high molecular weight aggregates to cellular membranes in all forms of cataracts.

These alterations lead to the formation of light-scattering foci that interfere with the normal transmission of light through the lens, ultimately causing reduced transparency and visual impairment.

LENS PHYSIOLOGY

Active transport mechanisms in the lens epithelium move ions, amino acids, and other metabolites. Water movement in the lens is governed by the movement of ions or osmotically active substances. Disruption of normal water movement can lead to rapid cataract formation, as seen in some cases of poorly managed diabetic ketoacidosis.

The lens actively accumulates certain substances like ascorbic acid (vitamin C) from the aqueous humor. Recent identification of specific ascorbic acid transporters in lens epithelial cells provides insight into how the lens maintains its antioxidant defenses.

Maintenance of proper lens hydration and transparency requires careful regulation of ion concentrations and osmotic gradients across lens membranes. Dysfunction of regulatory mechanisms, whether from metabolic disorders, trauma, or other causes, can rapidly lead to lens opacification.

LENS BIOCHEMISTRY

The unique biochemical composition of the lens is critical for maintaining its transparency and refractive properties. Key biochemical features include:

- *Crystallins:* The major structural proteins of the lens, comprising up to 90% of total lens protein. There are three main families:
  1. α-*crystallins:* Function as molecular chaperones to prevent protein aggregation
  2. β-*crystallins:* Contribute to lens refractive index
  3. γ-*crystallins:* Highly concentrated in lens nucleus and important for lens transparency

  Crystallins undergo various post-translational modifications with age, including oxidation, deamidation, and truncation. These changes can lead to protein aggregation and cataract formation.

- *Cytoskeletal proteins:* Maintain lens fiber cell shape and organization. These include:
  - Beaded filaments (phakinin and filensin)
  - Spectrin
  - Actin
- *Membrane proteins:* Critical for lens fiber cell structure and function. Major proteins include:
  - *Aquaporin 0 (MIP)*: Forms water channels
  - *Connexins*: Form gap junctions for intercellular communication
- *Antioxidant systems*: Protect lens from oxidative damage. Key components are as follows:
  - Glutathione
  - Ascorbic acid
  - Superoxide dismutase
  - Catalase
- *Metabolic enzymes*: Support lens energy production and maintain redox balance. These include:
  - Glycolytic enzymes
  - Pentose phosphate pathway enzymes
  - Glutathione peroxidase and reductase

CATARACT

Cataract (seeing through a waterfall) is a common eye condition characterized by the clouding of the normally clear lens of the eye, leading to a gradual decline in vision quality. This clouding occurs when proteins in the lens begin to break down and clump together, causing the lens to become opaque and interfering with the passage of light to the retina.

Pathophysiology of Cataract Formation

Several key mechanisms contribute to cataract formation are as follows:[2]
- *Osmotic stress*: Seen in diabetic and galactosemic cataracts, where accumulation of sugar alcohols (sorbitol or galactitol) creates an osmotic gradient drawing water into lens fibers. This causes cellular swelling and disrupts the normally tight packing of lens fibers, creating light-scattering discontinuities.
- *Protein aggregation*: In aging lenses and nuclear cataracts, crystallin proteins combine to form large aggregates capable of scattering light. These aggregates may exist free in the cytoplasm or bound to cell membranes.
- *Oxidative stress*: Oxidative damage from reactive oxygen species can:
  - Deactivate sulfhydryl-dependent enzyme systems
  - Protein aggregation through the formation of protein-protein disulfide bridges
  - Change lens color by forming chromophores
  - Disrupt membrane structure

  Glutathione plays a crucial role in protecting the lens from oxidative damage.

- *Metabolism*: While aberrant lens metabolism has long been suspected as a causative mechanism in cataract formation, there is surprisingly little evidence supporting this in humans. Studies of cataractous lens epithelium have often found relatively normal metabolic activity.

  In older human lenses, there is little metabolic activity in the cortex and nucleus, even in clear lenses. The declining ability of the lens to metabolically resist oxidative damage appears to be a more significant factor than overall metabolic dysfunction. Recent research has focused on the lens's ability to accumulate dietary antioxidants. For example, studies have shown that lycopene, a dietary carotenoid, can accumulate in the lens and help offset osmotic and oxidative stress. This suggests that dietary factors may play a role in maintaining lens health and potentially slowing cataract progression. The lens's unique metabolic properties—including its reliance on anaerobic glycolysis in fiber cells and its high concentrations of antioxidants—make it an intriguing subject for metabolic studies. However, the relationship between lens metabolism and cataract formation remains an area of ongoing research and debate.

Symptomatology of Cataract

- *Visual changes*: The most prominent signs of cataracts involve changes in vision. Blurry or cloudy vision is typically the initial symptom of cataracts. People with cataracts may feel like they are looking through a foggy window or a piece of wax paper. This blurriness can affect both near and distance vision, making it difficult to read, watch television, or recognize faces.

  As cataracts progress, individuals may experience a gradual fading or yellowing

of colors. The world may appear less vibrant, and distinguishing between different shades, particularly blues and purples, can become challenging.
- *Light sensitivity and glare*: Increased sensitivity to light is another common symptom of cataracts. People may find bright lights uncomfortable or even painful. Glare from sunlight or artificial light sources like headlights can be particularly bothersome, often causing halos or starbursts to appear around lights. This can make driving at night particularly challenging and hazardous.
- *Changes in visual acuity*: Cataracts can cause frequent changes in eyeglass or contact lens prescriptions. Interestingly, some individuals may experience a temporary improvement in their near vision, known as "second sight," secondary to the increase in optical indices of nucleus post sclerosis, rendering additional plus refractive power to the lens. However, this improvement is usually short-lived and followed by a decline in both near and distance vision.
- *Difficulty with low-light conditions*: Many people with cataracts report increased difficulty seeing in low-light situations. This can manifest as poor night vision, making activities like driving at night or reading in dimly lit rooms more challenging. Centrally located cataracts such as posterior subcapsular or posterior polar cataracts are notoriously famous for having better vision in dim light as more light from peripheral clear area enters the eye in a dilated pupil in low light but can render the patient temporarily blind if some bright light such as headlight of incoming vehicle constricts the pupil.
- *Double vision and distortions*: In some cases, cataracts can cause monocular double vision, where a person sees a double image in one eye. This symptom can be particularly disorienting. Additionally, some individuals may experience distortions in their vision, such as straight lines appearing curved.
- *Progression of symptoms*: It is important to note that the progression of cataract symptoms can vary significantly from person to person. Some individuals may experience a rapid decline in vision, while others may have only minor visual disturbances for years. The type of cataract can also influence the specific symptoms experienced. For example, posterior subcapsular cataracts often cause more problems with glare and reading vision, while nuclear cataracts typically affect distance vision more than near vision.

Classification of Cataract

- *Morphological classification*: Based on the location of cataract opacity (nuclear, cortical, and posterior subcapsular).
- *Etiological classification*: Based on the etiology, the cataract can be classified as congenital, age-related, complicated (secondary to any other eye disease), traumatic (secondary to trauma), metabolic (secondary to systemic metabolic imbalance such as diabetes, myotonic dystrophy, etc.), or drug-induced (most commonly steroid).
- *Based on maturity of the cataract*: Immature, mature, and hypermature.
- *Lens opacities classification system III (LOCS III)*: Standardized grading system using photographic standards, it is the most commonly and objective scale of cataract grading. The cataractous lens of the patient is compared to the standard photograph to visually match the pigmentation of the cataract, the amount

of cortical and subcapsular cataract and subsequently assign the grade of cataract.

Management of Cataract with Phacoemulsification

Proposed in 1965 by Dr Charles Kelman

"The author will find a way to remove cataract through a tiny incision eliminating the need for hospitalization and dramatically shortening the recovery period"

—**Dr Kelman in his proposal for research grant**

It is based on ultrasonic drill used by dentists. Other ideas Dr Kelman toyed with were electronic toothbrush, rotating devices, meat grinders, butchering devices, micro-blenders, etc.[3]

First phacoemulsification surgery was performed in 1967, it took 4 hours with ultrasound time being 61 minutes and then patient was left aphakic as intraocular lenses (IOLs) had just been proposed by Ridley and were not popularized.

Journey of Phaco

Phaco has been in continuous development in 1967 and is still evolving. It is one of the highly individualized surgeries; the technique depends vastly on the expertise of operating surgeon and steps are modified to suit the patient's need and condition. Small incision cataract surgery (SICS) is one such modification that branched out from evolution of phaco.

Phacoemulsification is a unique blend of electronics and surgical skills. To understand the phaco one needs to understand the machine and also the surgical techniques involved.

Phaco console: It is the computer which controls all phaco parameters. Power, vacuum, and flow rate settings fed into console. Settings represent maximum level of the parameter achievable. The amount to be delivered is then modulated with foot pedal.

Controlling the machine with foot pedal

Foot pedal **(Fig. 1 and Table 1)** comprises:
- *Central part*: It has two indentations for three positions.
- *Sidekicks*: It is the flip switch along the central part which when flipped reverses the flow in central tip and causes release of aspirated material. It is used to release accidental aspiration of other ocular tissues.

Dual-linear control of foot pedal: A relatively newer concept in control is dual-linear foot pedal **(Fig. 2)** in which the linear control of vacuum is provided along with phaco power. This is made possible with linear motion in vertical direction (known as pitch) and in horizontal direction (known as yaw). It is upon surgeon's wish to endow functionality in whichever direction he/she wants, conventional positions being vacuum in pitch and phaco power in yaw, with additional vacuum power in yaw.

Components of Phacoemulsification Machine

Phacodynamics: The various functions of the phacoemulsification machine **(Fig. 3)** and their interconnected functions are as follows:
- Ultrasound power and its modulation
- *Fluidics*: Deals with irrigation of anterior chamber, aspiration of emulsified material, and dissipating heat generated by the phaco tip.

Ultrasonic power:

It is calculated as *Power = Frequency × Stroke length*
- Frequency of tip is the rate at which the phaco tip oscillates. It is fixed for a particular machine but ranges from 15 to 49 kHz across the range of machines.

Lens Embryology and Growth

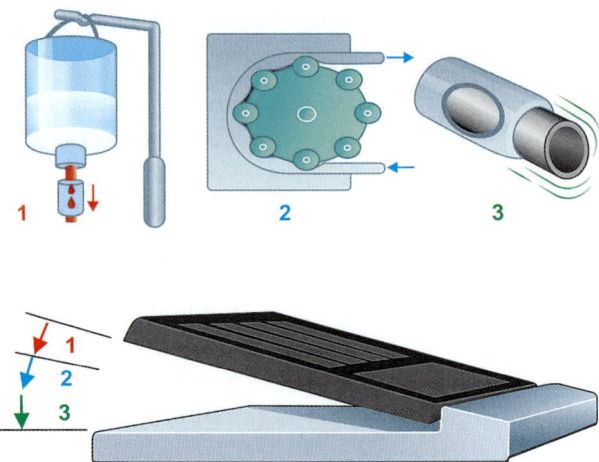

Fig. 1: Foot pedal with its positions and corresponding functions: (1) Irrigation (plunger slides away from tubing); (2) Irrigation and aspiration (I and A), (pump head begins to rotate); (3) Irrigation, aspiration, and phacoemulsification (ultrasound power is active).

TABLE 1: Positions and features of the phaco foot pedal.

Positions	Feature
0	Resting (no fluid flows)
1	Irrigation (plunger slides away from tubing)
2	I and A (pump head begins to rotate)
3	I + A and phaco power (ultrasound power is active)

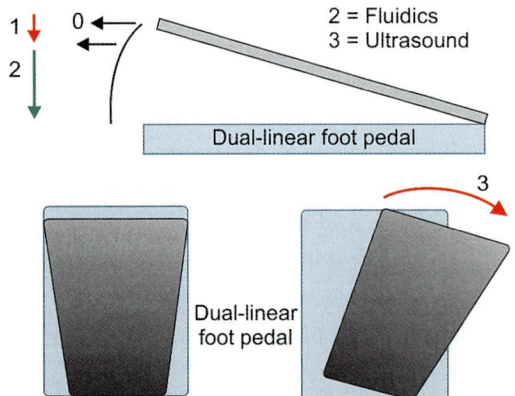

Fig. 2: Dual-linear foot pedal, demonstrating linear control of vacuum along with phaco power, achieved through vertical motion (pitch) and horizontal motion (yaw).

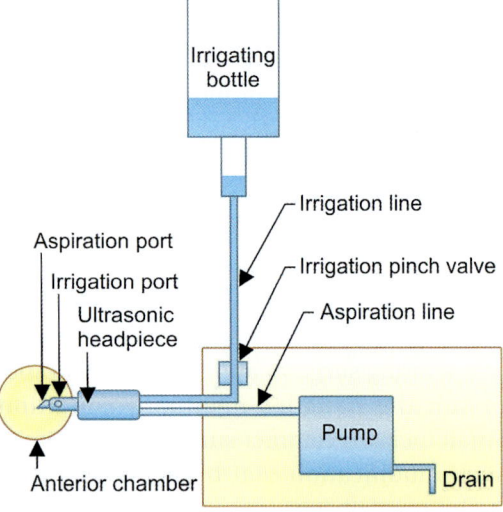

Fig. 3: Diagrammatic illustration of the components of a phacoemulsification machine.

- Stroke length is the length where the tip travels during the oscillation. It is denoted in percentage of maximum length the tip can travel. It is the only parameter that can be altered for modulation of ultrasound power.

Phaco handpiece: The instrument that converts electric power from the phaco machine into ultrasound and delivers the energy into anterior segment by the phaco tip. It also houses the facility of irrigation and aspiration. The conversion of energy happens by transducer. The transducers are based on two different principles:
1. *Magnetostrictive*: Application of external magnetic field on ferrous material increases or decreases its size, causing movements. These movements are made into ultrasonic range. It was very heavy and required a stabilization tripod and thus went out of fashion very early. Its advantage is contact-free excitation and has longer lifespan. Main disadvantages are that it has low efficiency with higher heat production causing tissue burn.
2. *Piezoelectric*: Crystals are excited by voltage difference to create high frequency movements in ultrasonic range. *This is the only type in use nowadays.* Its advantage is higher efficiency with lesser heat production; it also has low mass allowing the ease of movement. The main disadvantage is that it has shorter life.

Phaco tip: It is made up of titanium and oscillates at preset frequency to cause emulsification. It also has aspiration orifice located on the distal extremity while other features such as angulation, diameter, and shape are variable. The tip is covered with a sleeve that insulates and protects the sclerocorneal tissue from thermal and mechanical damage. It also has two irrigation orifices located 180° apart on silicon sleeve.

There are various types of tips, based on angulation of tip, shape of the tip, and angulation of bevel **(Fig. 4)**. Kelman tip **(Fig. 5)** is angulated just proximal to the aspiration orifice and allows for torsional movements of the tip. Cobra head is the flared tip which allows for a greater hold on the nucleus fragment. Anti-blocking suction (ABS) tip allows for control of surge due to presence of an extra aspiration orifice. The bevel angulation is from 0 to 45° **(Fig. 6)**. The steeper the bevel, the better is its grasping power. The slanter it is, the better is its cutting power.

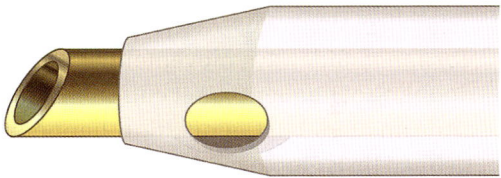

Fig. 4: Mackool phaco tip.

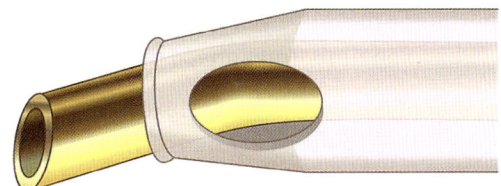

Fig. 5: Kelman phaco tip.

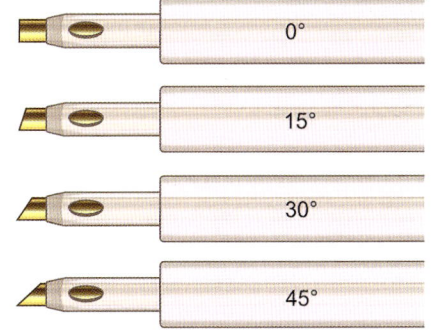

Fig. 6: Anti-blocking suction (ABS) tip with varying bevel angulations ranging from 0 to 45°.

Phaco power delivery: It is usually denoted by stroke length percentage, i.e., percentage of maximum stroke length the tip travels. 100% power is usually 3/1000th of an inch movement of tip.

Thumb rule for the power required to emulsify the nucleus is:

(Grade of nucleus × 15) + 25

Types of phaco tip movements are as follows:
- *Linear*: Movement of tip is only in the axis of handpiece. It only provides cutting action in a single axis.
- *Torsional*: Sideways movements causing doubling of frequency as it cuts both ways and thus less heat generation happens. Kelman tip is employed in this movement.
- *Elliptical*: It allows for an elliptical movement of the tip creating a larger direct cutting effect.

Duration of power delivery of the phaco determines the duty cycle, i.e.,

(Phaco on time/Total phaco time) × 100

Amount of power delivered: Maximum power is determined by stroke length. The machine is preset to the highest power desired and then further controlled by foot pedal.

The linear or surgeon mode is where the gradient of pressure on foot pedal gives the amount of power delivered by the tip. The foot gradient (FG) refers to the distance the foot pedal is pressed (measured in millimeters) to produce a specific amount of phaco energy.

To give an example: If the total foot pedal excursion from IAP_0 to IAP_{max} is 10 cm (100 mm) and the maximum preset phaco energy is 100%, the FG is calculated as:

FG 100 mm/100 1 unit power per 1 mm of excursion

Now, if maximum preset phaco power is charged to 50%:

FG 100 mm/50 1 unit power per 2 mm of excursion

Various methods of energy delivery in linear mode **(Table 2)** are as follows:
- *Constant (DC-100%)*: The phaco power being delivered is continuous whenever the foot pedal is pressed. Most heat is generated in this mode. It is commonly used in the trenching.
- *Pulse (DC-50%)*: The tip moves for half second and rests for half second for every second the foot pedal is pressed.
- *Hyperpulse (DC-20, 33, and 60%)*: Patented as WhiteStar by AMO, it provides a very rapid change in phaco on and off mode of various duration, reducing heat production so much that it is popularly

TABLE 2: Advantages and disadvantages of various methods of energy delivery in linear mode.

Mode	Advantages	Disadvantages	Applications
Continuous	Simple	Repels nuclear material, increase wound temperature	Sculpting
Pulse	Less increase in wound temperature	Can repel nuclear material	Segment removal
Burst	• Less increase in wound temperature • Holds material well		Chopping
Hyperpulse	• Followability with long off cycle • Cool with long off cycle		Sculpting bimanual small incision

known as cold phaco with maximum temperature being 55° Celsius.
- The Burst mode employs the gradient of foot pedal to decrease the time duration between two pulses of energy, and subsequently becoming continuous mode at full throttle.
- *Hyperburst mode*: It gives micropulses of burst mode.
- *Occlusion*: Machine varies the power and duration whenever the tip gets occluded to prevent the postocclusion surge. Mostly implied in emulsification of sticky epinucleus.

Effects of power delivery:
- *Direct impact/Jackhammer phenomenon*: It is the direct mechanical effect of phaco tip movement.
- *Cavitation energy*: There are the micropockets of steam produced by the tip movement produced when the tip moves backward which are of high energy and they burst further causing breaking of nucleus.
- *Acoustic shock waves*: This is the effect of ultrasonic waves causing mechanical effect farther away from the tip.

Fluidics: It deals with the following:
- Removal of the emulsified material
- Maintaining the grip during emulsification
- Maintenance of AC
- Dissipation of the heat energy produced at the tip

Components of fluidics
- *Continuous inflow*:
  - Usually, a bottle of BSS hanged; inflow is passive gravity dependent, also affected by tubing size and sleeves. Maintaining a bottle height of 3 ± 1 feet ensures a safe IOP while providing adequate fluid to the eye.
  - Newer machines now have gravity independent of inflow system.
- *Continuous outflow/aspiration*: It happens through various pump mechanisms, and through leakage through incision sites. It is also affected by diameter of phaco tip, tubing diameter, and machine settings.

Outflow pumps: The thumb rule of vacuum required is again based on the grade of nucleus being dealt with, i.e.,

$$(\text{Grade of nucleus} \times 20) + 80$$

The vacuum can be generated by:
- *Peristaltic pump (Fig. 7)*: The rotation of the rollers by the pump pinches the soft, silicon tubing, creating a negative pressure by squeezing the fluid out of the tube. Vacuum buildup occurs only when the tip becomes occluded. Flow rate and vacuum can be set independently in a peristaltic system by the speed of rollers.
- *Venturi pump (Fig. 8)*: The swift movement of a compressed gas creates a negative suction force, i.e., the vacuum, inside a closed chamber (cassette). This vacuum is then directly transmitted to the handpiece. Flow rate is a fixed fraction of the vacuum generated. This process is controlled by the foot pedal.
- *Quattro pump*: The Quattro pump works on the principle of active irrigation and aspiration, where both are measured,

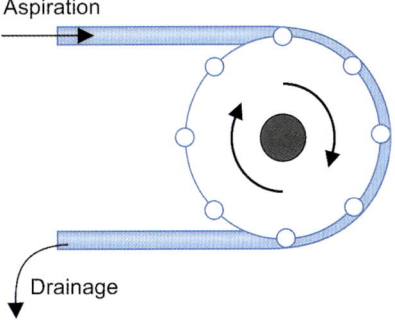

Fig. 7: Diagram of a peristaltic pump.

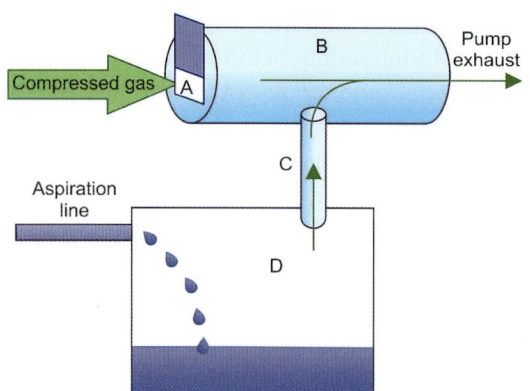

Fig. 8: Diagram of a Venturi pump.

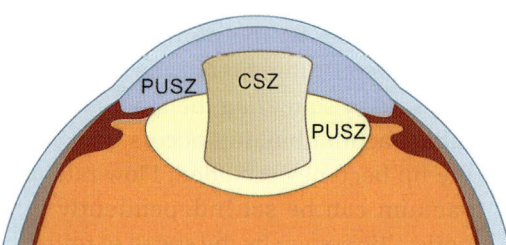

Fig. 9: Central safe zone (CSZ) and peripheral unsafe zone (PUSZ).

and any mismatch in the amount of fluid is compensated by active infusion, maintaining the anterior chamber.

Terminologies in fluidics
There are two zones **(Fig. 9)**:
1. *Central safe zone (CSZ)*: The CSZ is a surgical concept, not an anatomical structure. It refers to an area within the boundaries of the continuous curvilinear capsulorhexis (CCC), vertically bounded by the cornea at the top and the posterior capsule at the bottom. This zone provides the maximum available space within the AC. All aspiration procedures, including nuclear, epinuclear, or cortical material removal, should occur within this zone. As nuclear pieces and cortical matter are extracted, they should be brought to the CSZ for safe aspiration. As more nuclear material is removed, the safety margin and available space within the CSZ increase.
2. *Peripheral unsafe zone*: It is the region outside the CSZ, within the anterior segment of the eye. It goes close to other ocular structures and use of phaco power of vacuum can cause damage to iris or angle or posterior capsule or zonules and ciliary body.

Zones of followability: The pressure gradient at the phaco tip creates eddy currents from the infusion orifice to the phaco tip. This region, influenced by the fluid dynamics, is termed the zone of followability.
- *Area of highest followability*: The region directly in front of the phaco tip, where aspiration is most efficient.
- *Areas of poor followability*: The anterior chamber angle and the capsular fornices, where aspiration is less effective.
- *Areas of no followability*: Fragments located near the side port or the main wound, where fluid leakage occurs, preventing fragments from being drawn into the tip.

Rise time: Rise time refers to the duration required for the machine to reach the maximum preset vacuum after occlusion is achieved. In a Venturi system, the rise time is typically rapid and linear, primarily determined by the highest preset vacuum level. In contrast, in a peristaltic pump, the rise time is influenced by the flow rate of the machine. A higher flow rate generally results in a shorter rise time, although this relationship is not perfectly linear.

Surge: Surge refers to the sudden withdrawal of fluid from the AC that occurs after occlusion breaks. It is a critical limiting factor when selecting high vacuum or flow levels. Surge can lead to complications during phacoemulsification, and managing it is essential for maintaining intraocular pressure and ensuring surgical stability. Various methods to control surge are integrated into newer phacoemulsification machines, while some techniques can also be applied by the surgeon to minimize its occurrence.

Surge prevention by the machine is by virtue of:

Compliance: Property of the tubing to collapse, i.e., deform under pressure. Its extent depends on the thickness of the tube and is inversely proportional to it. In a peristaltic machine, high vacuum tubings and cassettes are used to decrease the compliance of the tubings thus preventing surge.

Venting: Venting refers to a mechanism (sensor) in the machine that detects an occlusion break and releases fluid into the system to compensate for the volume lost as the tubing reexpands. This process helps to prevent the aspiration of fluid from the AC **(Figs. 10A to C)**.

Anti-blocking suction tip: The ABS tip **(Fig. 11)** is a modified phaco needle featuring a 0.175-mm hole drilled into the shaft. When occlusion occurs at the tip, fluid flows into this hole, with the flow rate determined by the vacuum and flow settings. This modification ensures that some fluid flow is always present, preventing complete occlusion. To function properly, the ABS tip must be used with high vacuum tubing.

Partial-occlusion phacoemulsification: Micropulse phaco is employed to prevent total occlusion and mitigate surge. A 4-ms aspiration cycle is initiated until the nuclear fragment partially occludes the tip. Following this, a 4-ms burst of phaco energy is delivered to emulsify the fragment before it can fully occlude the phaco tip.

Smart tips: Sensors in the machines now sense the occlusion and vary the vacuum generated depending on the amount of occlusion and decrease the power as the occlusion is about to break.

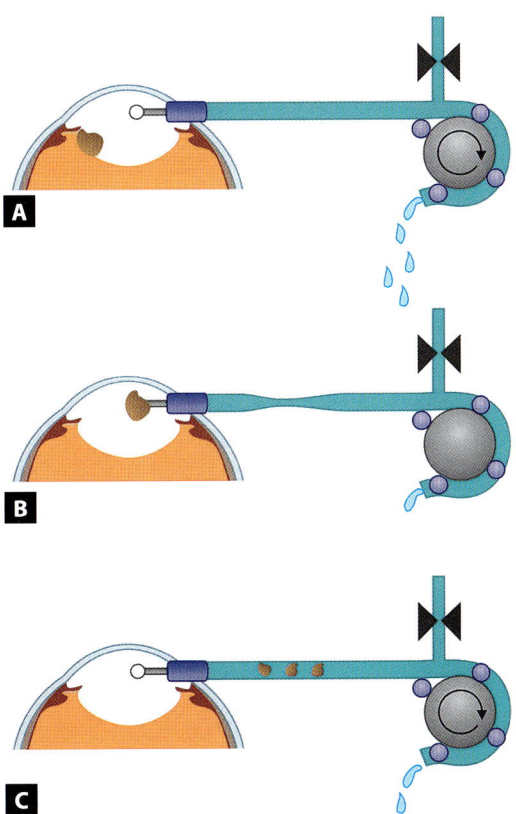

Figs. 10A to C: Diagrammatic representation of the venting mechanism in phacoemulsification.

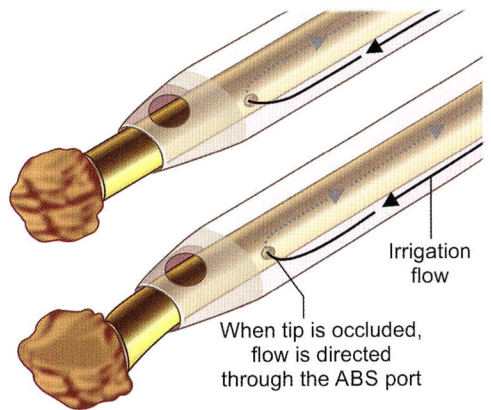

Fig. 11: Image of the anti-blocking suction (ABS) tip.

Surgeon's control of surge is by various methods by which the surgeon can himself/herself prevent the surge. These are by:
- Raising the bottle height to increase infusion
- Use of anterior chamber maintainer
- A thicker fluid increases the resistance and does not flow out easily.
- Use of ophthalmic viscosurgical devices (OVDs) **(Table 3)**

TABLE 3: Advantages and disadvantages of ophthalmic viscosurgical devices (OVDs).

Advantages of cohesive OVDs	*Disadvantages of cohesive OVDs*
Healon® (Abbott Medical Optics), Healon GV® (Abbott MO), Proviso® (Alcon), Amvisc® (Bausch and Lomb)	Healon® (Abbott Medical Optics), Healon GV® (Abbott MO), Provisc® (Alcon), Amvisc® (Bausch and Lomb)
Create, deepen, and maintain space in anterior chamber	They can come out of the eye easily as a whole during surgery or under intense vitreous pressure (specially in case of large incisions)
Clear vision, transparency	They are unwillingly removed during phacoemulsification
Ideal for flattening the anterior capsule to facilitate capsulorhexis	They do not stay attached to corneal endothelium
Ideal to open capsular bag for IOL insertion	Some have a high risk of postoperative IOP peaks if not completely removed (e.g., Healon® 5)
They mechanically enlarge and stabilize the size of the pupil	
Easy to remove at the end of procedure	
Advantages of dispersive OVDs	*Disadvantages of dispersive OVDs*
Vitrax® (Abbott Medical Optics), Viscoat (Alcon), and OcuCoat (Bausch and Lomb)	Vitrax® (Abbott Medical Optics), Viscoat (Alcon), and OcuCoat (Bausch and Lomb)
Ability to coat intraocular structures	Low viscosity dispersives do not maintain spaces well
They stay adhered to endothelium during the emulsification procedure (endothelial protection)	May have air bubbles inside or form microbubbles during surgery
They tend to stay in place during the fluidics of phacoemulsification surgery (high shear rates)	Difficult to remove completely at the end of procedure (risk of postoperative noninflammatory Tyndall in the anterior chamber)
They separate spaces (ability to partition spaces, surgical compartmentalization). They hold vitreous back in case of loose zonules or in case of a small hole in the posterior capsule)	Some may not be completely transparent or can see transparency reduced under ultrasonic waves
Ability to lubricate IOL and injector	They fragment into small pieces during irrigation and aspiration and this may obscure the visualization of posterior capsule during surgery
Removal of dispersive OVDs requires more effort at the end of procedure	

- *Practicing good foot pedal control*: Lifting the foot pedal to position I as occlusion breaks allows the piece to move on its own momentum, minimizing fluid withdrawal from the anterior chamber and reducing surge.
- By use of double-linear foot pedal which also has a linear mode for vacuum in addition to phaco power.

Selection of patients: For the beginners, the ideal case should be having moderate hardness and good fundal reflex. The following should be avoided in initial stages of learning:
- Deep set eyes
- Shallow AC
- Hazy cornea
- Nondilating pupil
- Brunescent cataract grade IV/V or very soft cataract
- Subluxated/dislocated lens
- Cataract in vitrectomized patient

ESSENTIAL SURGICAL STEPS

- Watertight entry wound
- Maintenance of AC
- Capsulorhexis
- Hydroprocedure
- Nucleus management
- Epinucleus management
- Cortex aspiration
- IOL implant
- Removal of OVDs

Wound Construction

Site: The choice of incision depends on surgeon's expertise, his/her ease, and preexisting astigmatism of the patient. Scleral incision is usually taken superiorly in astigmatic neutral zone **(Fig. 12)**. Clear corneal incision is popularly taken temporally as it allows for extra movement and negligible effect on astigmatism.

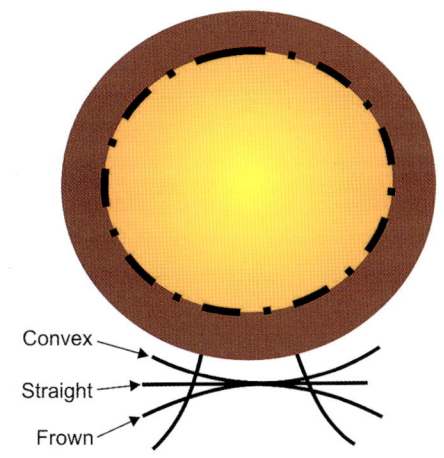

Fig. 12: Scleral incision taken superiorly in the astigmatic neutral zone.

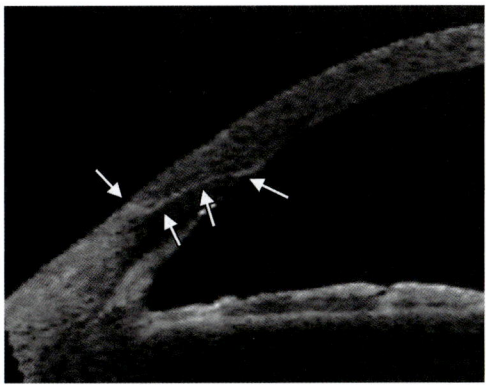

Fig. 13: Optical coherence tomography (OCT) image showing a triplanar wound.

Shape: The main incision should always be triplanar **(Fig. 13)** to ensure a watertight seal while side port entries are made uniplanar or biplanar.

Size: The size of the incision is determined by the surgical technique employed and the dimensions of the phacoemulsification tip being used.

Side port incisions: Small paracentesis limbal incision 1 mm wide, and 0.75 mm long, usually created 90° away from the main incision, using a 15–30° metal blade or a 1-mm diamond blade.

Capsulorhexis

It was developed by Neuhann and Gimbel in 1980s and is now the standard technique for planned anterior as well as posterior capsular opening. It is performed either with an Utrata forceps or a cystitome fashioned out from a 26G or an insulin needle. The choice of instrument depends on the surgeon's expertise as well as the cataract being dealt with. The shearing force is applied in tangential direction after raising a flap in continuous curvilinear manner, thus the name CCC **(Fig. 14)**.

Hydroprocedures

It is the use of water to create a plane between various layers of cataractous lens for better nucleus management.

- *Hydrodissection*: The injection of fluid into the cortical layer of the lens under the lens capsule to separate the lens nucleus from the cortex and capsule **(Fig. 15)**
- *Cortex cleaving hydrodissection*: A hydrodissection technique designed to cleave the cortex from the lens capsule and thus leave the cortex attached to the epinucleus, eliminating the need of cortical cleanup.
- *Hydrodelineation*: Separating the outer epinuclear shell from the central compact mass of inner nuclear material, the endonucleus, by the forceful irrigation of fluid into the mass of the nucleus.

Nucleus Management

It is the most essential step of phacoemulsification, i.e., the "emulsification" of "phako (lens)". Various techniques have evolved over the years to achieve a good and fast emulsification of the nucleus. The major techniques of which are as follows:

Divide and conquer: The phacoemulsification instrument is used to create a deep tunnel in

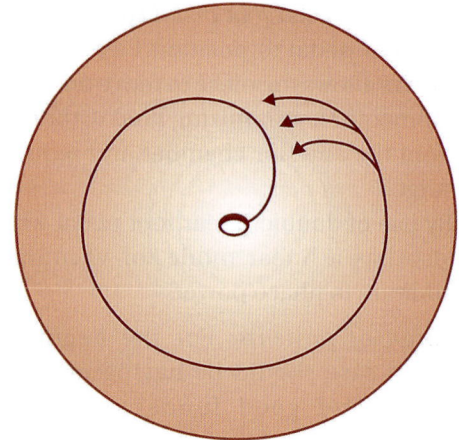

Fig. 14: Continuous curvilinear capsulorhexis (CCC) depicting the application of shearing force in a tangential direction.

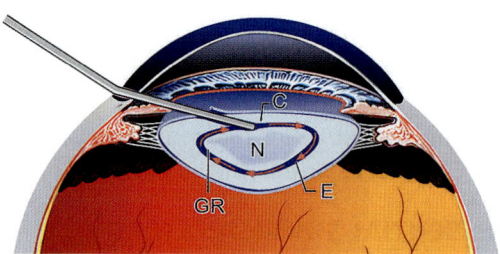

Fig. 15: Hydrodissection technique.

the center or the upper part of the nucleus. The nucleus is split into halves, sometimes fourths, and even occasionally into eighths. The steps are as follows:

- *Sculpting*: The process continues until a thin posterior plate of the nucleus remains.
- *Fracturing*: The posterior plate and nuclear rim are fractured for easier removal.
- *Wedge-shaped fragmentation*: A wedge-shaped section of nuclear material is broken away for emulsification.

Rotating: The remaining nucleus is rotated to facilitate further fracturing and emulsification.

It can be employed in:
- Classic four quadrant technique
- Trench divide and conquer
- Crater divide and conquer method

Phaco Chop

Kunihiro Nagahara first introduced the phaco chop technique in 1993. It also uses the lamellar structure of the nucleus to create radial fractures in the lens.

A high vacuum level is essential to achieve the necessary holding power for chopping. Depending on the size of the phaco needle, the vacuum should be set between 250 and 400 mm Hg. When using a peristaltic fluid pump, it is crucial to ensure that total occlusion of the phaco tip is achieved to reach the maximum preset vacuum level. With the vacuum set high, the phaco tip must be buried into the nucleus using phaco power (foot pedal position 3). Once full occlusion is achieved, the surgeon should back off the pedal to position 2, allowing the nucleus to be held by the high vacuum level while proceeding with the chopping technique.

The various methods for chopping the nucleus include:
- *Horizontal chop*: Where the two instruments move in horizontal plane in respect to each other during the emulsification. The original chopping technique, described by Nagahara, involves a horizontal chop. In this method, the phaco probe is embedded into the nucleus, and the Nagahara chopper is introduced beneath the capsulorhexis, moving toward the lens equator. Once positioned at the equator, the chopper is brought toward the phaco tip. The chopping action occurs as the chopper and phaco tip are moved together. After the initial chop, the two pieces must be separated by pulling the instruments apart. Typically, the surgeon will pull the chopper to the left while pushing the phaco probe to the right. Full separation of the pieces is necessary for their complete mobilization, allowing further chopping into smaller segments.
- *Vertical chop*: Where the two instruments move in vertical plane in respect to each other during the emulsification. In denser nuclei, vertical chopping proves to be an effective and safe technique. The phaco tip is embedded into the nucleus, and a high vacuum level is applied to secure it in place. The chopper is then positioned vertically at the center of the nucleus, within the boundaries of the capsulorhexis. Once both the chopper and phaco tip are fully embedded in the nucleus, the instruments are pulled apart—the chopper is moved to the left, and the phaco probe to the right—resulting in the separation of the nuclear halves. These halves can then be further subdivided into smaller segments and emulsified.
- *Tilt and chop*: When the nucleus is tilted with the help of chopper and the tip is introduced from one end to initiate emulsification. To reduce stress on the capsular bag, particularly in cases of pseudoexfoliation or trauma with zonular weakness, the nucleus can be tilted out of the bag. A larger capsulorhexis, around 5 mm or more, along with hydrodissection or viscodissection, helps in prolapsing the nucleus partially from the capsular bag. Once the nucleus is tilted outward, it becomes easier to position the chopper around the lens equator or even behind the nucleus. The chopper is then brought toward the phaco tip, and the instruments are pulled apart, effectively dividing the nucleus into two halves.

Stop and chop: This is a hybrid technique that combines elements of divide and conquer and phaco chop. In this technique, the trenching is first done to crack the nucleus into two pieces and then each piece is further chopped by any of the chopping methods. It produces less stress on the zonules as the initial cracking which produces the maximum stress is avoided by trenching but in lieu of higher amount of phaco time being used.

Epinucleus Management

The recommended settings are power of 20 ± 10%, flow rate of 30 ± 6, and vacuum of 250 ± 100 mm Hg. The vacuum is kept variable to prevent postocclusion surge in this stage. Chip and flip technique is utilized to achieve epinuclear plate removal.

Cortex Management

Cortex is aspirated either with coaxial irrigation aspiration technique or by bimanual method of irrigation aspiration. Bimanual method provides an effective and easy way to remove subincisional cortical matter.

Foldable Intraocular Lenses

The final step in phacoemulsification surgery involves the implantation of a foldable IOL into the capsular bag. It either is loaded into the injector in the OT or comes as preloaded syringes which can be inserted through main incision into the bag **(Fig. 16)**.

COMPLICATIONS OF PHACOEMULSIFICATION

Wound related: Premature entry, torn edges, and leaking wound

Capsulorhexis related: Run off rhexis, improper size, capsular tags, and wrong completion of rhexis.

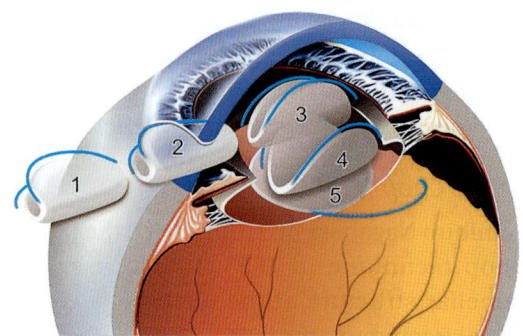

Fig. 16: Implantation of a foldable intraocular lens (IOLs).

- *Nucleus management related:*
  - *Inability of removal of nuclear fragment*: Soft cataract with high vacuum timings, hard cataract with low vacuum settings
  - Ultrasound energy dissipation to other tissue
  - Burrowing of the fragment
  - Milking
  - Chattering
  - Pieces in no followability zone
  - Zonular stress and dehiscence due to improper technique utilized in harder/softer nucleus.

Posterior capsular rupture (PCR): Extension of rhexis margin, direct injury, during hydrodissection, and occult PCR in posterior polar cataracts.

CONCLUSION

A comprehensive understanding of lens embryology, anatomy, physiology, and the principles of phacoemulsification is crucial for modern cataract surgery. From the intricate process of lens fiber development to the biomechanics of power modulation and fluidics, each aspect contributes to optimal surgical outcomes. Advances in surgical techniques and machine design have significantly improved precision and safety, enabling tailored approaches for diverse clinical scenarios. As cataract remains a leading cause of reversible blindness, continuous learning and innovation in lens biology and surgical execution are imperative. Mastery of these fundamentals empowers surgeons to deliver superior visual rehabilitation with minimal complications.

REFERENCES

1. Augusteyn RC. On the growth and internal structure of the human lens. Exp Eye Res. 2010;90(6):643-54.
2. Cvekl A, Vijg J. Aging of the eye: Lessons from cataracts and age-related macular degeneration. Ageing Res Rev. 2024;99:102407.
3. Kelman CD. Phaco-emulsification and aspiration. A new technique of cataract removal. A preliminary report. Am J Ophthalmol. 1967;64(1):23-35.

CHAPTER 3

Physiology of Eye and Vision

Mary Stephen, Kalyan Basa, Karthikeyan Mahalingam

INTRODUCTION

Human eye works in accurate manner to produce a clear image. Numerous factors play a crucial role to subserve the function. Few of the important factors include uniformity of ocular surface, transparent nature of cornea and lens, and rigidity of eye sclera's structure which is maintained by the intraocular pressure (IOP).

The eyeball has two divisions (1) anterior and (2) posterior segment **(Fig. 1 and Video 1)**. Anterior segment is further divided into anterior and posterior chamber, which is filled by clear fluid with ionic constituents almost similar to plasma.

ANTERIOR SEGMENT BARRIERS AND ITS CLINICAL SIGNIFICANCE

Blood aqueous barrier is the capillary network arrangement formed by nonpigmented epithelium of ciliary body. It is a relatively impermeable structure. Breach in the blood aqueous barrier of any etiology can lead to entry of large molecular weight compounds and inflammatory cells into the anterior segment. Evidence of anterior chamber cells, flare, formation of hypopyon (inflammatory), and plasmoid aqueous is due to break in blood aqueous barrier often due to inflammation and alteration in capillary permeability.[1]

Aqueous Humor Formation

The formation involves three mechanisms which are diffusion, active secretion, and ultrafiltration **(Fig. 2 and Video 2)**. Diffusion involves movement of small lipid soluble components and ions to pass along their concentration gradient across cell membrane of ciliary epithelium. Active secretion is the

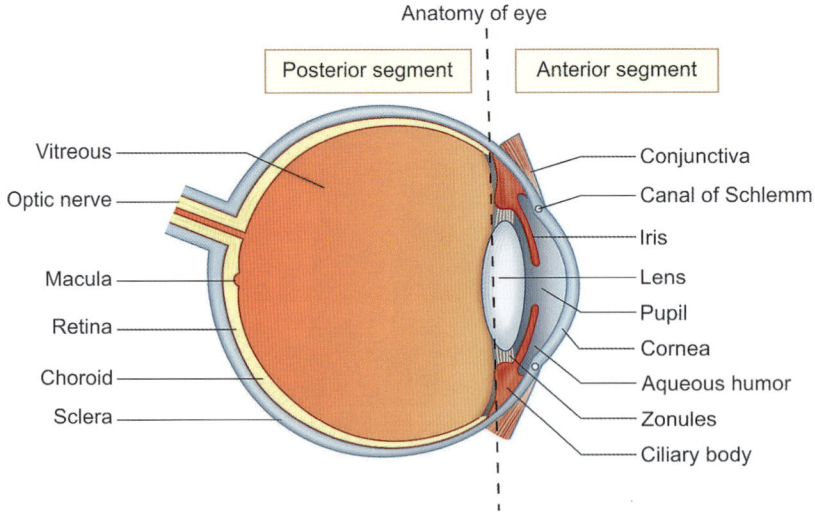

Fig. 1: Diagrammatic representation of basic ocular anatomy with anterior and posterior segment structures.

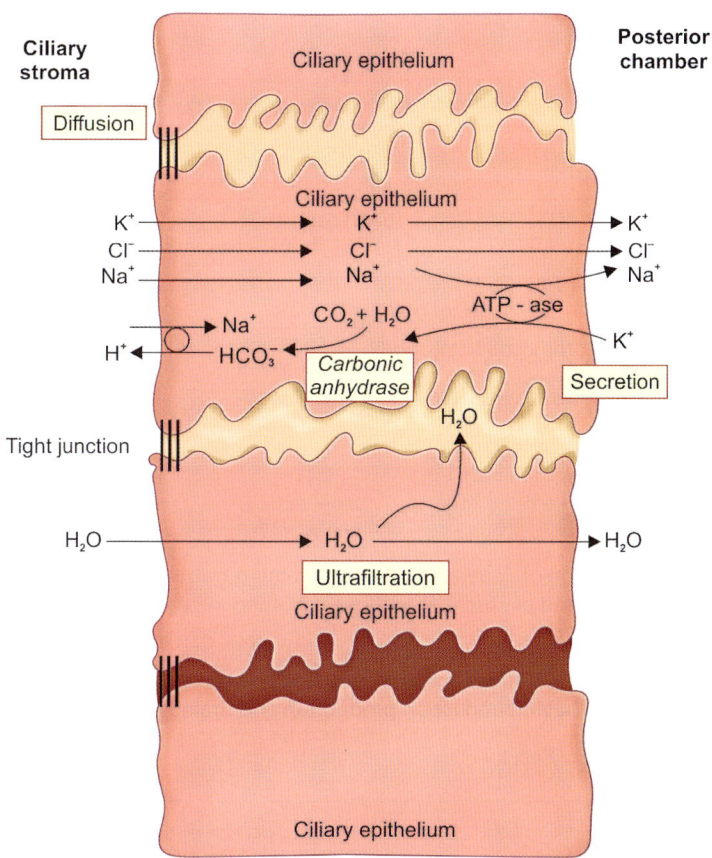

Fig. 2: Schematic representation of the aqueous humor formation explaining the three mechanisms (diffusion, ultrafiltration, and active secretion).

major contributor (around 95%) with ions of sodium and bicarbonate which are actively transported across ciliary epithelium. This active transport creates osmotic gradient and draws water with it. Hydrostatic pressure from blood flow moves water and small molecules through fenestrated capillaries. The complete mechanism remains unclear. The aqueous humor secreted into the posterior chamber has diluted concentration of plasma constituents because of limited passage across blood aqueous barrier.

Aqueous humor dynamics: Aqueous circulation is required for both intraocular pressure regulation and metabolic processes. Since the ciliary area is where the majority of the fluid forms, it reaches posterior chamber from the ciliary plexus and flows through pupil into anterior chamber. The drainage of aqueous humor is via trabecular and uveoscleral outflow pathways **(Video 3 and Fig. 3)**.[2,3]

Intraocular Pressure

The normal intraocular pressure of the human eye ranges from 10 to 21 mm Hg. This pressure is vital to maintain the globe structure. Intraocular pressure can be measured by various noninvasive techniques. Noncontact tonometer is commonly used for

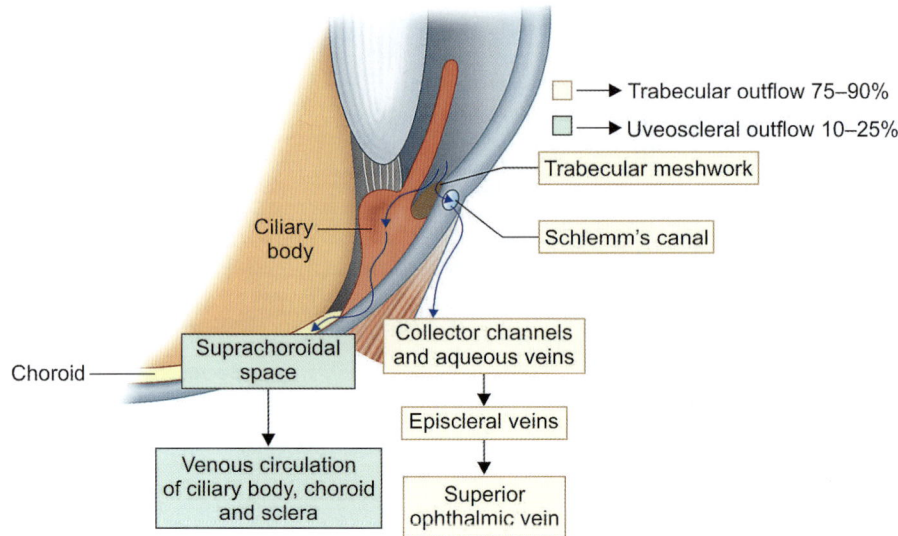

Fig. 3: Schematic representation of aqueous outflow explaining trabecular outflow explained in yellow boxes and uveoscleral outflow explained in green boxes.

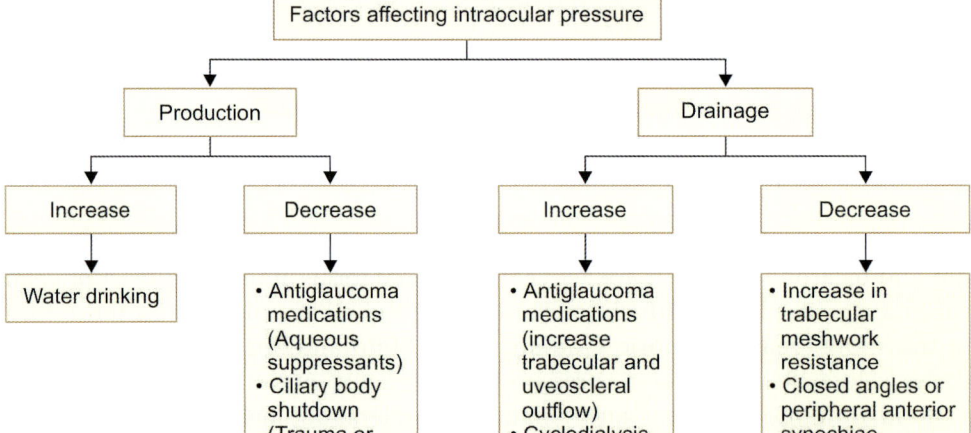

Flowchart 1: Factors affecting the intraocular pressure including the factors having impact on production and drainage.

mass screening and Goldmann applanation tonometer is the ideal tool for accurate intraocular pressure measurement. Resistance at the level of trabecular pathway is the common cause for elevated intraocular pressure. Defective drainage due to pre-trabecular and post-trabecular pathways including elevated episcleral venous pressure also can lead to increased intraocular pressure, leading to a form of chronic progressive optic neuropathy called glaucoma. Numerous factors alter the intraocular pressure explained in **Flowchart 1**.

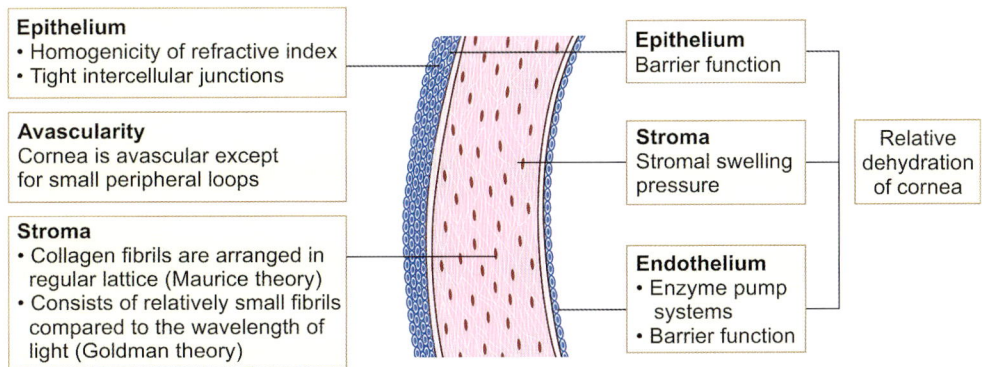

Fig. 4: Schematic figure explaining the factors maintaining corneal transparency.

Metabolism

Vascularized tissue of eye has same metabolism as other body tissues. The cornea needs very little energy to maintain its transparency and cellular regeneration. Corneal metabolism and factors maintaining corneal transparency are explained in the **Video 4 and Figure 4**. Although the lens's metabolism is fairly complex, it can be made simpler to provide an overview in the **Video 5**.

BASIC PHYSIOLOGY OF VISION AND WALD'S VISUAL PATHWAY

Creating a sharp image of a stimulus on the retina's surface is the eye's function. Cornea and lens are the major refractive surfaces and cornea contributes to two-thirds of total refractive power of eye. The lens is what allows us to perceive objects at all distances by further refracting the light rays that enter our eyes. The reflex ciliary muscle action causes the ocular lens to change form, becoming flatter for distant objects and more spherical for near ones. The pupillary size is regulated for various light intensities by a reflex contraction of sphincter pupillae, in bright environment and dilatation by dilator pupillae, in dark environment. The retinal ganglion cells in the human eye are about a million in number. On the other hand, there are about 125 million photoreceptors. At the fovea, retinal ganglion cells are numerous with reduction in number toward the periphery and so visual sensitivity in fovea is highest.

The optic disc is said to be the blind spot as no visual sense is produced for a visual stimulus. When light strikes the retina, it triggers two vital processes: (1) electrical and (2) photochemical.

The rods and cones' pigments are affected by the photochemical alterations. The pigment that has been studied the most is rhodopsin, or visual purple, which is present in significant amounts in rods. Related pigments have also been found in the rods of different animal species, and three distinct pigments appear to be connected to the foveal cones. Rhodopsin is a type of chromoprotein. This photochemical reaction is what starts the visual process and produces the electrical potential changes that travel from the bipolar cells to the ganglion cells and ultimately to the brain via the optic nerve fibers. Although the exact makeup of the pigments in the cones is still unknown, it is most likely that each one responds differently to the various wavelength bands in the spectrum that are interpreted as red, green, and blue.

Flowchart 2: Flowchart representing the Wald's visual cycle, explaining the break and formation of rhodopsin with light stimulus.

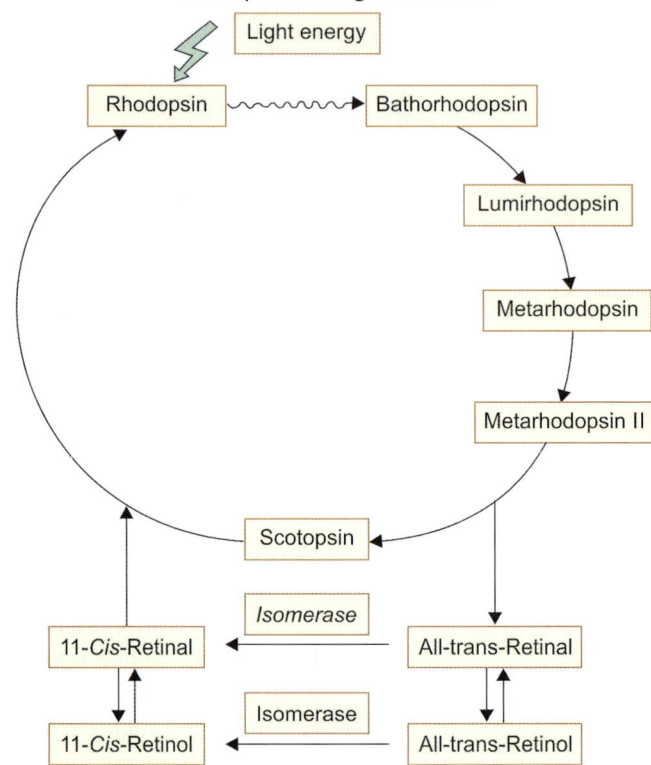

Walds' Visual Cycle

Rhodopsin is the visual pigment in the outer segment of rods that gives us scotopic vision—the capacity to see in the dark.[4] The chromophore of rhodopsin is 11-cis-retinal, which is ensconced in a single peptide transmembrane protein known as opsin by three distinct chemical bonds. The rhodopsin cycle has been explained in brief in **Video 6** and **Flowchart 2**.

Color Vision

This ability enables humans to discern between various colors that are stimulated by light with various wavelengths. Color vision is a function of cones and colors can only be perceived in an illuminated environment. When exposed to extremely low levels of light, the dark-adapted eye perceives nothing but black.

Three pigments found in many cones preferentially absorb light wavelengths that correspond to the colors red, green, and blue on the spectrum. Normal color vision is trichromatic.

Theories of color vision are as follows:
- Young–Helmholtz trichromatic theory
- The Hering opponent theory, now updated by Hurvich and Jameson
- Edwin Land's theoretical model of color vision

BINOCULAR VISION AND STEREOPSIS

The visual cortex combines the images from both eyes to form what is perceived as a single image. The object of interest falls on the fovea and the surrounding objects falls onto corresponding retinal points, giving us the clear image. Horopter is an imaginary line in space, representing external projection of corresponding retinal points. Actually, from two distinct two-dimensional retinal images from the two eyes, the brain creates a three-dimensional vision of the outside world. This occurs because there is an area in space (Panum's fusional area) on each side of the horopter that is still inside the "limits" of fusion which will be viewed without any blur. Human brain tends to suppress the image outside this fusional area.[5]

Three components or grades of binocular single vision are as follows:
1. Simultaneous binocular perception (**Fig. 5**)
2. Fusion (**Fig. 6**)
3. Stereopsis (**Fig. 7**)

The above components of binocular single vision have been explained in **Video 7**.

VISUAL PATHWAY

The photoreceptors, rods, and cones are the end organ of neurosensory retina. First order neurons of the visual pathway are bipolar cells with their axons. The retina's ganglion cells form the second order neurons and terminate in lateral geniculate body. Cell fibers which transmit impulses to the occipital lobe (visual cortex) constitute third order neurons. The visual pathway and defects are explained in the **Video 8 and Figure 8**.

Broadly speaking, fibers originating from peripheral regions of the retina enter the optic nerve's peripheral portion, while fibers from regions of the retina close to the optic disc reach the nerve's central section. These fibers retain their relative positions all the way back to the chiasma. On the other hand, macular area fibers function differently. Fibers from

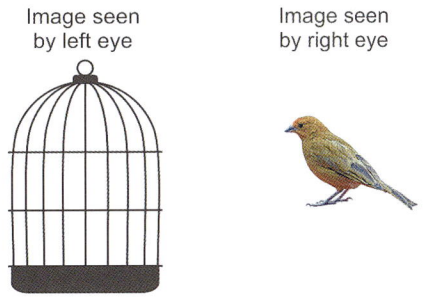

Simultaneous perception is the ability to see two dissimilar objects simultaneously

Fig. 5: Simultaneous binocular perception is represented by two dissimilar objects (cage in one eye and bird in one eye) seen by individual eyes appears as singe image (bird inside the cage).

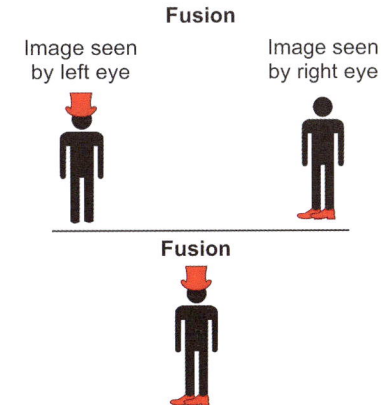

Fusion is the ability to produce a composite picture from two similar pictures, each of which is incomplete in one small detail

Fig. 6: Fusion is represented by ability of human eyes to fuse two similar images (one image with hat and other image with shoe) with minor difference to form a single composite image (image with both hat and shoe).

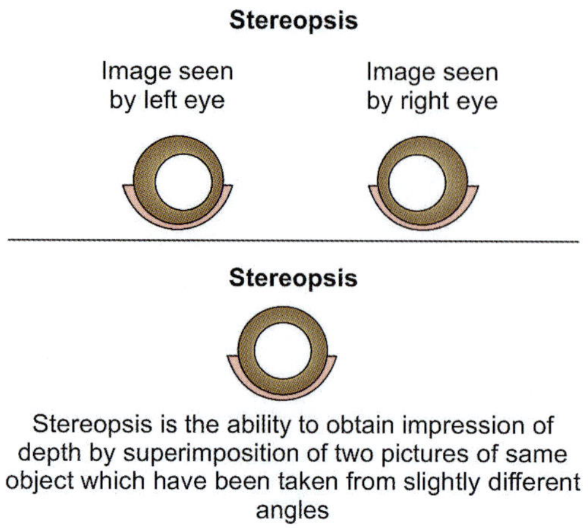

Stereopsis

Image seen by left eye   Image seen by right eye

Stereopsis

Stereopsis is the ability to obtain impression of depth by superimposition of two pictures of same object which have been taken from slightly different angles

Fig. 7: Stereopsis is the ability to obtain depth by superimposition of two images of same objects taken at slightly different angle (bucket handle orientation).

the macula form the papillomacular bundle and rest of retina converge as nasal and temporal fibers. They enter the nerve from its exterior, dispersing over a triangular-shaped region with the apex pointing toward the nerve's center. These papillomacular fibers quickly become more centrally positioned, eventually locating themselves all in the center. When the nerve fibers are traced even farther back, there is a partial decussation where the temporal fibers enter the optic tract of the same side and reach the dorsal half of the lateral geniculate bodies, while the nasal fibers cross in the chiasma. The fibers get terminated into the calcarine fissure and visual cortex.[6,7]

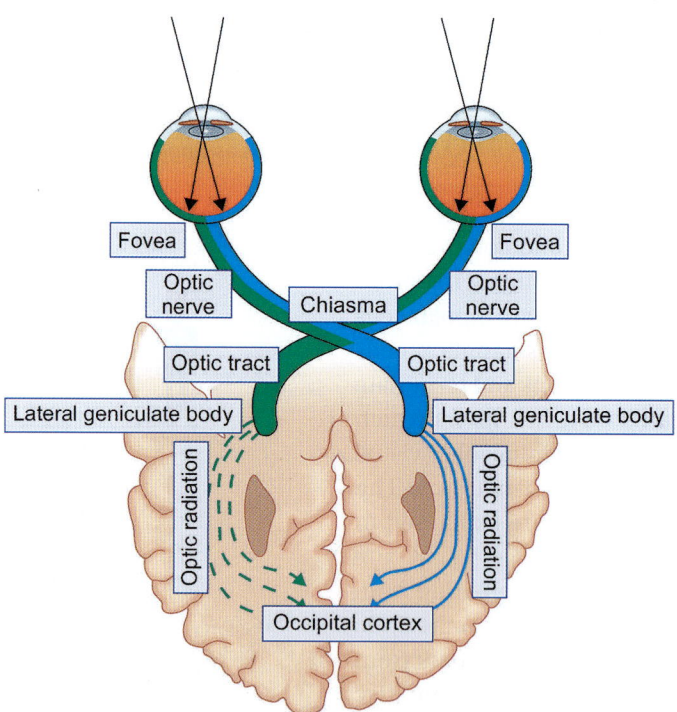

Fig. 8: Schematic representation of visual pathway starting from the light rays falling in retina till visual cortex. Retinal fibers are divided into nasal (decussate to opposite side) and temporal (passes in same side) go through optic nerve to reach optic chiasma and optic tract. From lateral geniculate body via optic radiations, the fibers will reach the occipital lobe.

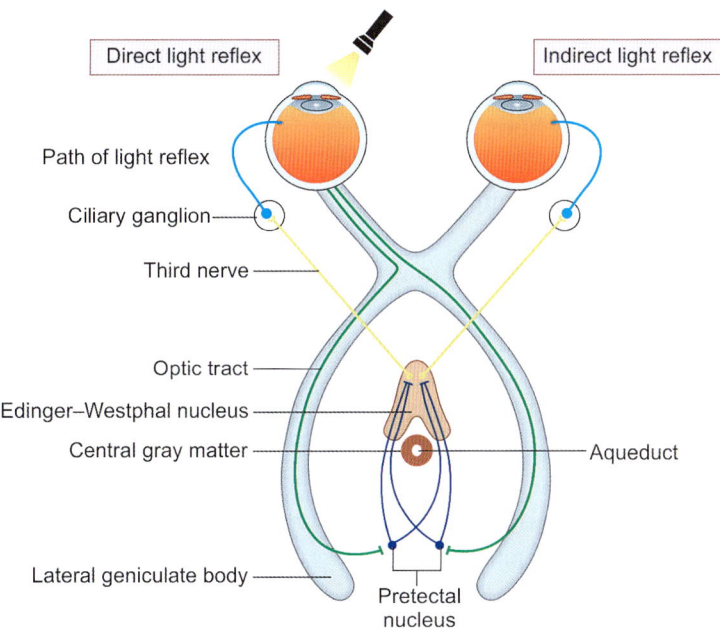

Fig. 9: Schematic representation of pupillary reflex, where in once light falls on the photoreceptors, the impulse passes through optic nerve, optic tract to reach pretectal nucleus from there both sides of Edinger–Westphal nucleus gets stimulated which via ciliary ganglion tends to cause pupillary constriction in both eyes resulting in both direct and consensual light reflex.

PUPILLARY PATHWAY AND REFLEX

Two important muscles playing an important role for pupillary reflex are sphincter pupillae and dilator pupillae, which are of neuroectodermal in origin. Pupil constriction is called miosis, due to sphincter pupillae contraction and pupil dilation is called mydriasis, due to dilator pupillae action. Through the third cranial nerve, the cholinergic parasympathetic system supplies the sphincter pupillae. The fibers begin on the floor of the Sylvius aqueduct in the Edinger–Westphal nucleus. The fibers come out of it and travel via the midbrain to the orbit through the third nerve's major trunk. The fibers leave the inferior oblique muscle and run as short root of ciliary ganglion. The nerve continues as short ciliary nerve and reaches the iris by passing through inner ocular coats.[8]

Constriction of pupil with light constitutes *direct light reflex* and constriction of other eye pupil constitutes *indirect (consensual) light reflex*. Photoreceptors are the starting point of the light reflex. Light reflex pathway has been explained in **Video 9 and Figure 9**.

The near reflex is a phenomenon that happens when one looks at anything close by. It is mostly triggered by the body's response to convergence, but accommodation also plays a role. The reflex is initiated by contraction of medial rectus muscle.

The *psychosensory reflex* causes the pupil to dilate on sensory and psychic inputs.

VIDEO LEGENDS

Video 1: Video demonstrating the parts of the eye.
Video 2: Video explaining the mechanism for aqueous humor formation.

Video 3: Video explaining the aqueous humor outflow. The aqueous humor is produced from nonpigmented epithelium of ciliary body and pass through posterior chamber into anterior chamber via pupil. With aqueous convection current, the aqueous humor produced pass to the angle and involves in two drainage pathways. Conventional trabecular pathway, where via trabecular meshwork pass through Schlemm's canal and drains to venous circulation. Uveoscleral outflow passes along the surface of iris and uveal tissue to pass through suprachoroidal space and drains to venous circulation.

Video 4: Self-explanatory video explaining the major factors which play a crucial role in maintaining corneal transparency and metabolism. The individual layers are explained in detail.

Video 5: Self-explanatory video of the lens metabolism and the various pathways which provides nutrient support to the lens.

Video 6: Video explaining the break of rhodopsin with light into opsin and retinal which then joins to form rhodopsin after passing through a cyclical change.

Video 7: Video demonstration of the three components of binocular single vision. Simultaneous binocular perception is represented by two dissimilar objects (cage in one eye and bird in one eye) seen by individual eyes which appear as single image (bird inside the cage). Fusion is represented by ability of human eyes to fuse two similar images (one image with hat and other image with shoe) with minor difference to form a single composite image (image with both hat and shoe). Stereopsis is the ability to obtain depth by superimposition of two pictures of same objects taken at slightly different angle (bucket handle orientation).

Video 8: Videographic representation of visual pathway starting from the light rays falling in retina till visual cortex. Retinal fibers are divided into nasal (decussate to opposite side) and temporal (passes in same side) go through optic nerve to reach optic chiasma and optic tract. From lateral geniculate body via optic radiations, the fibers will reach the occipital lobe. The various levels of damage in visual pathway are represented in the video. Damage of same side optic nerve results in total blindness of that side, lesion at optic chiasma leads to bitemporal hemianopia, with homonymous hemianopia in lesion posterior to optic chiasma.

Video 9: Videographic representation of the pupillary pathway where in light falls on the photoreceptors, the impulse passes through optic nerve, optic tract to reach pretectal nucleus from there both sides of Edinger–Westphal nucleus gets stimulated which via ciliary ganglion tends to cause pupillary constriction in both eyes resulting in both direct and consensual light reflex.

CHAPTER 5

Refraction Part 2

Zain Khatib

This chapter delves deeper into astigmatism and cylindrical powers. The video presents a comprehensive, step-by-step approach to performing retinoscopy for various types of refractive errors, including simple, compound, and mixed astigmatism. Additionally, it explains how to derive the final subjective acceptance from the retinoscopy cross, providing viewers with a thorough understanding of the process.

a. *Astigmatism:* Conceptual understanding
b. Detailed subjective refraction
c. Simple and compound myopic and hyperopic astigmatism, mixed astigmatism

Kindly scan the QR code below to access the online Videos.

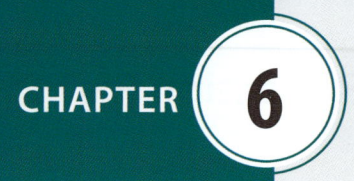

CHAPTER 6

Basic Concepts Related to Strabismus

Zain Khatib

Strabismus is often a challenging topic for many ophthalmologists to fully understand. Concepts such as the horopter, diplopia, and abnormal retinal correspondence necessitate a strong visual understanding for effective comprehension. This chapter explores these essential topics, providing a solid foundation for understanding strabismus and its complexities.

a. Axes and angles in the human eye
b. Binocular vision, retinal correspondence and squint
c. Concept of horopter
d. Concepts of confusion and diplopia
e. Fusion and fusional reserves
f. Abnormal retinal correspondence
g. Compensatory head posture

Kindly scan the QR code below to access the online Videos.

CHAPTER 7

Evaluation of a Case of Squint

Zain Khatib

This chapter discusses the various tests required to be done in a case of strabismus, focusing mainly on concomitant strabismus. Each test is discussed in detail with live examples and optical diagrams to aid in explanation.

a. Cover tests
b. Understanding the optics of prisms
c. Prism bar cover tests and other tests done with prisms
d. Sensory adaptation tests
e. Tests for fusional vergences
f. Tests for accommodation and convergence
g. Examples of cases of concomitant squint

Kindly scan the QR code below to access the online Videos.

Strabismus

Gunjan Saluja

BASICS OF STRABISMUS

Strabismus is the misalignment of the visual axis of two eyes.

Relevant Anatomy

See **Table 1**.

LAWS GOVERNING EXTRAOCULAR MOVEMENTS

Hering's Law of Equal Innervation

According to this law, the corresponding or "yoke" muscles get equal and simultaneous innervation aiding in motor coordination between the two eyes and binocular movement.

Sherrington's Law of Reciprocal Innervation

During binocular movement, the direct antagonist receives equal and simultaneous inhibition of innervation allowing opposing muscle to relax. For example, in levo version, the left lateral rectus gets excitatory stimulus and the left medial rectus gets simultaneous and equal inhibitory stimulus.

TABLE 1: Origin, insertion, nerve supply, and actions of extraocular muscles.

Extraocular muscle	Origin	Insertion	Nerve supply • All extraocular muscle except 4th and 6th are supplied by 3rd cranial nerve	Action
Superior rectus (SR)	All the rectus muscles originate from the annulus of Zinn located in the lesser wing of sphenoid	7.7 mm from limbus superiorly	Superior division of 3rd nerve	Elevation
Inferior rectus		6.5 mm from limbus inferiorly	Inferior division of 3rd nerve	Depression
Medial rectus		5.5 mm from limbus medially		Adduction
Lateral rectus		6.9 mm from limbus laterally	Abducens	Abduction
Superior oblique	Lesser wing of sphenoid	Passes beneath SR Anterior end 12–14 mm behind limbus Posterior end 17–19 mm behind limbus	Trochlear nerve	• Intorsion • Depression in adduction
Inferior oblique	Orbital surface of maxilla	• Inserts posterior to the equator inferolaterally • Posterior to lateral rectus	Inferior division of 3rd nerve	• Extorsion • Elevation in adduction

REFERENCES

1. Freddo TF. A contemporary concept of the blood-aqueous barrier. Prog Retin Eye Res. 2013;32:181-95.
2. Goel M, Picciani RG, Lee RK, Bhattacharya SK. Aqueous humor dynamics: a review. Open Ophthalmol J. 2010;4:52-9.
3. Civan MM, Macknight AD. The ins and outs of aqueous humour secretion. Exp Eye Res. 2004;78(3):625-31.
4. Tsin A, Betts-Obregon B, Grigsby J. Visual cycle proteins: Structure, function, and roles in human retinal disease. J Biol Chem. 2018;293(34):13016-21.
5. Blake R, Wilson H. Binocular vision. Vision Res. 2011;51(7):754-70.
6. Patel SC, Smith SM, Kessler AT, Bhatt AA. Imaging of the Primary Visual Pathway based on Visual Deficits. J Clin Imaging Sci. 2021;11:19.
7. Shields MB, Kanski JJ. Shields' Textbook of Glaucoma, 5th edition. Philadelphia: Lippincott Williams and Wilkins; 2018.
8. Adler S, McGowan FX. Adler's Physiology, 3rd edition. Philadelphia: Elsevier; 2016.

Refraction Part 1

Zain Khatib

This chapter on refraction focuses on the fundamental principles of refraction and retinoscopy. Retinoscopy, an age-old technique in ophthalmology, is best understood with the help of visual aids and diagrams. In this video, we will explore key concepts related to these topics, accompanied by clear illustrations to enhance understanding and make the material more accessible.

a. Basics of retinoscopy
b. Understanding working distance error
c. Understanding optics of retinoscopy movements
d. Basic subjective refraction
e. Cycloplegia and wet retinoscopy

Kindly scan the QR code below to access the online Videos.

Concept of Binocular Vision and Stereopsis

Grades of Binocular Vision

- *Simultaneous macular perception*: It is the ability to perceive two dissimilar objects simultaneously that are being projected to corresponding retinal points.
- *Fusion*: Ability of two eyes to fuse similar looking objects with slight dissimilarity
- *Stereopsis*: It is the highest grade of binocular vision and is the ability to differentiate between two closely kept objects.

CLINICAL EVALUATION

Relevant history in a case of squint:
- *Age of onset:* Congenital or acquired
- History of birth trauma, ICU stay [retinopathy of prematurity (ROP)—causing pseudostrabismus], low birth weight, and milestones (divergent squint)
- *Onset:*
  - 4–6 months—infantile
  - 2 years—accommodative esotropia
- Progression and course
- History of use of glasses
- Amblyopia treatment received if any
- Any previous strabismus surgery
- *Other examination:*
  - Visual acuity—unaided or with glasses
  - Fixation—central, steady, or maintained
  - Head posture—usually associated with paralytic squint or with pattern strabismus

  Anomalous head posture can be facing turn (in horizontal limitation of movement and nystagmus) **(Fig. 1)**, chin lift (in vertical deviations), and head tilt (in patients with torsional deviation)

  Aim of anomalous head posture is to avoid diplopia by turning the head in the direction of action of paralytic muscle.

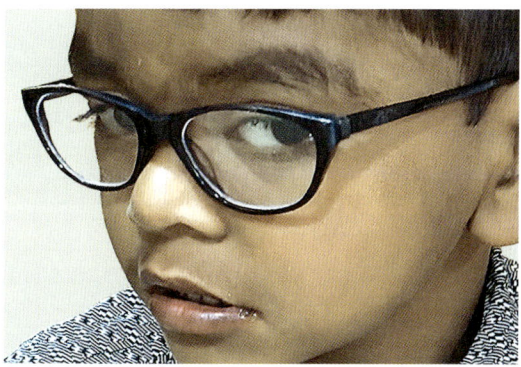

Fig. 1: Anomalous head posture, head turn in a patient of nystagmus.

- Extraocular movements—observe both uniocular (ductions) and binocular movements (versions) **(Video 1)**
- Hirschberg pupillary reflex test **(Fig. 2)**
- Grading of ocular motility **(Fig. 3)**
- Cover test **(Video 2)**
- Uncover test **(Video 3)**
- Krimsky test and prism bar cover test **(Video 4)**
- Near point of convergence (NPC) **(Video 5)**, measured with the help of RAF rule
- Near point of accommodation (NPA) **(Video 5)**
  Normal NPA varies according to age
  A complete ocular evaluation of anterior and posterior segment should be performed.

Sensory Evaluation of Strabismus (Video 6)

AC/A ratio: AC/A ratio is the ratio of accommodative convergence to accommodation **(Table 2)**.

Esodeviation

Esodeviation is an inward deviation of the eyeball.

True versus pseudoesotropia: Pseudoesotropia—Appearance of esotropia but no refixation movement is noted on cover test.

36 Strabismus

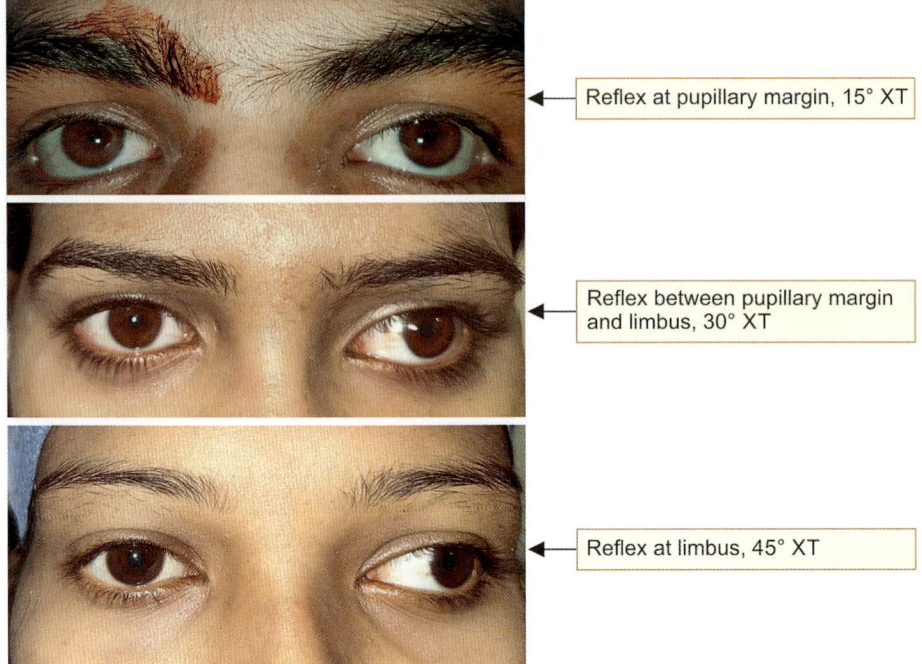

Fig. 2: Hirschberg pupillary light reflex (not the location of pupillary reflex), at the pupillary margin suggest 15°, between pupillary margin and limbus suggest 30°, and at the limbus suggest 45°.

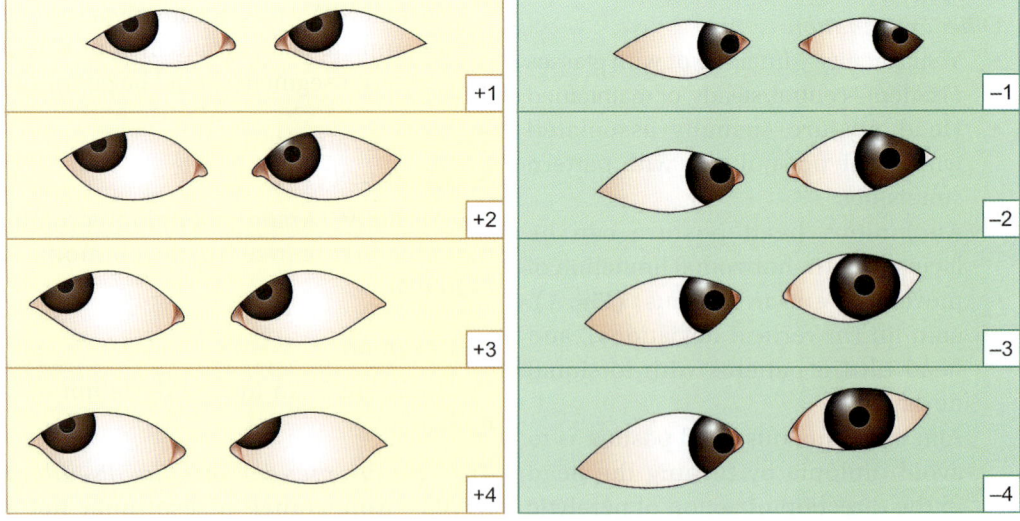

Fig. 3: Grading of ocular motility (overaction and underaction).

TABLE 2: Tests for binocularity and stereopsis at distance and near.

Test for binocularity	Test for stereopsis	
	Distance	Near
Worth four dot test (Fig. 4)	FD2 test (Frisby Davis distance test)	Randot—Vectographic (Fig. 6)
Bagolini-striated glasses	Distance Randot	TNO—Anaglyph
After image test, synaptophore (Fig. 5)		Lang's—Panographic

$$\text{Heterophoria method AC/A} = \frac{\text{IPD} + \text{Deviation for near} - \text{Deviation for distance}}{\text{Diopters of accommodation}}$$

$$\text{Gradient method AC/A} = \frac{\text{Deviation with lens} - \text{Deviation without lens}}{\text{Power of lens used}}$$

Note: "−" sign is used for exodeviations and "+" for esodeviations

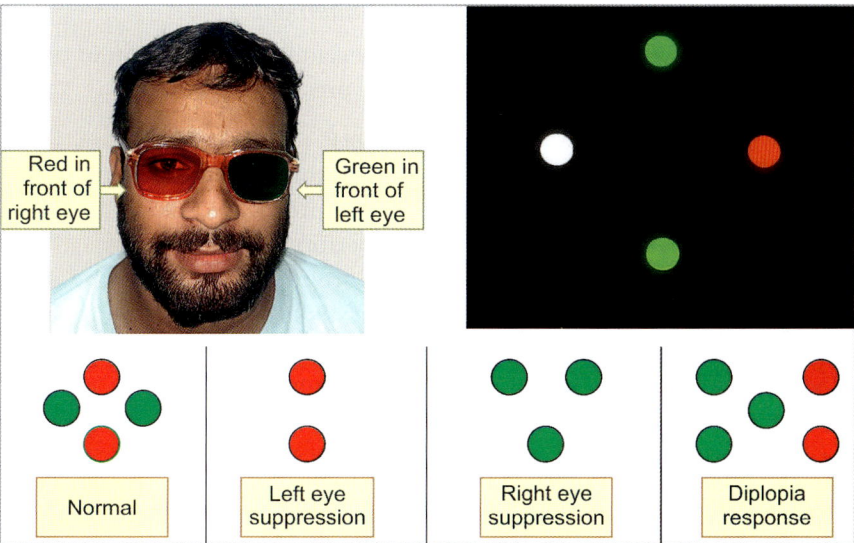

Fig. 4: Worth four dot test.

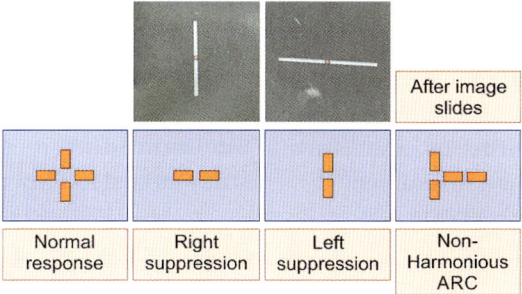

Fig. 5: After image test.

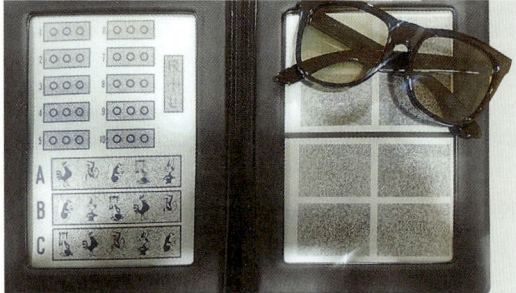

Fig. 6: Randot stereoacuity.

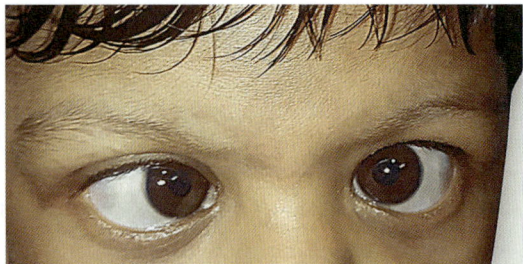

Fig. 8: Infantile esotropia. Note the onset is at 4–6 months of age with large angle of strabismus.

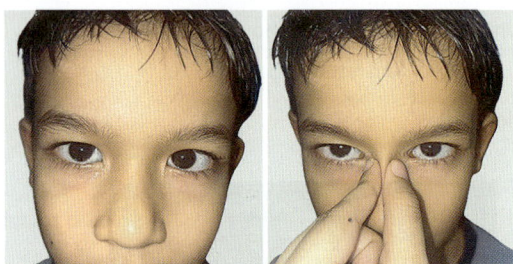

Fig. 7: Epicanthal fold with pseudoesotropia.

Causes:
- Epicanthal fold **(Fig. 7)**
- Large telecanthus
- Euryblepharon
- Large palpebral aperture

CLASSIFICATION
- Infantile esotropia
- Accommodative esotropia
- Microtropia
- Cyclic esotropia
- Sensory esotropia
- Consecutive esotropia

Infantile Esotropia

Infantile esotropia is characterized by the following **(Fig. 8)**:
- Onset at 4-6 months of age (term congenital esotropia is a misnomer)
- Large angle esotropia >30 PD
- Free alternate cross fixation
- Asymmetric optokinetic nystagmus
- No significant refractive error

- Not associated with mental deficit
- Associated with inferior oblique overaction in 66%, dissociated vertical deviation in 50%, and nystagmus in 33%.[1]

Management

Full cycloplegic correction of refractive error to be prescribed.

Surgery
- Bilateral medial rectus recession or unilateral recession resection to be performed.
- Careful examination and correction of associated inferior oblique overaction, dissociated vertical deviation, and nystagmus.

Accommodative Esotropia
- Accommodative esotropia results from uncorrected refractive error
- Blurred image acts as a stimulus for accommodation that is accompanied by convergence.
- Further poor fusional divergence results in esotropia **(Fig. 9)**.

Classification and management of accommodative esotropia has been summarized in **Flowchart 1**.

Microtropia
- Heterotropia less than five prism diopters associated with anomalous retinal

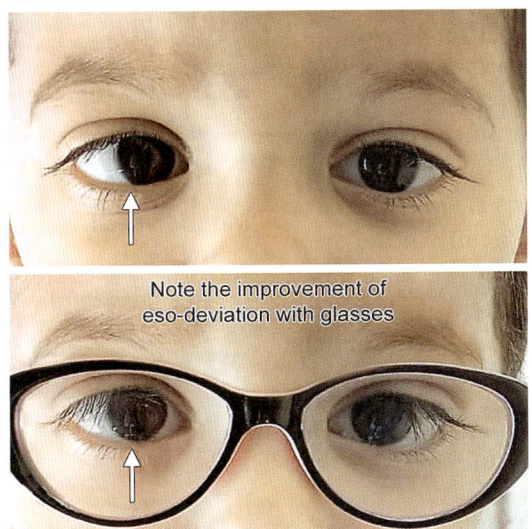

Fig. 9: Accommodative esotropia, note correction of squint with glasses alone.

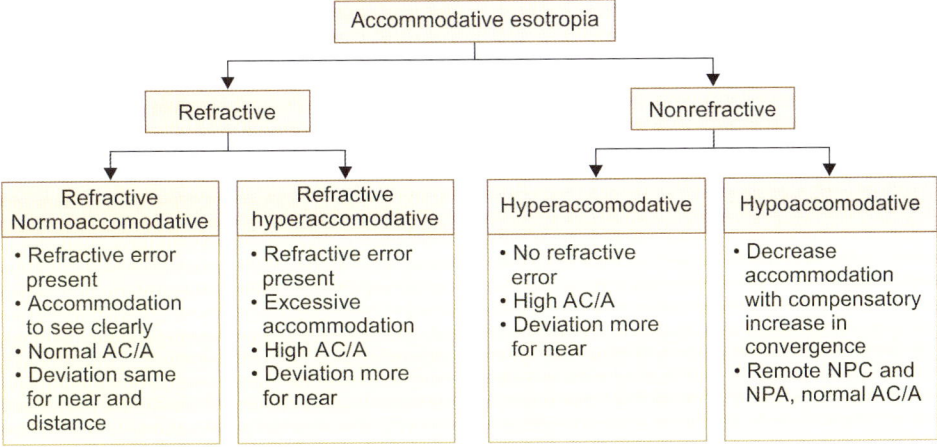

Flowchart 1: Classification of accommodative esotropia based on refractive and nonrefractive mechanisms.

(NPA: near point of accommodation; NPC: near point of convergence)

correspondence, partial stereopsis, and mild amblyopia
- Microtropia can be primary (related to strong dominance of fixating eye) or consecutive (after surgical correction of large angle heterotropia).

Diagnosis
- Bagolini-striated glass
- Four prisms base-out test **(Video 7)**
- Foveo-foveal test of Cuppers

Management of microtropia aims to treat amblyopia, done with occlusion

Cyclic Esotropia

- Cyclic change of deviation, with cycles lasting for 24–48 hours
- Orthophoria on nonsquint days with large angle esodeviation on squint days
- Exact etiopathogenesis is not known, can be due to low visual acuity in one as in cases of retinitis pigmentosa and traumatic aphakia. Also reported with ocular myositis, Graves' disease, craniofacial surgeries, and after brachytherapy.[2]

Management: Surgery is planned according to the deviation on the squinting days.

Acute Concomitant Esotropia

- Acute onset esotropia without any limitation of extraocular movements
- Associated with diplopia and normal binocular vision

Types have been summarized in the **Table 3**.

Sensory Esotropia

Early onset unilateral loss of vision results in esotropia **(Fig. 10)**

Consecutive Esotropia

- Esotropia appearing after surgery for exotropia
- Common in children undergoing surgery for intermittent exotropia
- Causes of consecutive esotropia in accordance with various steps have been summarized in **Table 4**.

Management

- Forced duction test (FDT) should be made free by carefully dissecting scar tissue

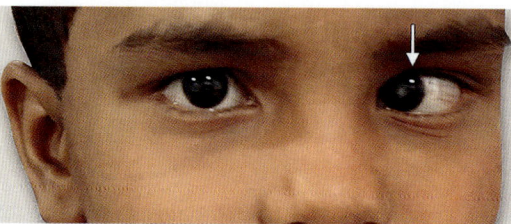

Fig. 10: Sensory esotropia in left eye due to congenital cataract.

TABLE 4: Causes of consecutive esotropia at various surgical stages.

Preoperative	• *Age:* Uncooperative patient • Errors in the measurement of deviation
Intraoperative	• Wrong measurements in caliper • Tight resection sutures
Postoperative	• Lost lateral rectus • Increase in axial length • Formation of pseudotendon

TABLE 3: Classification, pathogenesis, and management of acute concomitant esotropia*.

Types	Pathogenesis	Management
Type 1: Swan	Hyperopia with high accommodative convergence	Cycloplegic refraction
Type 2: Franceschetti	Esophoria manifestation to Esotropia triggered by illness, emotional, psychological stress, excessive near work	• Cycloplegic refraction • Reduce screen time • Avoid excess near work • Eye drop homide • Botox/surgical intervention for persistent esotropia
Type 3: Bielschowsky	Associated with myopia	

*Acute concomitant esotropia can be associated with large number of CNS disorders making neuroimaging essential

- Conjunctival recession should be performed to free FDT
- In cases of slipped lateral rectus, exploration with advancement of lateral rectus should be performed.

EXODEVIATION

Exotropia is an outward deviation of the eyeball, that can be concomitant or inconcomitant

True versus Pseudoexotropia

Appearance of exotropia with no movement on cover test.

Causes
- Hypertelorism
- Positive angle kappa

- Dragged macula due to foveal scarring as in retinopathy of prematurity

Convergence types
Refer to **Flowchart 2**.

True Exotropia

Exotropia classification
Infantile exotropia:
- Rare and usually associated with neurological abnormalities
- Freely alternating
- Lack of binocularity

*Intermittent divergent squint (**Fig. 11**) (IDS):*
- Exotropia is intermittently controlled by the convergence.
- Low birth weight, maternal smoking, and monozygotic twins are at an increased risk

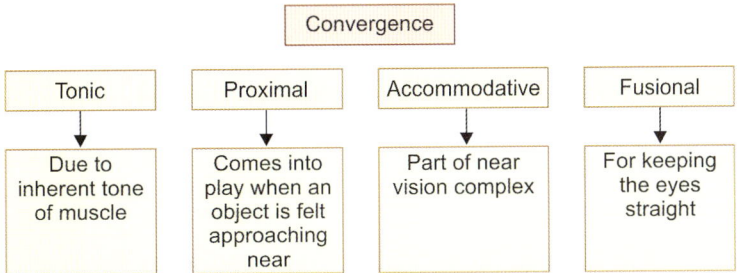

Flowchart 2: Types of convergence and their functional significance.

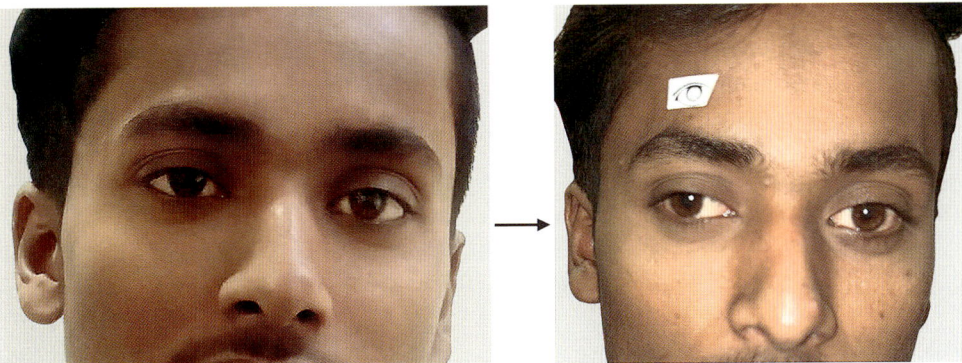

Patient is intermittently able to maintain the eye straight

Fig. 11: Intermittent divergent squint.

Table 5 shows the Calhounz staging of intermittent divergent squint.

Management of IDS
Refer to **Flowchart 3 and Table 6**.

Sensory Exotropia
Vision loss in one eye can lead to exodeviation.

Pattern Strabismus
- Pattern squints are horizontally comitant vertically incomitant squint **(Video 8)**.
- The following patterns can be observed:

> *A pattern*: Difference in deviation in upgaze and downgaze >10 PD

> *V pattern*: Difference in deviation in upgaze and downgaze >15 PD

> *X pattern*: Exodeviation in both upgaze and downgaze

TABLE 5: Calhounz staging of intermittent divergent squint.

Stage	Near	Distance
1	Orthophoria	Exophoria
2	Exophoria	Intermittent exodeviation
3	Intermittent exodeviation	Exotropia
4	Exotropia	Exotropia

Management
Refer to **Flowchart 4**.
- Anatomical factors such as plagiocephaly causing desagitalization of trochlea can also be associated with pattern strabismus.
- In patients with pattern strabismus but no oblique overaction, shifting of horizontal

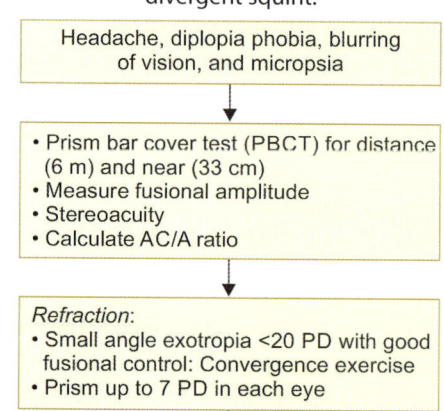

Flowchart 3: Management of intermittent divergent squint.

(PD: prism diopters)

TABLE 6: Classification of exodeviation based on AC/A ratio and corresponding management.

Type	Deviation	AC/A	Management
Convergence insufficiency	Deviation for near > deviation for distance (>10 PD)	Low AC/A	Bilateral MR resection
True divergence excess	• Deviation for distance > deviation for near • Difference persists even after occlusion/ +3D	• High AC/A • Due to proximal convergence	• Bilateral LR recession • May need +3 glasses for near
Basic	Deviation for near = deviation for distance	Normal AC/A	Bilateral LR recession/LR recession + MR resection
Simulated divergence excess	• Deviation for distance > deviation for near (>10 PD) • Difference disappears after occlusion for 30 min/+3D	• High AC/A • Due to tenacious proximal fusion	Bilateral LR recession/LR recession + MR resection

Flowchart 4: Classification and management of A and V patterns in strabismus.

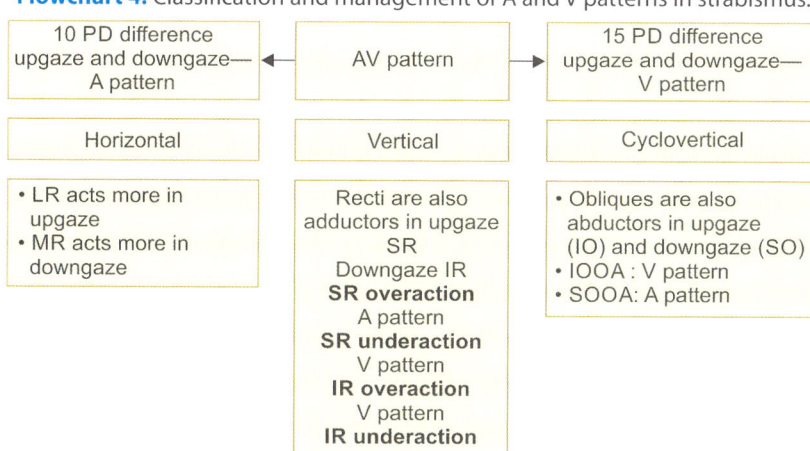

(IOOA: inferior oblique over-action; IR: inferior rectus; LR: lateral rectus; MR: medial rectus; PD: prism diopters; SOOA: superior oblique over-action; SR: superior rectus)

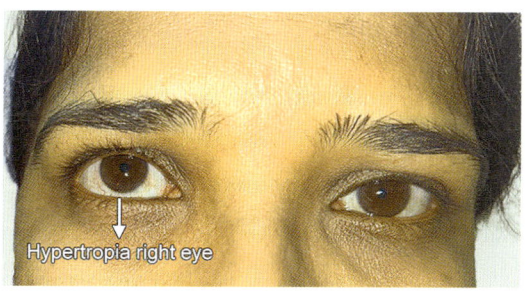

Fig. 12: Dissociated vertical deviation.

Flowchart 5: Clinical approach and management of dissociative vertical deviation (DVD).

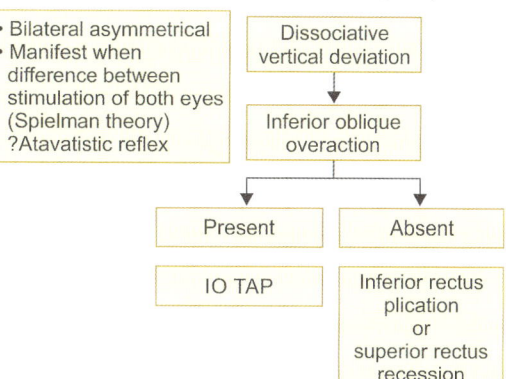

(IO TAP: inferior oblique total anterior positioning)

recti can be planned (MR toward apex and LR toward base).

Dissociated Vertical Deviation (Fig. 12)
Refer to **Flowchart 5**.

Noncomitant Squint
- Incomitant strabismus is the misalignment of visual axis that varies in different gaze.
- Incomitant squint can be paralytic or restrictive.

Paralytic squint
- Paralytic squint can result from the paralysis of 3rd, 4th, or 6th cranial nerve.
- The neurological causes can be supranuclear, nuclear, internuclear, or fascicular.
- Paralytic squint can be due to the following etiologies:
  • Congenital—following birth trauma
  • Trauma
  • Compression by intracranial mass/aneurysm
  • Ischemic causes—hypertension and diabetes

Clinical characters of paralytic squint:

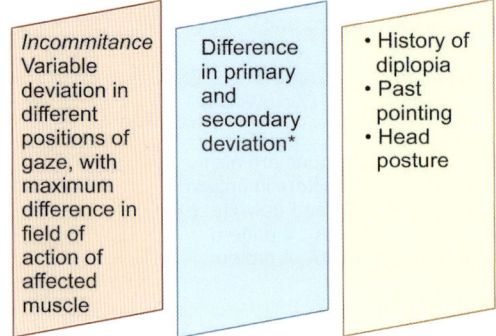

*Primary deviation is deviation measured with normal eye fixing. Secondary deviation is measured with affected (deviated paralytic) eye fixing. As it takes more innervation for the paralytic eye to take up fixation, secondary deviation is usually more than primary deviation.

Phases of paralytic squint:

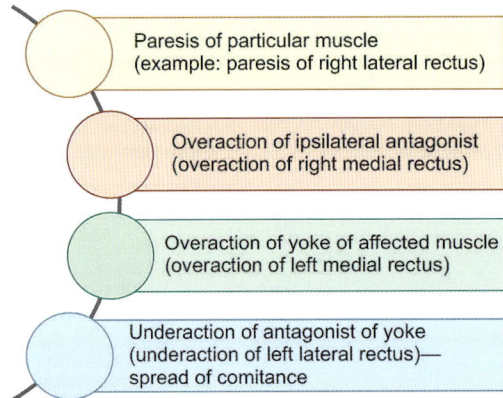

The various phases of paralytic squint can be documented with the help of Hess chart **(Video 9)**.

Third nerve palsy: Third nerve supplies superior rectus (SR), inferior rectus (IR), medial rectus (MR), inferior oblique (IO), and levator palpebrae superioris (LPS), hence, third nerve palsy causes loss of action of these muscles causing the eye to be fixed in down and out position **(Fig. 13)**.

Management of third nerve palsy
Refer to **Flowchart 6**.

Fourth nerve palsy (Fig. 12):
Management of fourth nerve palsy:
Refer to **Flowchart 7**.

Bilateral involvement is seen usually in patients with closed head trauma, with >10° of cyclodeviation. Cyclodeviation can be measured by subjective or objective methods.
- Subjective methods include synaptophore, using after image slides and Double Maddox rod **(Video 13)**
- Objective method includes indirect ophthalmoscope and fundus photography

Sixth nerve palsy (Video 14)

Management of sixth nerve palsy:
Refer to **Flowchart 8**.

Restrictive squint
In restrictive squint, the amount of limitation of movement is much more than deviation **(Fig. 14)**.

Duane's retraction syndrome (Video 15)

Refer to **Flowchart 9**.

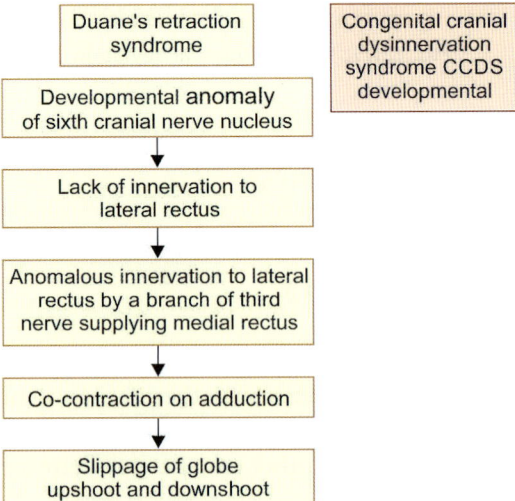

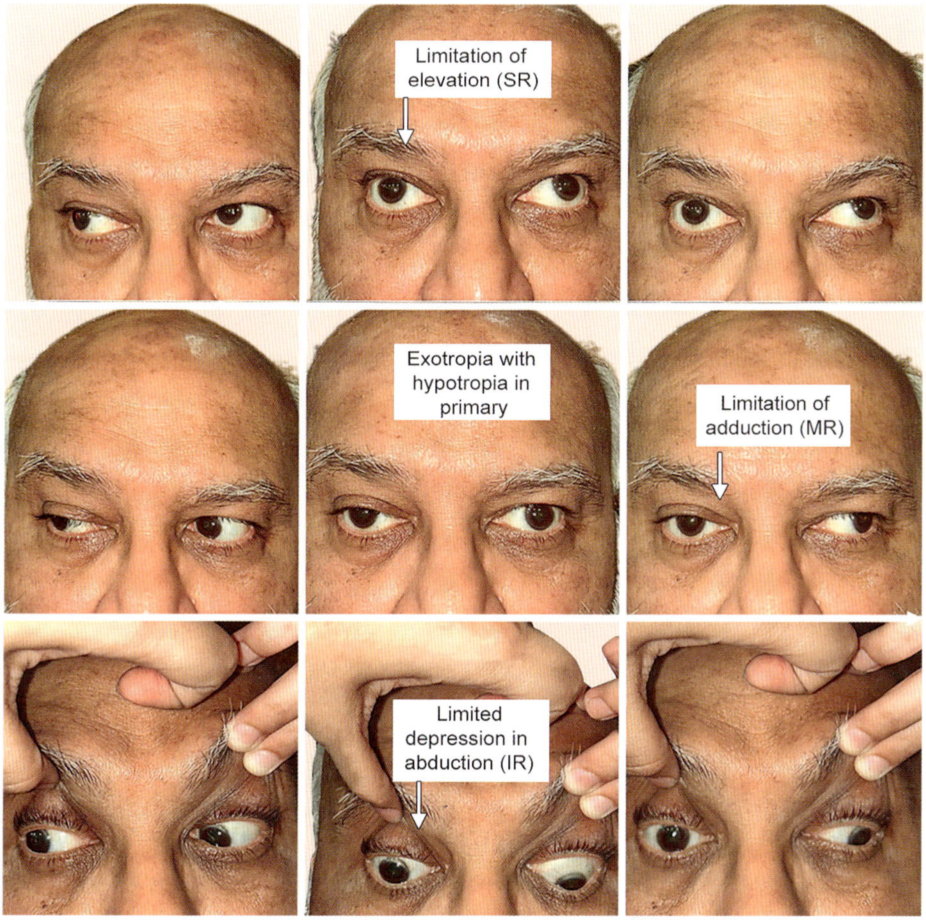

Fig. 13: Third nerve palsy.

Flowchart 6: Management of third nerve palsy.

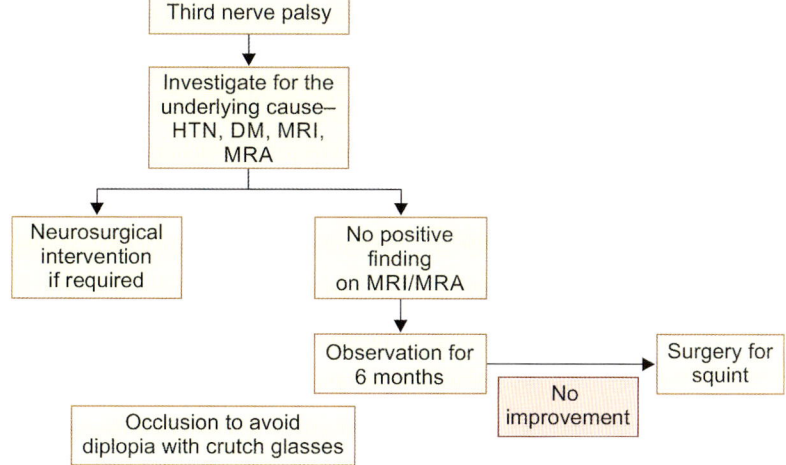

Contd...

Strabismus

Contd...

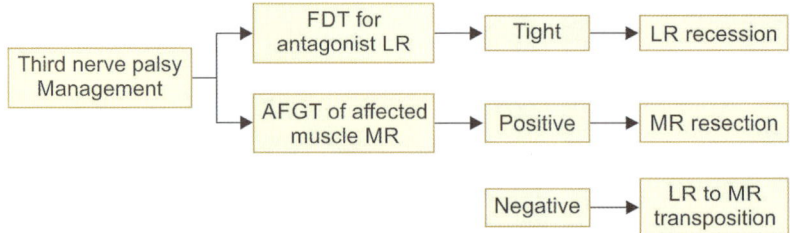

Note: Forced duction test and AFGT (Refer to **Flowchart 6**)
(AFGT: active force generation test; DM: diabetes mellitus; FDT: forced duction test; HTN: hypertension; LR: lateral rectus; MR: medial rectus; MRA: magnetic resonance angiography; MRI: magnetic resonance imaging) **(Videos 10 and 11)**

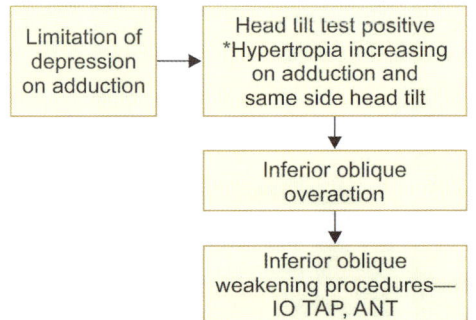

Flowchart 7: Management of fourth nerve palsy.

*Head tilt test **(Video 12)**
(IO ANT: inferior oblique antero-nasal transposition; IO TAP: inferior oblique total anterior positioning)

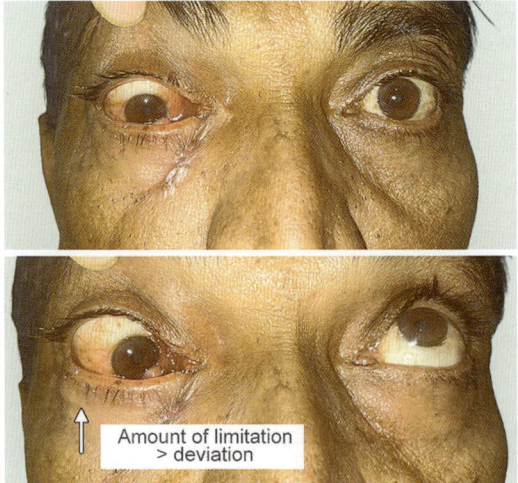

Fig. 14: Restrictive squint.

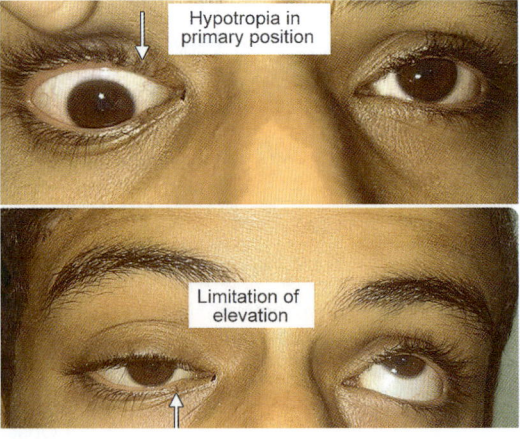

Fig. 15: Monocular elevation deficit.

Flowchart 8: Management of sixth nerve palsy.

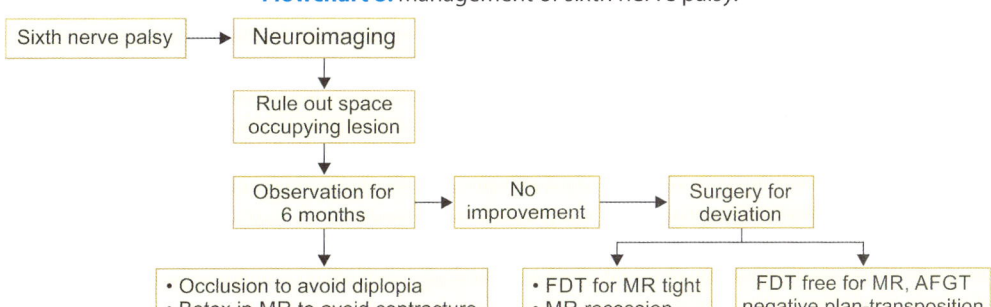

Flowchart 9: Management of Duane's retraction syndrome.

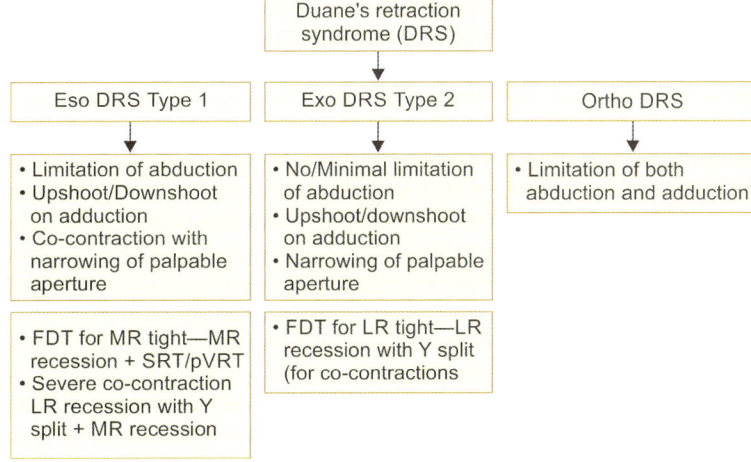

Myopic strabismus fixus:
Etiology: Exact etiology is not known **(Fig. 16)**.

Various Suggested Etiologies of Strabismus Fixus

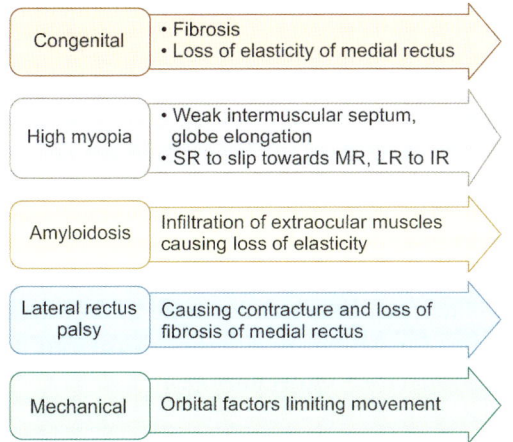

Evaluation and management
Refer to **Flowchart 10**.

Brown's syndrome: Also known as superior oblique sheath syndrome **(Video 16)**.

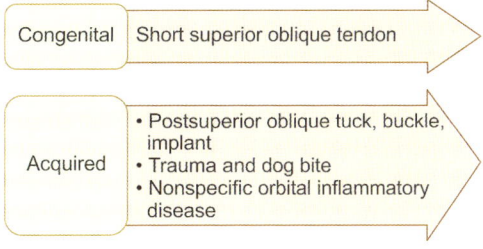

Flowchart 10: Evaluation and management of heavy eye syndrome.

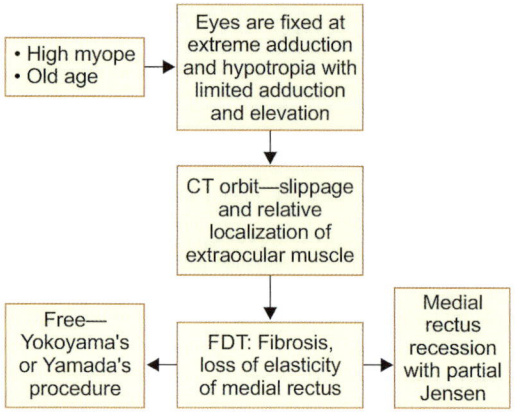

Flowchart 11: Evaluation and management of monocular elevation deficiency (MED).

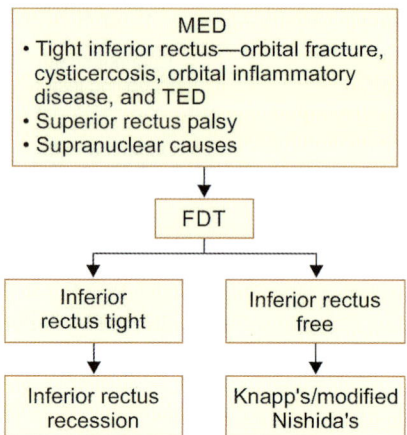

TABLE 7: Differential diagnosis of vertical strabismus with limited elevation in adduction.

Features	Brown's syndrome	Inferior oblique paresis	Primary superior oblique overaction
Clinical examination	Limitation of elevation on adduction	Limitation of elevation on adduction, associated with superior oblique overaction	Overdepression on adduction
Pattern	Y pattern	A pattern	A pattern
Forced duction test for superior oblique	Positive	Negative	Negative

Shortening of superior oblique tendon by congenital or acquired causes results in limitation of elevation in adduction.

Clinical features: Brown's syndrome can be mild, moderate, or severe.
- *Mild:* No hypotropia in primary
- *Moderate:* Hypotropia in adduction
- *Severe:* Hypotropia in primary
  - Brown's syndrome can be associated with superior oblique overaction (Brown's plus)
  - Limitation of elevation on adduction
  - Forced duction test for superior oblique is tight.
  - Slippage of globe on elevation results in Y pattern

Differential diagnosis:
See **Table 7**.

Management
- Superior oblique sheathectomy
- Superior oblique tenotomy and tenectomy
- Superior oblique expander surgery
- Lengthening of superior oblique tendon

MONOCULAR ELEVATION DEFICIT

See **Flowchart 11** and **Figure 15**.

Amblyopia

Unilateral or bilateral decrease in the visual acuity for which no organic cause can be attributed (*See* **Flowchart 12**).

Video 5: Measurement of near point convergence and near point accommodation using RAF rule. (measured with the help of RAF rule) Near point of convergence is the nearest point at which the target appears double. Normal NPC is 8–10 cm. Near point of accommodation is the nearest point at which target appears blurred.
Video 6: Synaptophore.
Video 7: Four prism base-out test for microtropia.
Video 8: V-pattern.
Video 9: Diplopia charting and Hess chart.
Video 10: Forced duction test.
Video 11: Active force generation test.
of prism till no refixation movement is obtained.
Video 12: Superior oblique palsy and head tilt test.
Video 13: Torsion evaluation.
Video 14: Sixth nerve palsy.
Video 15: Duane's retraction syndrome.
Video 16: Brown's syndrome.

REFERENCES

1. von Noorden GK, Campos EC. Exodeviations. In: von Noorden GK, Campos EC (Eds). Binocular Vision and Ocular Motility: Theory and Management of Strabismus. St. Louis: Mosby; 2002. pp. 356-376.
2. Garg SJ, Archer SM. Consecutive cyclic exotropia after surgery for adult-onset cyclic esotropia. J AAPOS. 2007;11(4):412-3.
3. Haggerty H, Richardson S, Hrisos S, Strong NP, Clarke MP. The Newcastle Control Score: a new method of grading the severity of intermittent distance exotropia. Br J Ophthalmol. 2004;88(2):233-5.

CHAPTER 9

Ocular Surface Disorders

Ritu Singh

INTRODUCTION

Ocular surface disease (OSD) is common in the general population, mainly due to lifestyle changes and increased digital device use. It often significantly impacts the quality of life (QOL) for those affected.

Ocular surface disease includes dry eye disease (DED), eyelid disorders, and conjunctivitis. It typically involves multiple factors affecting the corneal and conjunctival epithelium, as well as the lacrimal and meibomian glands.

DRY EYE DISEASE

The International Dry Eye Workshop (DEWS) DED as a condition affecting the ocular surface that involves multiple factors, marked by a disruption in tear film homeostasis and associated with ocular symptoms, with key contributing factors such as tear film instability, perosmolarity, inflammation, damage to the ocular surface, and neurosensory abnormalities.

Clinical Manifestations

- Symptoms of DED consist of a burning feeling, itching, redness, dryness, a feeling of a foreign object in the eye, and blurry vision.
- Signs include conjunctival hyperemia, corneal staining with fluorescein **(Fig. 1)**, and decreased tear break-up time (TBUT).

Diagnosis

Severity can be subjectively assessed using questionnaires such as ocular surface disease index (OSDI), standard patient evaluation of eye dryness (SPEED), and 5-item dry eye questionnaire (DEQ-5). Objective assessment includes the following:

Quantitative Tests

Tear meniscus height assessment.

Schirmer test: This test is performed using Whatman paper number 42 **(Fig. 2)**.

Qualitative Tests

- Tear film break-up time (TBUT) test
- Noninvasive break-up time (NIBUT)
- Ocular surface staining

Management

Artificial tears: Apart from established medications such as carboxymethylcellulose (CMC), hydroxypropyl methylcellulose (HPMC), polyethylene glycol (PEG), sodium

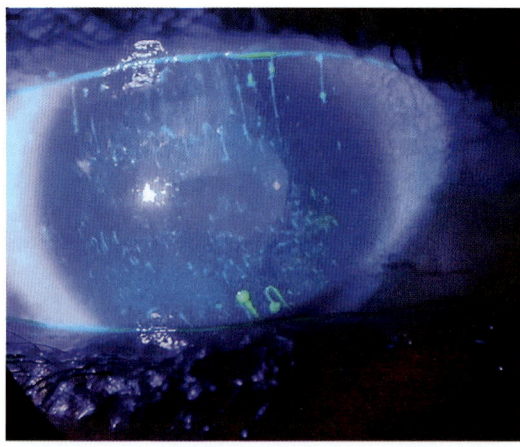

Fig. 1: Corneal staining with fluorescein viewed through a cobalt blue filter on a slit-lamp microscope. The image depicts filamentary keratitis resulting from chronic severe dry eye disease (DED).

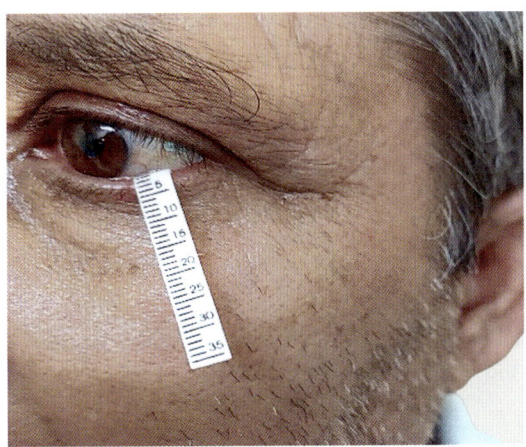

Fig. 2: Schirmer test strip placed in inferior fornix at the junction of medial two-thirds and lateral one-third of the lower lid.

hyaluronate, advances include preservative-free formulations and novel agents like lipid-based artificial tears that better mimic natural tear composition.

Perfluorohexyloctane eye drop (MIEBO) is the first topical formulation that addresses tear evaporation.

Anti-inflammatory agents: Systemic doxycycline and topical cyclosporine have shown promising results by acting upon inflammatory pathway. Newer treatments include lifitegrast (Xiidra), a lymphocyte function-associated antigen-1 (LFA-1) antagonist and emerging biologics such as anti-tumor necrosis factor-α (anti-TNF-α) agents.

- *Mucin secretagogues:* Diquafosol and rebamipide
- *Lifestyle modifications:* Increased use of wearable technology to monitor blink rates and provide reminders for ocular hydration.

Recent Advances

- *Scleral lenses:* These lenses create a fluid reservoir between the lens and the cornea, providing relief for severe dry eye patients.
- *Intense pulsed light (IPL) therapy:* This noninvasive treatment targets meibomian gland dysfunction, a common contributor to dry eye symptoms.
- *Interferometry:* Lipid layer thickness analysis by Lipiview
- *Matrix metalloproteinase-9 test:* InflammaDry
- *Tear osmolarity test*

CONJUNCTIVITIS

Definition and Types

Conjunctivitis refers to the inflammation of the conjunctiva, which can occur due to various factors, including infections, allergies, or irritants.

Clinical Manifestations

- *Viral:* Watery discharge, mild discomfort, and redness. Often associated with a recent upper respiratory infection or swollen lymph nodes.
- *Bacterial:* Thick, yellow or green discharge, more severe redness, and swelling.
- *Allergic* **(Fig. 3)***:* Itching, redness, and watery/ropy discharge. Often accompanied by other allergic constitutional symptoms.

Diagnosis

- *Clinical examination*: Based on symptoms and appearance
- *Culture and sensitivity*
- *Allergy testing:* Recent developments include specific immunoglobulin E (IgE) testing and conjunctival provocation tests to identify allergens more accurately.

Management

- *Viral:* Supportive care; topical steroids in subepithelial involvement

Ocular Surface Disorders

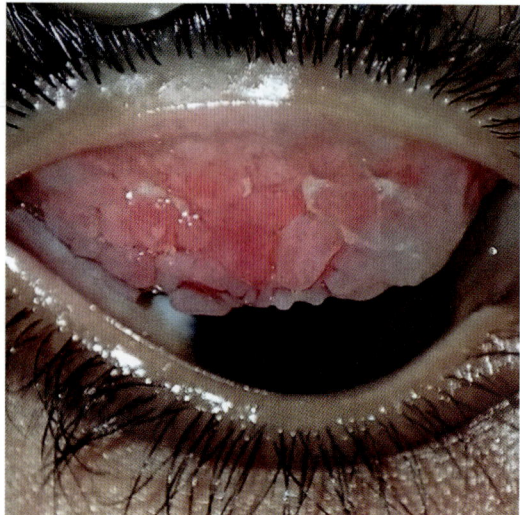

Fig. 3: Giant papillary conjunctivitis (excrescences seen on tarsal conjunctiva upon lid eversion).

- *Bacterial:* Topical antibiotics
- *Allergic:* Antihistamines, mast cell stabilizers, immunomodulators

BLEPHARITIS

Definition and Etiology

Blepharitis refers to the inflammation of the eyelid margins, commonly resulting from conditions such as seborrheic dermatitis or bacterial infections. Blepharitis can be categorized into two forms: (1) Anterior and (2) posterior.

Clinical Manifestations

- *Symptoms:* Redness, swelling, crusting, and itching of the eyelid margins
- *Signs:* Crusty debris at the eyelid margins and meibomian gland dysfunction **(Fig. 4)**

Diagnosis

Clinical history and examination: Identifying symptoms and examining eyelid margins.

Meibomian gland expression: To assess gland function, with recent advances including

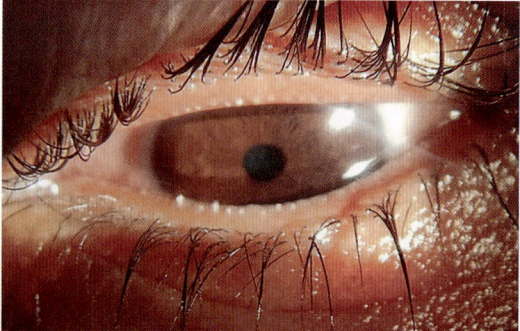

Fig. 4: Typical "toothpaste-like material" expressed in posterior meibomitis.

thermal pulsation devices that enhance meibomian gland function.

Management

- *Hygiene:* Warm compresses and eyelid scrubs; newer formulations include premoistened eyelid wipes with anti-inflammatory agents.
- *Topical antibiotics*
- *Anti-inflammatory agents:* Corticosteroids, cyclosporine A, and systemic doxycycline

Recent Advances

- *Intense pulse light therapy system:* A thermal pulsation system that provides deep heat and pulsatile massage to treat meibomian gland dysfunction.
- *Microbiome modulation:* Probiotics and other microbiome-modulating therapies are being researched for their potential to restore ocular surface health.

PTERYGIUM

Definition and Etiology

Pterygium is a benign growth of fibrovascular tissue (elastotic degeneration) that extends from the conjunctiva onto the cornea **(Fig. 5)**. It is often associated with prolonged exposure to ultraviolet (UV) light. Types include progressive and regressive.

Clinical Manifestations

- Important to differentiate from pseudo-pterygium by "probe test"

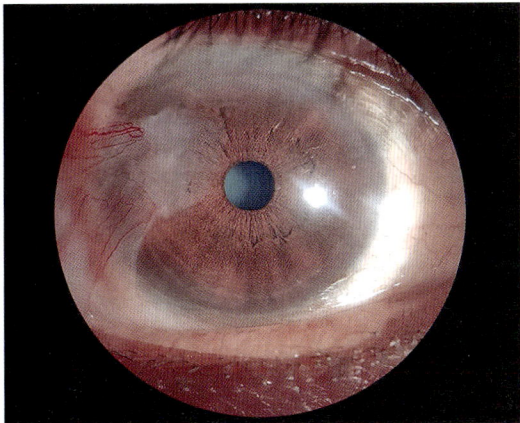

Fig. 5: Grade 2 nasal regressive pterygium.

- *Symptoms:* Eye irritation, redness, and foreign body sensation
- *Signs:* Triangular or wedge-shaped growth on the conjunctiva extending onto the cornea, which may cause astigmatism and vision problems.

Management

- *Observation:* For small and asymptomatic pterygia
- *Topical anti-inflammatory agents*
- *Surgical excision with autograft (Pterygium Extended Removal Followed by Extended Conjunctival Transplant/P.E.R.F.E.C.T) or amniotic membrane transplantation*
- Adjunctive use of mitomycin and 5-fluorouracil reduces the risk of recurrence

CHAPTER 10

Corneal Lacerations and Management Protocols

Sunandini Bose

INTRODUCTION

Ocular trauma is a significant contributor to monocular blindness in India, with an incidence rate estimated between 4.5 and 7.5%.[1,2] Corneal injuries are among the most frequent form of ocular trauma. Corneal penetrating wounds are because of sharp object with simple point of entry. Corneal lacerations can be of various sizes and shapes and can be partial thickness or full thickness in nature. Lacerations may range from straightforward linear cuts to intricate stellate patterns, and in some cases, they can affect the visual or pupillary axis. There can be tissue loss involved also. All these factors decide our choice of repair techniques and decide our clinical outcomes. Lacerations require urgent care and should be attended within 24 hours. The goal of wound repair is to have an anatomical integrity, restoration of function, attain a watertight wound, and reduce chances of microbial infection due to prolonged exposure of environment.

Ocular trauma can be broadly classified based on mechanism of injury into mechanical and nonmechanical. We will be discussing mechanical injuries only.

OCULAR TRAUMA CLASSIFICATION (FLOWCHART 1)[3,4]

The Birmingham Eye Trauma Terminology (BETT) system provides a structured classification for ocular trauma based on four parameters:
1. Type
2. Grade
3. Presence/absence of relative afferent pupillary defect (RAPD)
4. Extent/zone of injury **(Boxes 1 to 4)**

TYPE OF FOREIGN BODY

- *Toxic:*
  - *Metallic:*
    - *Magnetic:* Iron, steel, and nickel
    - *Nonmagnetic:* Copper, aluminum, mercury, and zinc
  - *Nonmetallic:* Vegetative matter
- *Inert:*
  - *Metallic:* Gold, silver, and platinum
  - *Nonmetallic:* Carbon, glass, porcelain, plaster, rubber, and stone

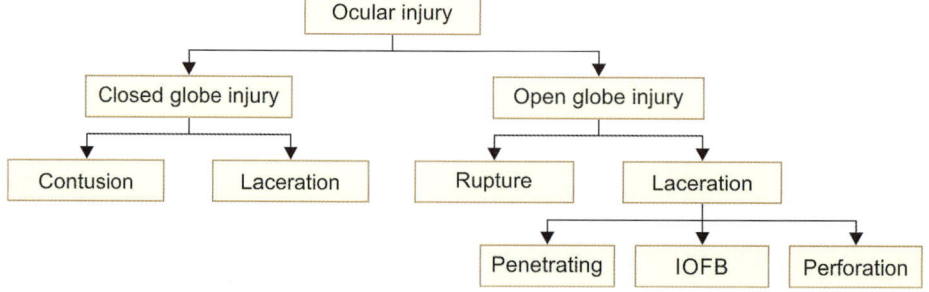

Flowchart 1: Classification of ocular trauma.[3]

(IOFB: intraocular foreign body)

Corneal Lacerations and Management Protocols

BOX 1: Open-globe injury classification.

Type
A. Rupture
B. Penetrating
C. Intraocular foreign body
D. Perforating
E. Mixed

Grade
Visual acuity
1. >20/40
2. 20/50 to 20/100
3. 19/100 to 5/200
4. 4/200 to light perception
5. No light perception

Pupil
Positive: Relative afferent pupillary defect present in the injured eye
Negative: Relative afferent pupillary defect absent

BOX 3: Closed-globe injury classification.

Type
A. Contusion
B. Lamellar laceration
C. Superficial foreign body
D. Mixed

Grade
Visual acuity
1. 2 = 20/40
2. 20/50 to 20/100
3. 19/100 to 5/200
4. 4/200 to light perception
5. No light perception[1]

Pupil
Positive: Relative afferent pupillary defect present in affected eye
Negative: Relative afferent pupillary defect absent in affected eye

BOX 2: Zones of injury in open-globe trauma. Zone I (red)—wound involvement is isolated to the cornea. Zone II (orange)—full-thickness wound involves the sclera no more posteriorly than 5 mm from the corneoscleral limbus. Zone III (blue)—full-thickness wound is posterior to zone II (Fig. 1).

Zone
Zone I: Isolated to cornea (including the corneoscleral limbus)
Zone II: Extends from the corneoscleral limbus up to 5 mm into the posterior sclera
Zone III: Positioned posterior to the anterior 5 mm of the sclera
Measurements are taken at a distance of 20 feet (6 meters) using a Snellen chart or a Rosenbaum near card, with corrective lenses and a pinhole if necessary. The test is conducted under bright lighting, with the other eye fully covered

BOX. 4: Injury zones in closed-globe trauma. Zone I (yellow) represents a superficial injury, affecting only the bulbar conjunctiva, sclera, or cornea. Zone II (red) extends into the anterior segment structures up to the posterior lens capsule, including the pars plicata. Zone III (blue) involves injury to one or more structures within the posterior segment (Fig. 2).

Zone
Zone I: External, involving only the bulbar conjunctiva, sclera, or cornea
Zone II: Anterior segment, including structures up to the posterior lens capsule and the pars plicata (excluding the pars plana)
Zone III: Posterior segment, involving structures located behind the posterior lens capsule

MANGEMENT

Patient's Examination and Preparation

It is crucial to meticulously ensure that no intraocular structures are exposed, while also minimizing any discomfort or pain for the patient.

A slit-lamp examination should be performed, along with visual acuity tests using a Snellen chart and near vision chart. A detailed examination is necessary, and a Seidel test should be conducted to rule out open- or closed-globe injuries **(Video 1)**.

- Orbit rim—rule out fracture
- Eyelids—laceration, canalicular tear, and tissue loss

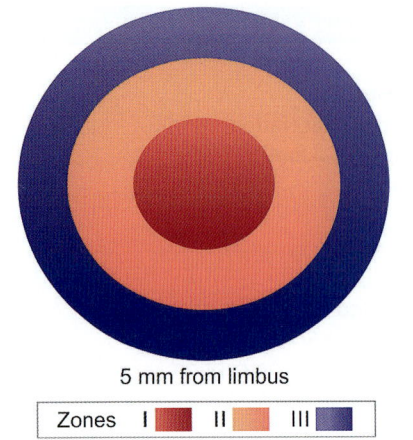

Fig. 1: Zones of injury in open-globe trauma.

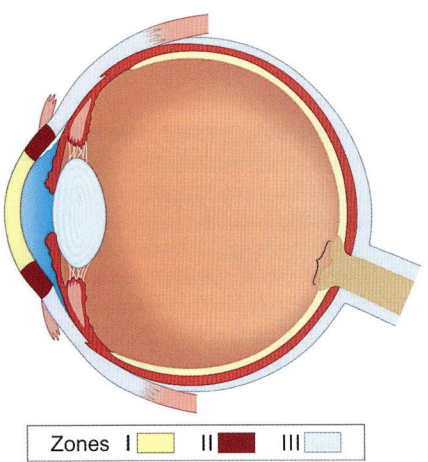

Fig. 2: Injury zones in closed-globe trauma.

- Extraocular muscle—rule out extraocular muscle entrapment and avulsion—partial or total.
- Conjunctiva—tear and subconjunctival hemorrhage
- Sclera—partial or full-thickness tear, area and dimension of tear, intraocular tissue, or vitreous protrusion
- Cornea—penetrating injury, lamellar laceration or full-thickness laceration, area and dimension of tear, visual axis involvement, intraocular tissue, or vitreous protrusion
- Iris—iris incarceration in wound and iridodialysis
- Anterior chamber (AC)—formed or not, hyphema and height, and vitreous in AC
- Lens—traumatic anterior lens capsule rupture, traumatic subluxation, and nucleus drop
- Vitreous—vitreous hemorrhage and expulsion
- Retina—retinal detachment, commotio retinae, and macular edema
- Choroidal detachment and choroidal hemorrhage
- Any signs of posterior scleral tear

While the patient awaits surgical repair, eye shield should be applied. Injection tetanus toxoid should be given if not given in last 6 months.

Imaging

- In the absence of a CT scan and due to financial constraints, plain X-rays [anteroposterior (AP) and lateral views] can be performed. X-rays help in identifying or ruling out intraocular and extraocular foreign bodies and in detecting orbital fractures.
- B-scan ultrasonography should be avoided in cases of a ruptured globe, as it poses a risk of vitreous expulsion and increases the chance of infection.
- *CT scan:* It is a noninvasive method to rule out foreign body, retinal detachment, vitreous hemorrhage, orbital wall fractures, and impacted chip of bone in tissue.
- *MRI:* It is useful in pregnant females.

Medical Management

Till the patient awaits surgery/corneal tear repair medical therapy should be started in form of eye drops and oral medications.
- Antibiotic eye drop—moxifloxacin/gatifloxacin/levofloxacin/ciprofloxacin

- Antifungal eye drop—natamycin
- Cycloplegic eye drop—homatropine and atropine
- Intraocular pressure (IOP) lowering drugs—β-blocker, α-2 agonist, and carbonic anhydrous inhibitor
- Topical steroids should be administered with caution, given the potential risk of infection.

Surgical Management

First and foremost, it is important to understand that no two lacerations are of the same nature and type. Even after years of training and doing multiple surgeries each laceration might land you in different situations.

Aim of Globe Repair

- Restoration of anatomic structure
- Watertight wound
- Prevent infection
- Restoration of smooth and optically effective refractive surface
- Reduce scarring
- Preservation of a spherical cornea to reduce astigmatism and improve contact lens fitting.
- Removal of foreign body
- Avoid uveal and vitreous incarceration
- Removal of disrupted lens and vitreous

Further discussed are the various techniques gathered with years of experience and book learning.

Anesthesia (Video 2—Subtenon Block)

Pediatric population, large tears with posterior margin not visible, uncooperative patient, mentally challenged patient, and general anesthesia should be the anesthesia of choice. General anesthesia also helps in patient's comfort, decreases chances of tissue expulsion from wound. Retrobulbar anesthesia and peribulbar anesthesia increase the vitreous pressure and should be used with caution. Subtenon anesthesia should be used with caution in scleral tear. Subtenon anesthesia is highly effective for corneal tears because it does not significantly increase pressure and can be easily topped up if needed **(Video 2)**.

Corneal Suturing Principles

While doing corneal suturing, one must remember to assess the wound length and depth, tissue loss, vitreous protrusion, choroid protrusion, lens status, and iris health.

Suture Material

- *Cornea:* 10-0 nylon, spatulated needle, may or not use double armed
- *Sclera:* 8-0 Vicryl, spatulated needle, may or may not use double armed

Equipment Needed

- Fumigated operation theater
- Microscope
- Sterile gown, gloves, eye drape sheet, and trolley cover
- Eye speculum, Lim's forceps, cyclodialysis spatula, straight forceps, corneoscleral scissor, curved forceps, needle holder, 15° side post blade, ophthalmic viscoelastic substance, balanced salt solution (BSS), sterile eye pad, eye shield, IV stand, IV line, bimanual cannulas or Simcoe cannula, and 5 mL syringe.
- In case of leak or small penetrating wound—cyanoacrylate glue and fibrin glue
- In case of tissue loss—donor cornea button
- In case of traumatic cataract with anterior lens capsule rupture—rhexis forceps, vannas scissor, vitrectomy probe ±, crescent knife, and 2.8 mm keratome knife.

Culture/debride laceration: It should be performed. It is also beneficial, if patient develops corneal infection or endophthalmitis. Care should be taken not to put undue pressure to prevent prolapse of tissue.

Partial thickness laceration: Inspect the laceration under an operating microscope. Clear out any debris under BSS with hydro cannula. Foreign bodies should be thoroughly searched under high magnification. Seidel test should be performed to confirm partial thickness depth of laceration, even if AC is formed. If positive treat as full-thickness laceration and treat as described below. If negative after clearing debris, manage with bandage contact lens (BCL) alone in case of shallow/not deep laceration. In case of deep laceration, putting suture should be considered in view of induced astigmatism after healing. Tissue adhesives, such as fibrin glue or cyanoacrylate glue, can be utilized, as both are equally effective and well-tolerated **(Video 3)**.[5,6]

Full-thickness laceration: The goal of corneal suturing is apposition of anterior and posterior margins without any overriding or underriding **(Fig. 3)**. Effects of suture placement for corneal lacerations. (1) For sharp perpendicular wounds, deep suture placement equidistant from the wound margins gives excellent wound approximation. (2) Shallow sutures create internal wound gape. (3) Full-thickness sutures may create a conduit for microbial invasion. (4) Sutures of unequal depth create wound override. (5) Sutures of unequal length create wound override. (6) For shelved lacerations, evenly spaced sutures are crucial, starting from the inner aspect of the wound, to ensure precise alignment and healing.

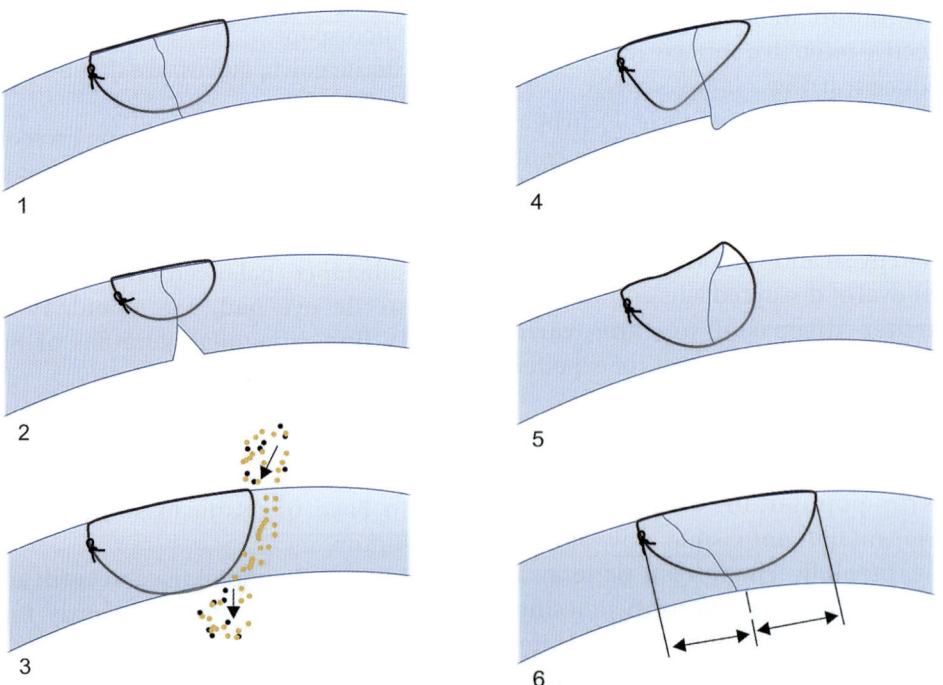

Fig. 3: Corneal suturing.

Laceration <2 mm: Tissue glue in the form of cyanoacrylate glue or fibrin glue with BCL can be used.[5,6] Multilayered amniotic membrane grafting has also shown good healing when done for corneal perforation cases along with fibrin glue or suturing technique.[7] Glue also helps in stopping epithelial invasion of the wound. Primary suturing in these cases can be avoided in view of induced astigmatism and should only be done if a watertight wound reconstruction is not possible. In case suturing is performed, long bites should be avoided, and small bites can be taken at equal distance. AC should be formed with viscoelastic substance or air depending upon the nature of tear and surgeon's experience. After repair, the wound should be checked for leak with a dry cotton-tipped bud or Seidel test can be performed. Intracameral antibiotic in the form of preservative-free moxifloxacin is injected to reduce chances of endophthalmitis (**Fig. 4**—glue BCL, **Fig. 5**—blue BCL with suture, and **Fig. 6**—laceration <2 mm)

Laceration >2 mm: If possible, drawing a cornea tear before attempting to repair is beneficial for mental preparation. Long sutures cause compression of wound and should be placed in periphery or limbus and shorter sutures should be placed in the center of cornea involving pupillary axis to avoid decreased vision due to scarring and astigmatism. Needle should pass 90% depth for proper apposition and no full-thickness sutures should be taken in view of creating track for leak and entry of microorganism. Repairing a corneal laceration should produce good apposition to the edges of laceration. Point to be noted is the suture length should be equal in both ends from posterior edge of laceration. A slip knot of 3-1-1 or 2-1-1 can be done for knot tying. Burying the knot is necessary to avoid foreign body sensation, neovascularization, infection, and loosening of suture. Keeping the loose ends short eases in burying the suture. Burying the suture should be done in

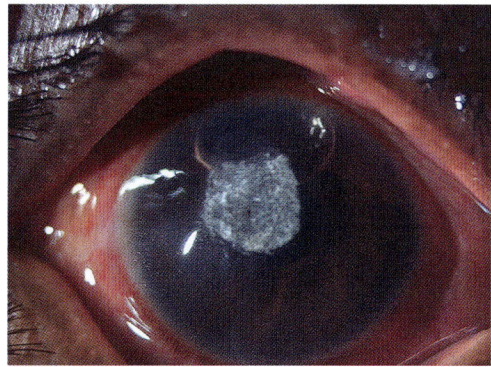

Fig. 4: Corneal laceration, repaired with cyanoacrylate glue, with placement of bandage contact lens.

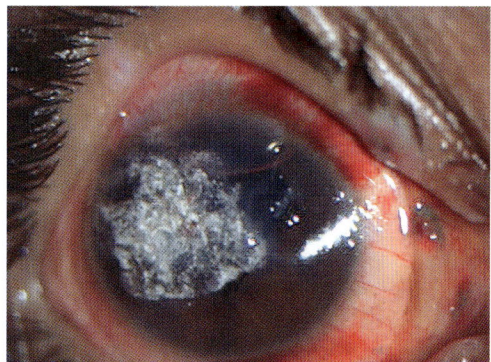

Fig. 5: Corneal laceration, repaired with cyanoacrylate glue and 10-0 nylon sutures with placement of bandage contact lens.

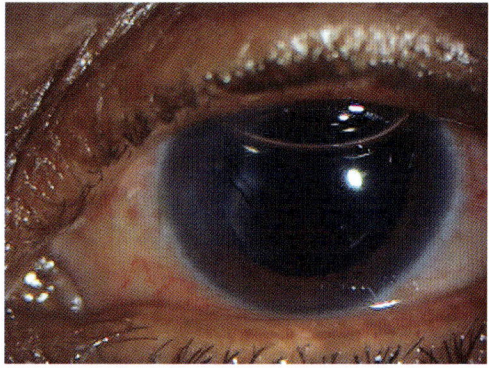

Fig. 6: Laceration less than 2 mm.

corneal stroma and after burying, the suture should be pulled to reverse direction for later easy removal. Long and tight bites of suture should be taken in cases of corneal edema of edges in laceration keeping in mind that once edema resolves, the sutures will get loose if not tightly placed **(Fig. 7)**. Suture knot burial. (1) Knot is trimmed short and rotated beneath the corneal surface using smooth forceps. (2) Direction of knot is reversed, leaving knot end away from corneal surface. (3) The knot is repositioned just beneath the corneal surface.

Suturing Techniques Based on Shape of Laceration

- *Linear laceration:* Suturing can be started from midpoint of the laceration although author prefers putting sutures at the edges of laceration first and then a single suture at the midpoint and then further sutures are places. Doing so helps in maintaining the proper anatomical curvature of the cornea or sclera. Suture placement should be perpendicular to the orientation laceration at the point suture (**Fig. 8A**—diagrammatic representation of linear laceration, **Fig. 8B**—clinical photo of linear laceration, **Fig. 9**—linear laceration with traumatic cataract, and **Fig. 10**—linear laceration).
- *Curvilinear laceration:* When the curvilinear laceration extends to the center of cornea, corneal vault should be maintained while suturing. Long, tight sutures at the periphery flatten the cornea and short, less tight suture and superficial suture at the center of the laceration (**Fig. 11A**—diagrammatic representation curvilinear laceration, **Fig. 11B**—clinical photo curvilinear laceration with peripheral long suture and center smaller suture, and **Fig. 12**—curvilinear with IOL).
- *Oblique laceration:* As depicted in the **Figure 3**, the suture needs to be equal length from the posterior aspect/margin of the tear. If not then anterior overriding will occur and excessive scarring, granulation tissue, poor wound healing, and astigmatism will happen. Tension of suture should be balanced otherwise cheese wiring from the shallow end will occur. In a case scenario of both perpendicular as well as shelved/oblique laceration, the perpendicular laceration should be closed first to get a better approximation for the shelve/oblique part. The knot should be buried in the shorter anterior part so to avoid cut through of corneal tissue during removal (**Fig. 13**—oblique laceration and **Fig. 14A**—oblique with traumatic cataract and **Fig. 14B**— oblique with IOL).

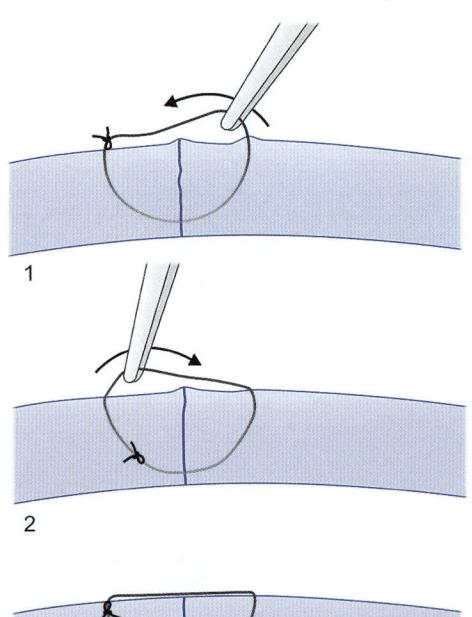

Fig. 7: Diagrammatic representation: Suture knot burial.

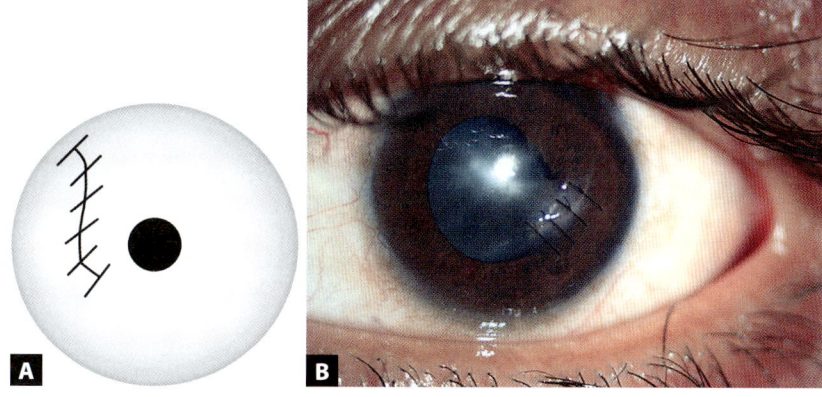

Figs. 8A and B: (A) Linear laceration; (B) Clinical photo of linear laceration.

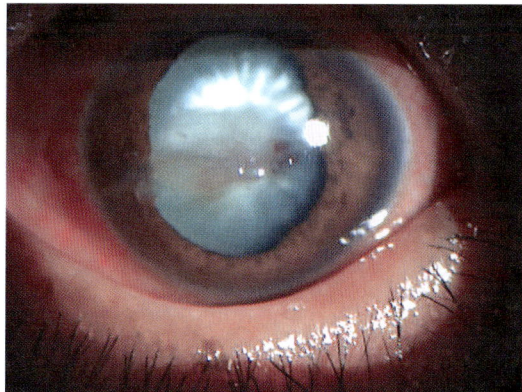

Fig. 9: Linear laceration with traumatic cataract.

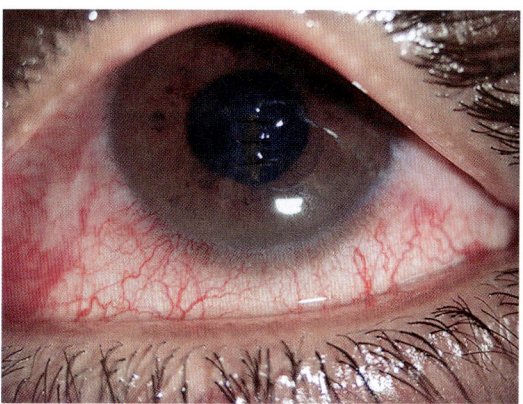

Fig. 10: Linear laceration.

- *Stellate laceration:* These are complex and challenging to deal with. The apex of the tear can be managed with a purse string suture or horizontal mattress suture. The purse string suture technique involves the use of a guarded diamond knife, calibrated to a depth of 0.3 mm, to create incisions in the normal corneal stroma, reaching half of the stromal thickness. Subsequently, a 10-0 nylon suture is threaded from the base of these incisions through the surrounding stroma and laceration, exiting through the adjacent incision until the apex is fully repaired on all sides. By tightening the suture, the apical edges are brought together, with the knot typically concealed within the stroma. The remaining linear sections of the wound can then be closed using standard methods **(Fig. 15)**.

Another form of stellate can be trivariate laceration. Where the three arms of the tear are held with long single sutures and the rest suturing is performed as usual **(Figs. 16A and B)**.

Corneoscleral laceration: The limbus should be repaired first for anatomic shape and then the cornea followed by the sclera. This avoids the tissue prolapse and stabilizes the globe **(Fig. 17)**.

Tissue loss: Minimal tissue loss can be managed with glue BCL after tear repair if

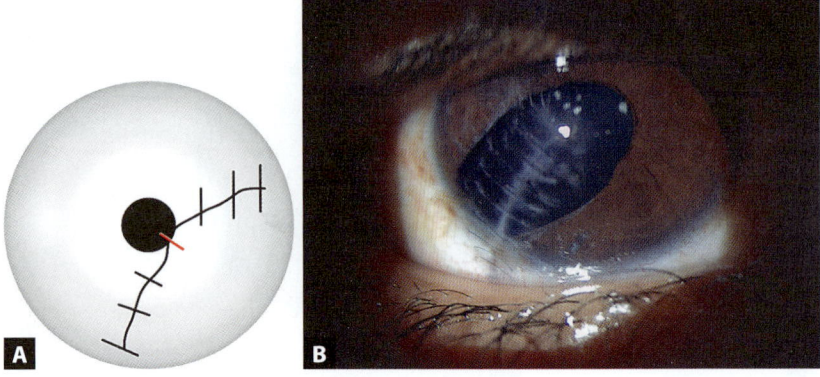

Figs. 11A and B: (A) A diagrammatic representation curvilinear laceration; (B) Clinical photo curvilinear laceration with peripheral long suture and center smaller suture.

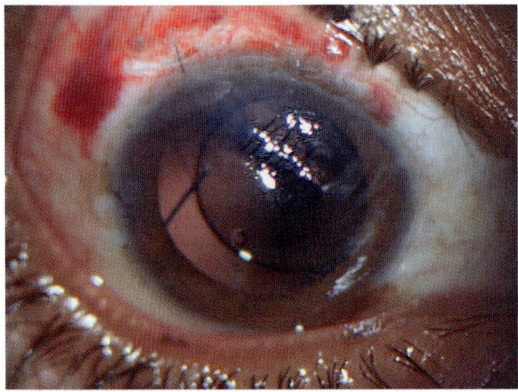

Fig. 12: Curvilinear with three piece IOL.

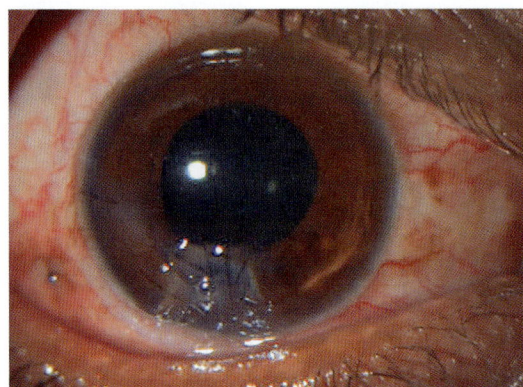

Fig. 13: Oblique laceration.

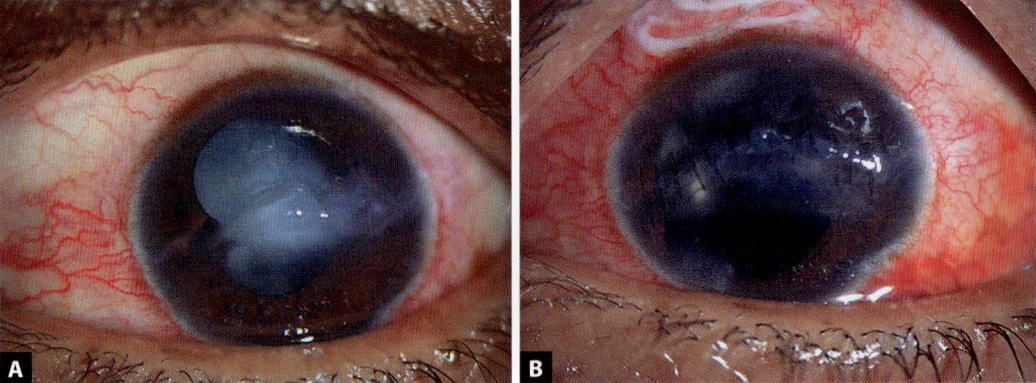

Figs. 14A and B: (A) Oblique with traumatic cataract; (B) Oblique with IOL SICS.

leak is present. Amniotic membrane grafting has also been shown to add to tectonic integrity and helps in tissue healing. Large area of tissue loss if donor cornea or sclera is available lamellar patch graft or even lamellar cornea autografting has been done. If tissue loss is beyond repair, penetrating keratoplasty can be performed in initial setting of after primary repair if donor corneal tissue is not available.

Traumatic cataract: Traumatic cataract should be removed in same sitting with or without IOL implantation depending upon the stability of the bag **(Figs. 18 and 19)**. Simple aspiration and cortical cleaning can be done after rhexis formation in younger age group. In case of nuclear sclerosis, after repairing is performed, a scleral tunnel can be made for nucleus prolapse and expression. If IOL is implanted, biometry of other eye should be taken and either three piece IOL or single piece IOL depending upon the health of zonules should be done **(Figs. 12 and 14B)**.

Decision to excise the iris or not depends upon the time since the injury and health of iris. If the iris has been prolapsed for >12 hours and the color is dull with gray-white discoloration, and excision can be performed **(Figs. 20A and B)**.

POSTOPERATIVE CARE

Depending upon the extent of injury, medication or follow-ups are maintained. Topical antibiotic eye drops, corticosteroid eye drops, cycloplegic eye drops, and lubricating eye drops should be given. In case of suspected vegetative matter or infective tear, corticosteroids should not be given. After the culture report, antibiotic eye drops/antifungal eye drops can be started accordingly.

Suture removal: It should be performed considering time since primary repair, astigmatism, healing rate, age of patient, and extent of injury. All sutures should not be removed together and alternative suture should be removed or those which are loose or very tight can be removed after healing is

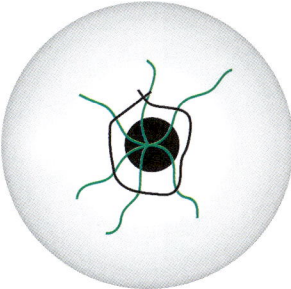

Purse string sutures—stellate laceration

Fig. 15: Stelate laceration.

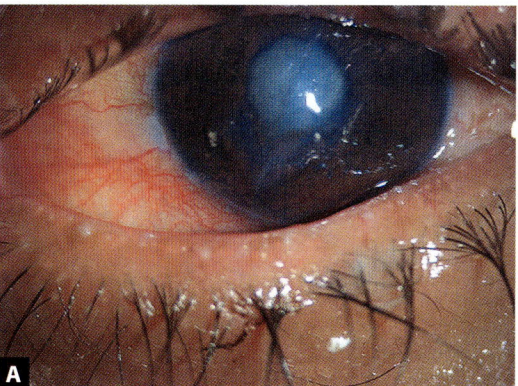
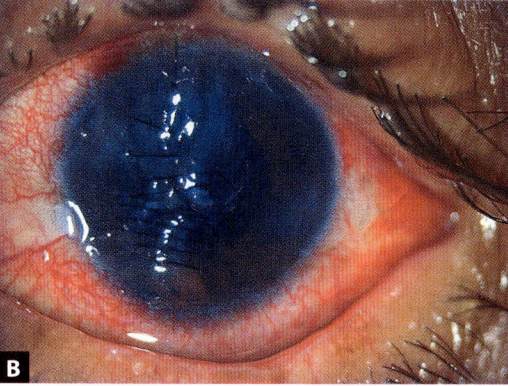

Figs. 16A and B: (A) Trivarate tear; (B) Trivarate tear repair.

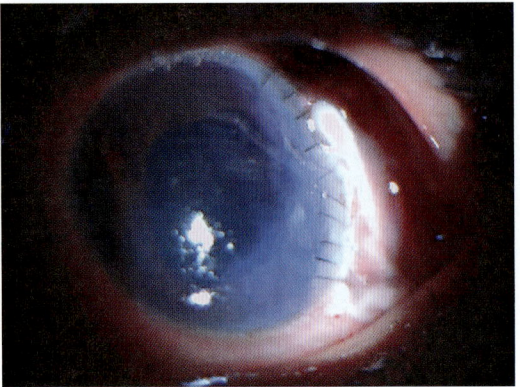
Fig. 17: Corneo scleral tear.

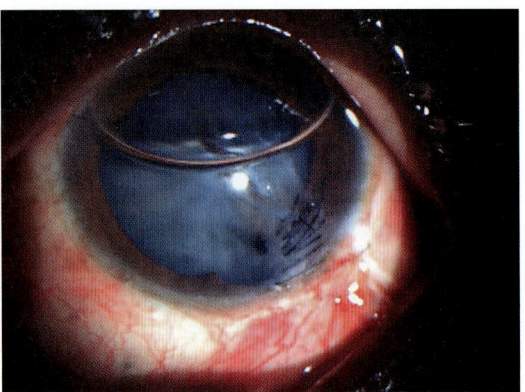
Fig. 18: Corneal peripheral tear with traumatic cataract with intact ALC.

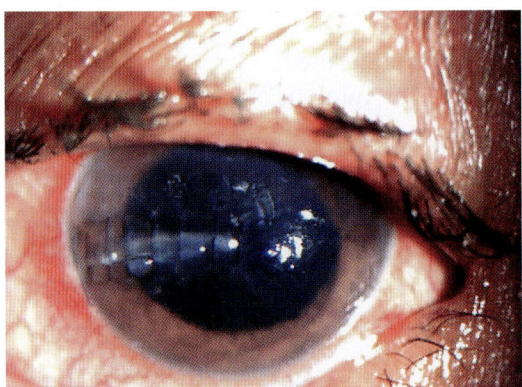
Fig. 19: Linear laceration repair with IOL.

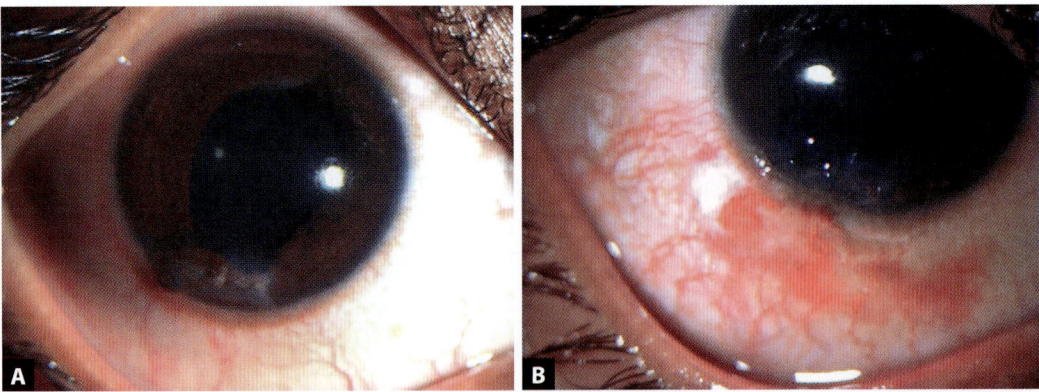
Figs. 20A and B: (A) Corneal tear with iris prolapse note the colour of iris; (B) Corneal tear repaired iris excised.

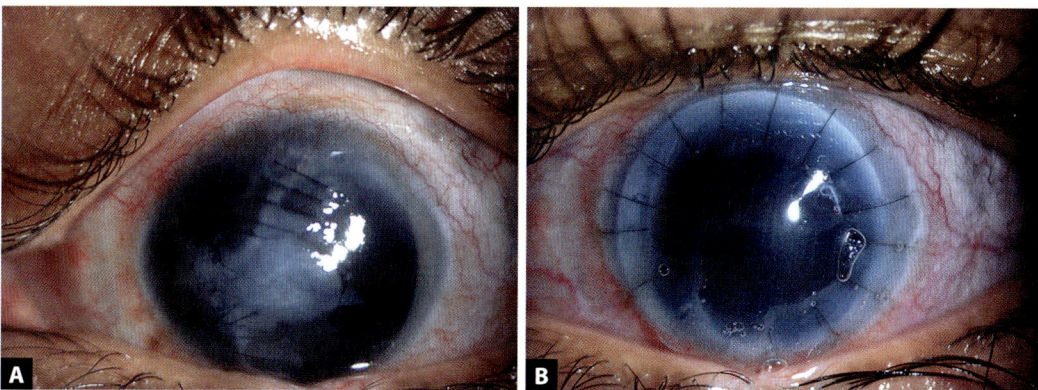

Figs. 21A and B: (A) Repaired corneal tear scarring; (B) Postcorneal tear opk.

complete. Corneal topography-guided suture removal can also be done.

Rigid gas: Permeable lenses, hybrid contact lenses, and scleral lenses represent outstanding noninvasive alternatives for enhancing patient vision and comfort, eliminating the need for further surgical intervention. In cases of excessive scarring, an optical keratoplasty can be performed to optimize visual potential **(Figs. 21A and B)**.

CONCLUSION

A corneal tear repair is work of art. Prompt treatment and management helps in saving the vision and anatomic integrity of the eye. Proper postoperative care and follow-up is required for complete visual rehabilitation. Public education regarding protective equipment is essential for minimizing accidents related to work or road activities.

VIDEO LEGENDS

Video 1: Siedel test-graft dehiscence
Video 2: Subtenon block
Video 3: Partial corneal tear with foreign body removal

REFERENCES

1. Nirmalan PK, Katz J, Tielsch JM, Robin AL, Thulasiraj RD, Krishnadas R, et al. Ocular trauma in a rural south Indian population: the Aravind Comprehensive Eye Survey. Ophthalmology. 2004;111(9):1778-81.
2. Krishnaiah S, Nirmalan PK, Shamanna BR, Srinivas M, Rao GN, Thomas R. Ocular trauma in a rural population of southern India: the Andhra Pradesh Eye Disease Study. Ophthalmology. 2006;113(7):1159-64.
3. Kuhn F, Morris R, Witherspoon CD, Heimann K, Jeffers JB, Treister G, et al. A standardized classification of ocular trauma. Ophthalmology. 1996;103:240-3.
4. Pieramici DJ, Sternberg P Jr, Aaberg TM Sr, Bridges WZ Jr, Capone A Jr, Cardillo JA, et al. A system for classifying mechanical injuries of the eye (globe). The Ocular Trauma Classification Group. Am J Ophthalmol. 1997;123(6):820-31.
5. Siatiri H, Moghimi S, Pourabdollah E, Rahimi F, Fallah M, Siatiri N. The efficacy of fibrin glue in corneal perforations. Iran J Ophthalmol. 2008;20:10-4.
6. Jhanji V, Young AL, Mehta JS, Sharma N, Agarwal T, Vajpayee RB. Management of corneal perforation. Surv Ophthalmol. 2011;56:522-38.
7. Hick S, Demers PE, Brunette I, La C, Mabon M, Duchesne B. Amniotic membrane transplantation and fibrin glue in the management of corneal ulcers and perforations: a review of 33 cases. Cornea. 2005;24(4):369-77.

CHAPTER 11

Keratoconus

*Sai Thaejesvi, Prasanna Venkatesh Ramesh, Shruthy Vaishali Ramesh,
Navaneeth Krishna MP, Ashik Azad, Pavithra P*

INTRODUCTION

Keratoconus is the most common corneal ectatic disorder, derived from the Greek word "keras" meaning cornea, and "conus" meaning cone—giving its word meaning of cone-shaped cornea **(Figs. 1 and 2)**. It is a bilateral, asymmetrical ocular disorder, which is characterized by gradually progressive thinning and subsequent steepening of the cornea. This manifests as decreased visual acuity in the patient and irregular astigmatism on clinical examination.[1]

EPIDEMIOLOGY

Keratoconus has a global prevalence of approximately 25 per 100,000 persons/year. The incidence is more among 20–30-year-olds, with the disease starting at puberty and reaching its peak in the third decade. There is no male-female predisposition, with both sexes being equally affected. There is a reported higher incidence among Asians in comparison to Caucasians.

ETIOPATHOGENESIS

Many processes have been proposed to explain the genesis of keratoconus.[2]

They include:

- *Genetic factors:* Polymorphisms in the lysyl oxidase (*LOX*) gene, responsible for crosslinking of collagen, which is involved in the biomechanical strength of the cornea, have been implicated. Other collagen genes which are associated with keratoconus include *COL5A1*, *COL4A3*, and *COL4A4*. Tissue remodeling genes such as matrix metalloproteinase (*MMP9*) have been linked to this disease process, as well as certain proinflammatory cytokines such as interleukins (*IL-1A* and

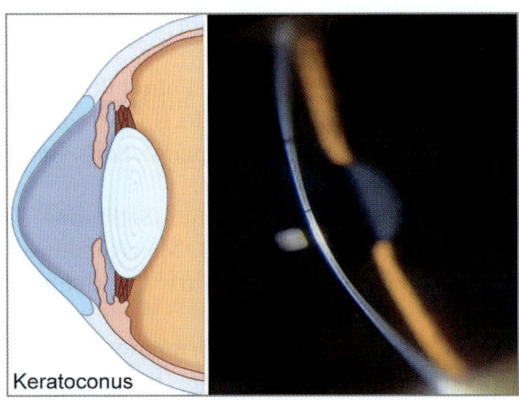

Fig. 1: Slit-lamp image of a cornea with keratoconus, demonstrating corneal thinning and conical protrusion, along with a schematic representation illustrating the abnormal corneal shape.

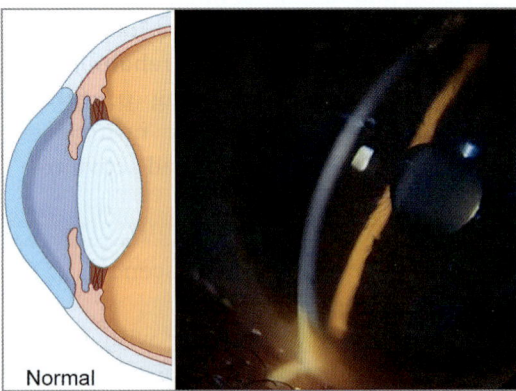

Fig. 2: Slit-lamp image of a normal cornea with a regular curvature and uniform thickness, accompanied by a schematic representation for comparison.

IL-1B genes) and transforming growth factor β-1 (*TGF-β1*) family of genes.
- *Eye rubbing:* Repeated, biomechanical friction created on the cornea by consistent eye rubbing, as seen in atopic disease and allergic keratoconjunctivitis, causes release of proinflammatory mediators, which induce proteolysis of collagen. This leads to irreversible weakening of the cornea, precipitating keratoconus.
- *Anomalous collagen:* Abnormally weak collagen, as implicated in certain connective tissue disorders, can also have an associated keratoconus.
- *Oxidative stress:* Keratoconus cases have been associated with reduced levels of antioxidants such as superoxide dismutase, glutathione, peroxidase, and catalase. Normally, these agents scavenge free radicals and prevent tissue damage.
- *Ultraviolet (UV) radiation:* Environmental UV radiation exposure causes accumulation of oxidative products, which weakens the cornea.
- *Hormones:* Presence of receptors for estrogen, progesterone, and androgens on corneal tissue explains the interplay of these hormones on the progression of keratoconus, especially in conditions such as polycystic ovarian disease (PCOD) and pregnancy. Thyroxine hormone has also been implicated.

CLINICAL CONDITIONS ASSOCIATED WITH KERATOCONUS

Associated Ocular Disorders
- Vernal keratoconjunctivitis
- Pellucid marginal degeneration
- Terrien marginal degeneration
- Fuch's corneal dystrophy
- Iridocorneal endothelial syndrome
- Aniridia
- Congenital cataract
- Retinitis pigmentosa
- Retinopathy of prematurity
- Leber tapetoretinal degeneration

Associated Systemic Disorders
- Down syndrome
- Marfan syndrome
- Ehlers–Danlos syndrome
- Osteogenesis imperfecta
- Neurofibromatosis
- Alagille syndrome

CLINICAL FEATURES

Symptoms
Typical presentation is in the late teens and 20s, with blurring of vision and history of frequent glass change. Patients may also show symptoms of associated allergic conjunctivitis and eye rubbing. Due to asymmetry of the disease, some patients may remain asymptomatic.

Signs
- Decrease in visual acuity
- Scissoring reflex on retinoscopy—due to irregular astigmatism
- Munson's sign—V-shaped protrusion of the lower lid on down gaze. Seen in advanced keratoconus, due to corneal protrusion **(Figs. 3A and B)**.
- Rizzuti sign—on throwing light on temporal limbus, sharply focused beam of light is seen on nasal limbus **(Fig. 4)**.
- On slit-lamp examination—corneal thinning and protrusion may be seen, most commonly seen in inferonasal quadrant. Scarring at the apex of the cone may be seen in advanced cases.
- Fleischer's ring is a ring of iron deposits seen at the base of the cone, best seen using cobalt filter light **(Fig. 5)**.
- Vogt striae—fine, vertical, and parallel lines seen in the posterior stroma at the

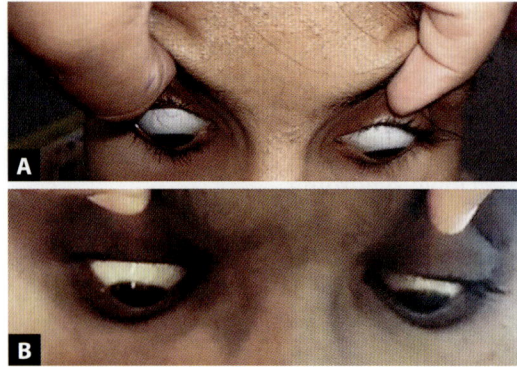

Figs. 3A and B: Clinical images demonstrating Munson's sign—V-shaped protrusion of the lower eyelid on downgaze due to corneal protrusion in advanced keratoconus.

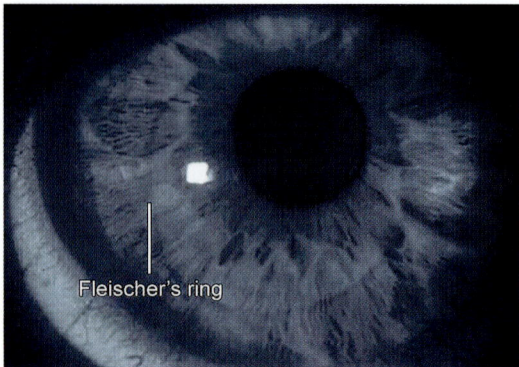

Fig. 5: Slit-lamp image demonstrating Fleischer's ring—iron deposition at the base of the cone in keratoconus, best observed using a cobalt blue filter.

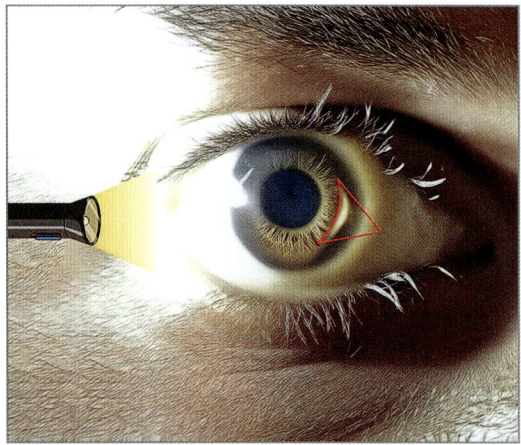

Fig. 4: Clinical image demonstrating Rizzuti's sign—conical reflection of light on the nasal cornea when a penlight is shone from the temporal side. A red triangular marking highlights the illuminated area on the nasal side.

apex of the cone. These lines disappear on appearance of external pressure.
- Charleaux oil droplet reflex—seen on retroillumination, and also with distant direct ophthalmoscopy
- Prominent corneal nerves
- Acute corneal hydrops—seen in advanced ectasia, characterized by sudden onset of pain, diminution of vision, and redness. It occurs due to imbibition of aqueous into the stroma, secondary to a break in the Descemet's membrane. It resolves with stromal scarring.

INVESTIGATIONS

- Placido disc—crowing of the mires along the steeper axis of the cornea
- Corneal topography—shows the presence of irregular astigmatism on axial maps. Diagnostic indices for keratoconus include Rabinowitz criteria and Massachusetts Eye and Ear Infirmary (MEEI) criteria.[3]
- Corneal tomography provides detailed information on anterior and posterior elevation maps, pachymetry, and the posterior corneal surface
- Corneal optical coherence tomography (OCT)—to detect focal thinning
- Corneal biomechanics—using ocular response analyzer
- Confocal microscopy

TREATMENT

- Spectacles—useful in early cases, to correct astigmatism.
- Contact lens—options include soft toric lens, rigid gas permeable (RGP) hard lens, bicurved hard lens, hybrid lens, and scleral lens

- *Surgical interventions:*
  - Corneal collagen crosslinking (CXL)—done using riboflavin combined with UVA radiation, to increase the formation of corneal covalent bonds and strengthen the weakened cornea.
  - Intracorneal ring segment—these are rings made of polymethyl methacrylate (PMMA), which are implanted on the cornea to correct the astigmatism.
  - Photorefractive keratectomy—using excimer laser ablation technique
  - Keratoplasty—done in advanced cases of keratoconus with apical scarring and in corneal hydrops. Options include penetrating keratoplasty and lamellar keratoplasty.[1]

RECENT ADVANCES IN KERATOCONUS MANAGEMENT

- Genetic screening—using buccal swab, to identify variants of *TFG-β1* and *LOX* genes which is implicated in the pathogenesis of keratoconus.
- Artificial intelligence is now being used in the diagnosis, grading, and early detection of keratoconus, on integration with tomography imaging techniques.
- New variants in cross-linking such as Epi-on CXL and IVMED-80 crosslinking
- Extracellular vesicles—uses mesenchymal stem cells for corneal reconstruction

REFERENCES

1. Bui AD, Truong A, Pasricha ND, Indaram M. Keratoconus Diagnosis and Treatment: Recent Advances and Future Directions. Clin Ophthalmol. 2023;17:2705-18.
2. Davidson AE, Hayes S, Hardcastle AJ, Tuft SJ. The pathogenesis of keratoconus. Eye (Lond). 2014;28(2):189-95.
3. Alqudah N. Keratoconus: imaging modalities and management. Med Hypothesis Discov Innov Ophthalmol. 2024;13(1):44-54.

CHAPTER 12

Posterior Polar Cataract

Lipi Mittal, Sandeep Choudhary, Mayank Sharma

INTRODUCTION

Posterior polar cataract (PPC) is a clinically significant cataract characterized by a round, discoid, and opaque opacity in the central posterior lenticular region. The condition is congenital in most cases, but may not affect vision until later in life. PPC is known for its increased risk of complications during cataract surgery due to its fragile posterior capsule, which can lead to capsular rupture. A detailed understanding of its anatomy, etiology, and surgical considerations is critical for optimal outcomes.

EPIDEMIOLOGY

Posterior polar cataracts are bilateral in 65–80% of cases, although unilateral cases are possible. They can be inherited as an autosomal dominant pattern, although sporadic cases have also been reported.[1] Although they are often detected during the second to fourth decades of life, some cases present earlier if significant visual impairment occurs.

ETIOLOGY AND PATHOPHYSIOLOGY

Posterior polar cataracts result from developmental abnormalities that occur during lens formation and are associated with the persistence of hyaloid artery remnants and tunica vasculosa lentis. Several genetic mutations have been associated with PPC, particularly in genes such as *PITX3* on chromosome 10q25, *CRYAB* on chromosome 11q22, and CTTP 1–5.[2]

CLINICAL FEATURES

Symptoms

Usually asymptomatic in early life, cataract progression can lead to symptoms such as:
- Progressive blurring of vision
- Glare and haloes
- Intolerance to light
- Reduced contrast sensitivity

Signs

On slit-lamp examination, PPC appears as round, white, and well-defined central opacity located at the posterior aspect of the lens **(Fig. 1)**. The opacity is located near or adherent to the posterior capsule. The overlying cortical fibers may remain transparent or develop opacities, depending on the stage of the cataract. A meticulous history is essential to assess any potential hereditary patterns.

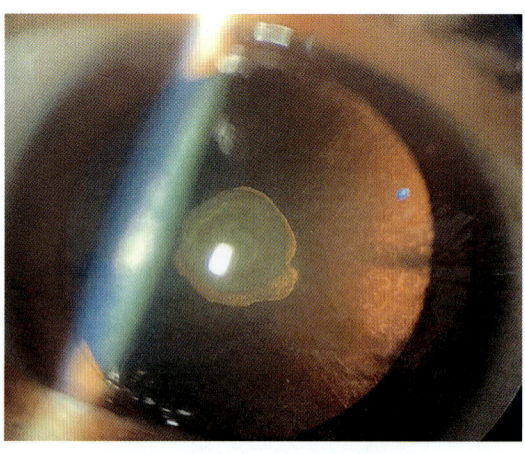

Fig. 1: Posterior polar cataract.

CLASSIFICATION OF POSTERIOR POLAR CATARACT

Schroeder's classification: It depends on the pupillary obstruction in the red reflex.[3]

Grade 1	A small opacity without any effect on the optical quality of the clear part of the lens
Grade 2	A two-third obstruction without other effect
Grade 3	Disc-like opacity in the posterior capsule surrounded by an area of further optical distortion. Only the dilated pupil shows a clear red reflex surrounding this zone
Grade 4	The opacity is occlusive; no sufficient red reflex is obtained by dilation of the pupil

Singh's classification:

Type 1	Posterior polar opacity associated with posterior subcapsular cataract
Type 2	Sharply defined round or oval opacity with a ringed appearance like an onion with or without grayish spots at the edge
Type 3	Sharply defined round or oval white opacity with dense white spots at the edge often associated with thin or absent posterior capsule
Type 4	Combination of the other and nuclear sclerosis

Duke and Elder's classification:[4]

Stationary type (most common)	Round and well-defined circular opacity with concentric rings on the central posterior capsule giving an appearance of bull's eye or onion peel (**Fig. 2**)
Progressive type	Whitish opacity at the posterior cortex in the shape riders with the feathery edges, it does not involve the nucleus

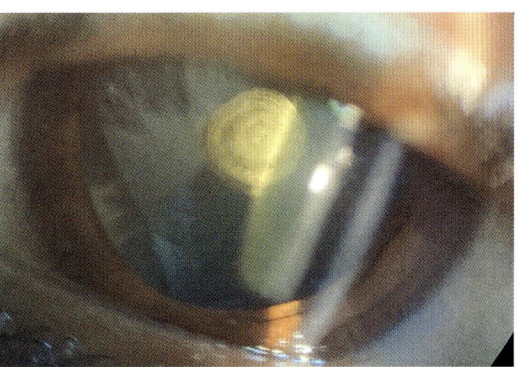

Fig. 2: Bull's eye or onion peel appearance.

Vasavada classification: It divides PPC into three distinct varieties:[5]

1. PPC with impending posterior capsular dehiscence
2. Preexisting posterior capsular dehiscence with PPC
3. Spontaneous dislocation of PPC

ASSOCIATED CONDITIONS

Posterior polar cataract may occur in isolation or association with other ocular conditions, such as:

- Persistent fetal vasculature (PFV)
- Microphthalmia
- Anterior polar cataract
- Posterior lenticonus conditions such as Alport syndrome, and Lowe syndrome may occasionally be associated with PPC.

SURGICAL MANAGEMENT

Posterior polar cataract poses unique challenges during cataract extraction due to the fragile posterior capsule and its risk of rupture. Meticulous planning and surgical techniques are required to minimize complications.

Preoperative Considerations

- *Informed consent:* Patient counseling is of the utmost importance. The patient

should be counseled about the nature of the cataract and the chances of complications such as nuclear drop and posterior capsular rupture during surgery. They should be informed that there may be a need for posterior segment intervention intraoperatively and secondary intraocular lens (IOL) implantation at a later sitting. Some cases may require neodymium-doped yttrium aluminum garnet (Nd-YAG) capsulotomy due to persistent posterior capsular opacification that could not be removed during surgery.
- *Imaging:* Preoperative imaging, such as anterior segment optical coherence tomography (OCT), may help to assess the integrity of the posterior capsule.

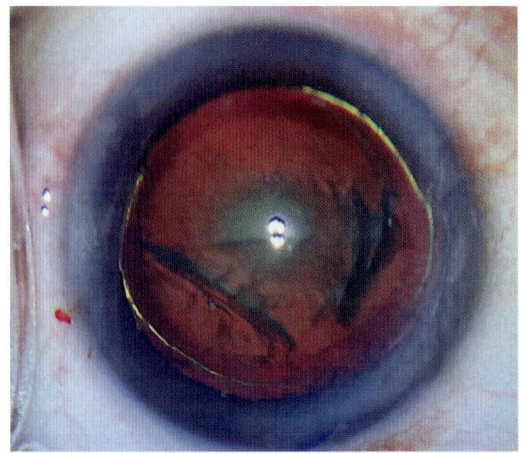

Fig. 3: Golden ring formation: Sign of successful hydrodelineation.

Surgical Techniques

- *Capsulorhexis:* An adequate size of approximately 5–5.5 mm continuous curvilinear capsulorhexis should be constructed. A small rhexis increases the hydrostatic pressure hampering the epinucleus and cortical removal while a larger rhexis does not allow IOL implantation in the sulcus, if needed.
- *Hydro procedures:* Traditional cortical cleaving hydrodissection is avoided because of increased hydraulic pressure leading to posterior capsular rupture. Hydrodelineation is preferred to separate the nucleus from the epinucleus, keeping the posterior capsule intact.

The inside-out delineation technique[6] is described for PPC with advanced nuclear sclerosis. Here, the trench is sculpted and a right-angled cannula is directed perpendicularly into the lens fibers through one of the trenched walls at an appropriate depth. Golden ring formation is an indicator of successful delineation **(Fig. 3)**. Rotation of the nucleus should be avoided.

- *Phacoemulsification:* Low fluidics and controlled phaco power are essential. A closed chamber technique should be followed to minimize the anterior chamber fluctuation and posterior capsule bulging.
- *Nucleus and cortical removal:* The nucleus and epinucleus should be removed cautiously, avoiding excess stress on the posterior capsule. A slow-motion phaco technique, using lower vacuum and aspiration rates, is often recommended.

Various nucleotomy techniques have been described:
- The phaco chop technique is used in harder PPC cases to minimize the stress on the posterior capsule. Before removing the phaco probe, the viscoelastic substance should be injected through the side port to maintain the anterior chamber.
- Phaco aspiration can be performed in softer cases
- *Lambda technique:* The nucleus is sculpted in lambda shape followed by a crack along the arms and then removing the central quadrant first. This technique prevents stretching of the posterior capsule.[7]

- *Inverse horseshoe technique:* After sculpting, the distal portion of the nucleus is divided and the viscoelastic substance is injected to lift the two portions of the nucleus forming a visco scaffold underneath, hence helping in hemidissection of the nucleus without causing much stretch on the posterior capsule.[8]
- *The reverse bloom technique consists of the following three steps:*
  1. Nucleus removal without disturbing the integrity of the posterior capsule
  2. Peeling of the cortical matter in an outside-in fashion (like reverse blooming of the flower)
  3. Gentle separation of the polar attachment from the capsule.

Epinucleus removal (layer-by-layer technique): Viscodissection is a preferred technique where the viscoelastic substance is injected in-between the cortex and the capsule and the epinucleus is gently peeled off. It is important to leave the central portion intact until the last stage of separation **(Fig. 4)**.[9]

Cortical matter removal should be performed at the lower bottle height where the cortical matter is removed tangentially rather than centrally, minimizing the pulling of the cortex. Capsular polishing should be avoided in all cases. In the case of posterior

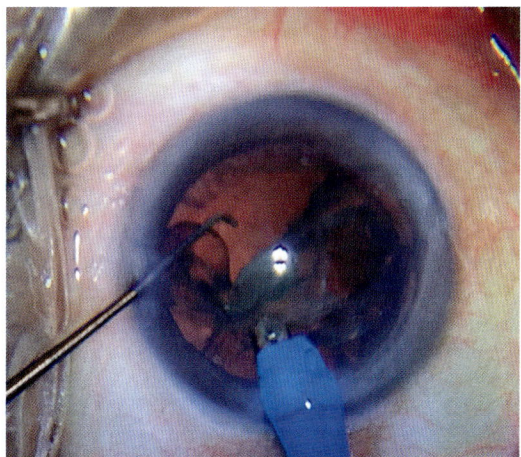

Fig. 4: Separation and aspiration of the epinuclear material layer by layer leaving the central portion intact until last stage.

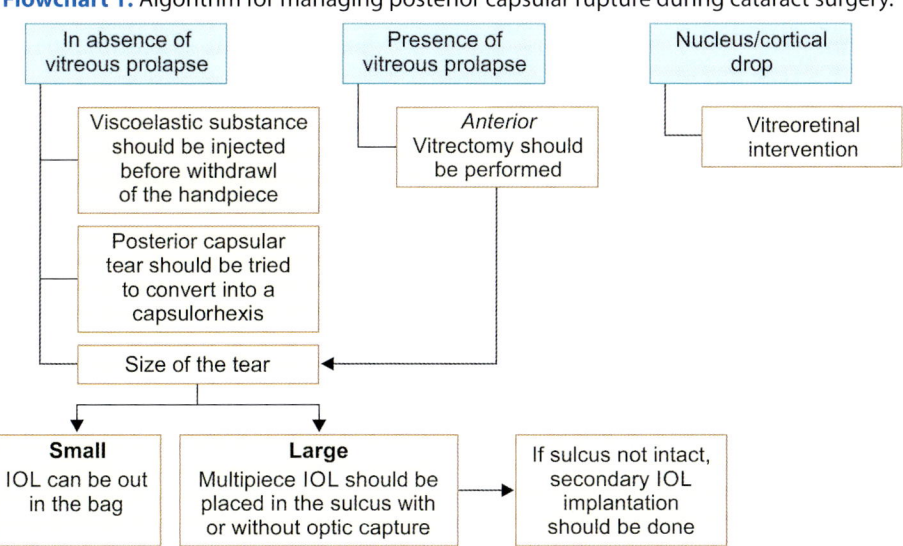

Flowchart 1: Algorithm for managing posterior capsular rupture during cataract surgery.

plaque, it should be left behind and Nd-YAG laser capsulotomy should be done later.

- *Intraocular lens implantation:* A foldable IOL can be implanted in the bag, if the posterior capsule remains intact. In case of posterior capsular rupture, IOL implantation in the ciliary sulcus or secondary IOL implantation may be required.
- *Handling a posterior capsular rupture* **(Flowchart 1)**.

COMPLICATIONS

Intraoperative	Postoperative
• Posterior capsular dehiscence	• Cystoid macular edema
• Nucleus drop	• IOL decentration
• Cortical drop	• IOL drop
• Aphakia	• Secondary glaucoma
• Vitreous prolapse	• Fibrinous uveitis
	• Retinal detachment

CONCLUSION

Posterior polar cataracts pose a unique surgical challenge due to their inherent nature. Understanding the risks associated with PPC and preparing for the complications can improve the visual outcome and rehabilitation.

REFERENCES

1. Yamada K, Tomita HA, Kanazawa S, Mera A, Amemiya T, Niikawa N. Genetically distinct autosomal dominant posterior polar cataract in a four-generation Japanese family. Am J Ophthalmol. 2000;129(2):159-65.
2. Gurnani B, Kaur K. Posterior Polar Cataract. 2023 Jun 11. In: StatPearls [Internet]. Treasure Island (FL): StatPearls Publishing; 2025.
3. Schroeder HW. The management of posterior polar cataract: the role of patching and grading. Strabismus. 2005;13(4):153-6.
4. Vasavada AR, Raj SM, Vasavada V, Shrivastav S. Surgical approach to posterior polar cataract: a review. Eye. 2012;26(6):761-70.
5. Vasavada A, Singh R. Phacoemulsification in eyes with posterior polar cataract. J Cataract Refract Surg. 1999;25(2):238-45.
6. Vasavada AR, Vasavada VA. Managing the posterior polar cataract: an update. Indian J Ophthalmol. 2017;65(12):1350-8.
7. Lee MW, Lee YC. Phacoemulsification of posterior polar cataracts—a surgical challenge. Br J Ophthalmol. 2003;87(11):1426-7.
8. Salahuddin A. Inverse horse-shoe technique for the phacoemulsification of posterior polar cataract. Can J Ophthalmol. 2010;45(2):154-6.
9. Vajpayee RB, Sinha R, Singhvi A, Sharma N, Titiyal JS, Tandon R. 'Layer by layer' phacoemulsification in posterior polar cataract with pre-existing posterior capsular rent. Eye (Lond). 2008;22(8):1008-10.

CHAPTER 13

Pediatric Cataract

Rajat Kapoor, Bhavatharini M

DEFINITION

A *pediatric cataract* is the opacification of the crystalline lens in children, which can impair vision. It may be congenital (present at birth or within the first year after birth) or may develop during childhood. It is one of the leading causes of treatable childhood blindness.[1-3]

TYPES OF PEDIATRIC CATARACT

- *Congenital cataracts:* Present at birth, often related to genetic factors, intrauterine infections, or metabolic disorders **(Fig. 1)**
- *Developmental cataracts:* Develop during childhood, usually due to trauma, steroid use, or systemic diseases. Most common cause being idiopathic **(Fig. 2)**
- *Acquired cataracts:* Result from trauma, uveitis, systemic diseases (e.g., diabetes), or drug toxicity (e.g., steroids) **(Figs. 3 and 4)**
- *Syndromic cataracts:* Associated with systemic conditions such as Down syndrome, Marfan syndrome, and galactosemia **(Figs. 5 and 6)**

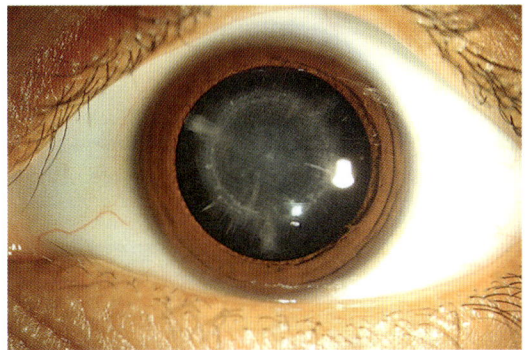

Fig. 2: Developmental/lamellar cataract.

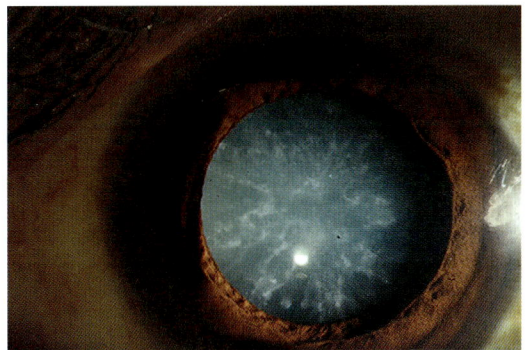

Fig. 3: Rosette cataract in a patient with blunt trauma.

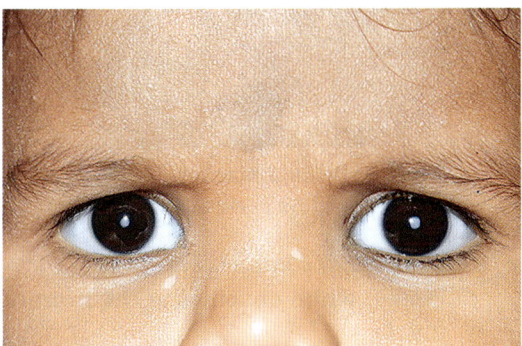

Fig. 1: Bilateral congenital cataract in a 2-year-old child.

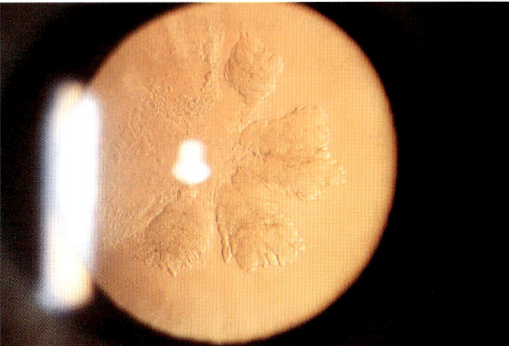

Fig. 4: Rosette cataract in a patient with blunt trauma as seen on retroillumination.

Pediatric Cataract

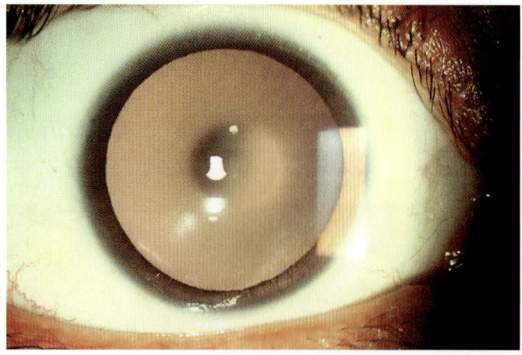

Fig. 5: Oil droplet cataract in a patient of galactosemia.

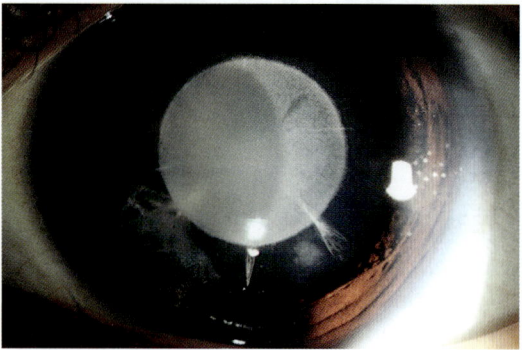

Fig. 7: Nuclear cataract.

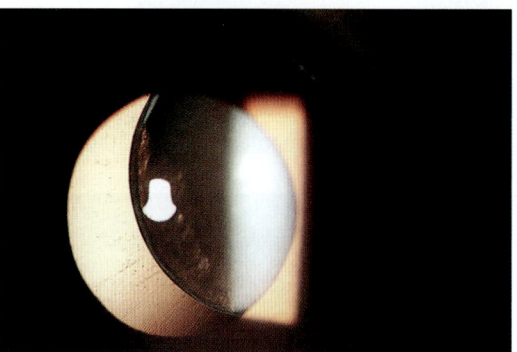

Fig. 6: Superotemporal lens subluxation in a patient of Marfan's syndrome.

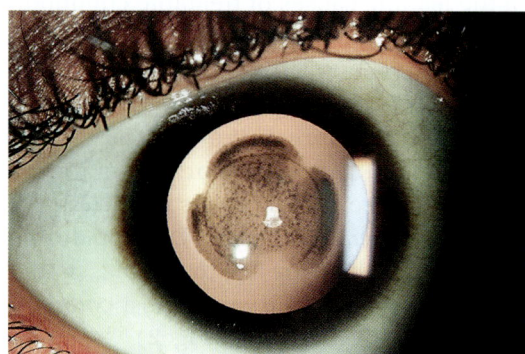

Fig. 8: Lamellar cataract.

MORPHOLOGY

- *Nuclear cataract* (**Fig. 7**):
    - Opacification of the central part of the lens (nucleus)
    - Often dense and associated with visual impairment from birth
- *Lamellar (zonular) cataract* (**Fig. 8**):
    - Involves the layers of the lens surrounding the nucleus
    - Common in metabolic disorders and usually bilateral
- *Posterior subcapsular cataract* (**Figs. 9 and 10**):
    - Located at the back of the lens capsule
    - Can affect near vision more than distance vision

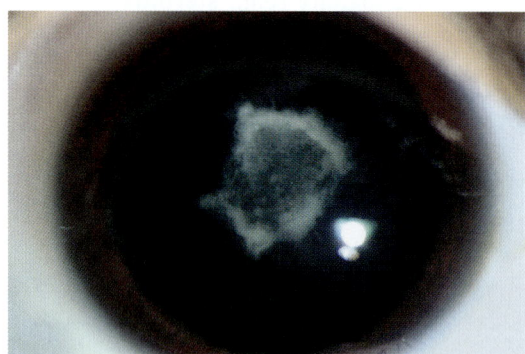

Fig. 9: Posterior subcapsular cataract on diffuse illumination.

- *Anterior polar cataract* (**Fig. 11**):
    - Small, white opacities at the front of the lens
    - Often less visually significant unless large and dense

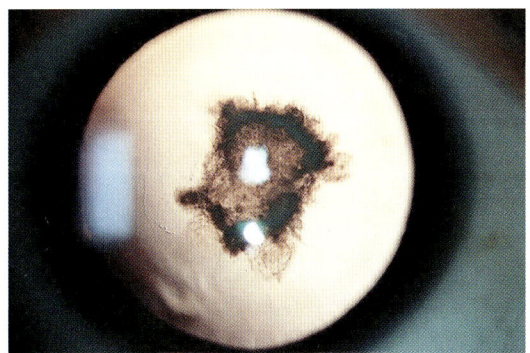

Fig. 10: Posterior subcapsular cataract on retroillumination.

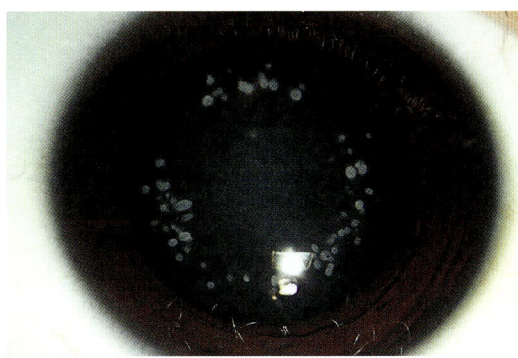

Fig. 13: Cerulean (blue dot) cataract.

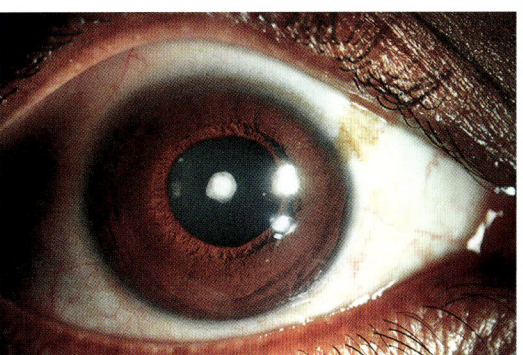

Fig. 11: Anterior polar cataract.

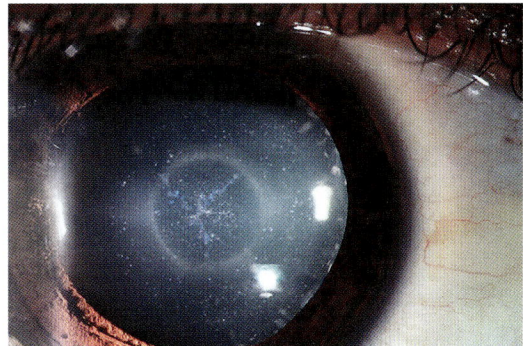

Fig. 14: Punctate lens opacities.

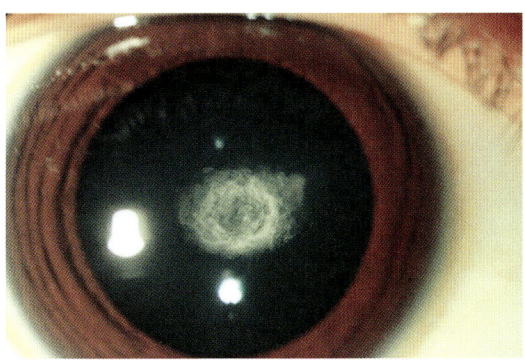

Fig. 12: Posterior polar cataract.

- *Posterior polar cataract (Fig. 12):* Opacity at the posterior pole of the lens, often associated with a dehiscence of the posterior lens capsule, leading to surgical complications
- *Cerulean (blue dot) cataract (Fig. 13):*
  - Small, bluish opacities scattered throughout the lens
  - Usually nonprogressive and has minimal impairment in visual acuity
- *Miscellaneous:*
  - Punctate lens opacities **(Fig. 14)**
  - Sutural **(Fig. 15)**
  - Coralliform **(Fig. 16)**
  - Wedge shaped **(Fig. 17)**
  - Anterior lenticonus **(Fig. 18)**
  - Posterior lenticonus **(Fig. 19)**
  - Membranous cataract **(Fig. 20)**
  - Persistent hyperplastic primary vitreous (PHPV) cataract **(Fig. 21)**

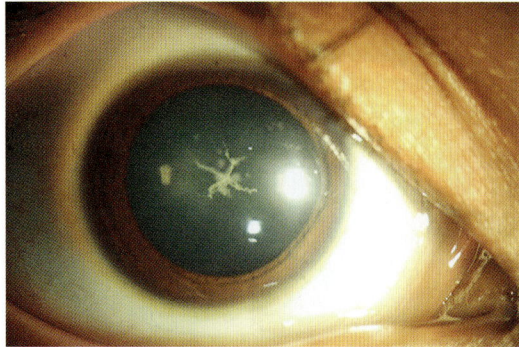

Fig. 15: Sutural cataract.

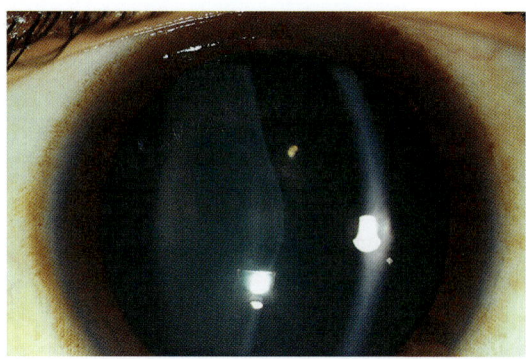

Fig. 18: Anterior lenticonus.

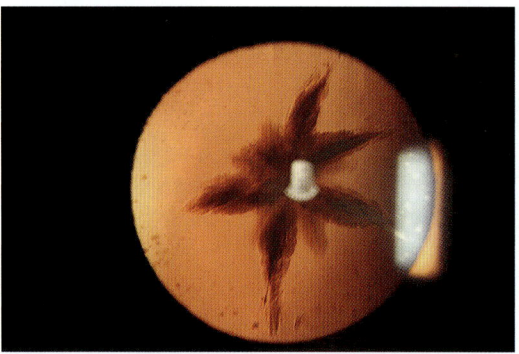

Fig. 16: Coralliform cataract on retroillumination.

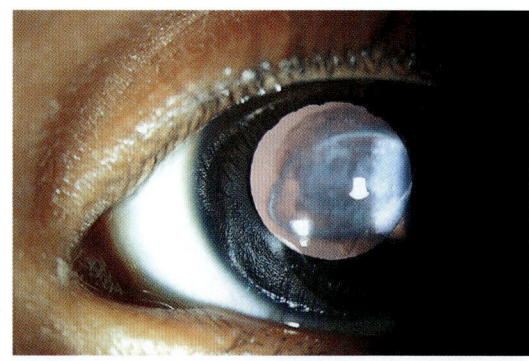

Fig. 19: Posterior lenticonus.

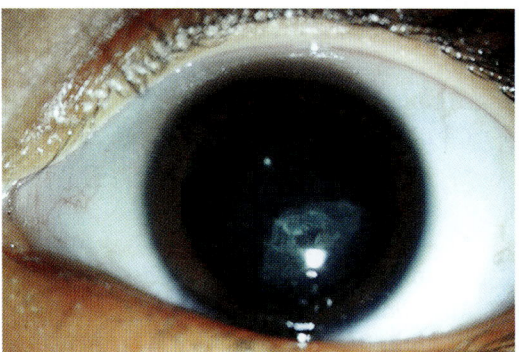

Fig. 17: Wedge-shaped cataract.

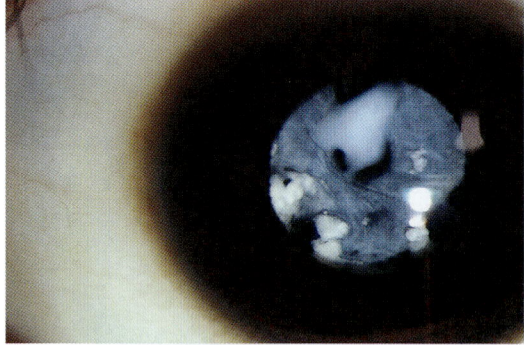

Fig. 20: Membranous cataract.

EVALUATION OF PEDIATRIC CATARACT

- *Initial presentation:* Parents often notice leukocoria (white reflex in the eye), photophobia to light, ocular misalignment, abnormal eye movements (nystagmus), or abnormal eye size (microphthalmos and buphthalmos).[4]
- *History taking:* A detailed history covers age of onset, family history, prenatal infections (TORCH), trauma,

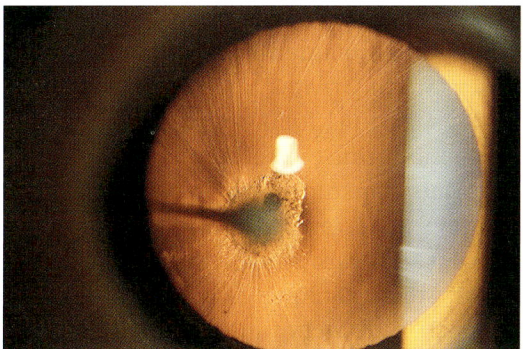

Fig. 21: Persistent hyperplastic primary vitreous (PHPV) cataract.

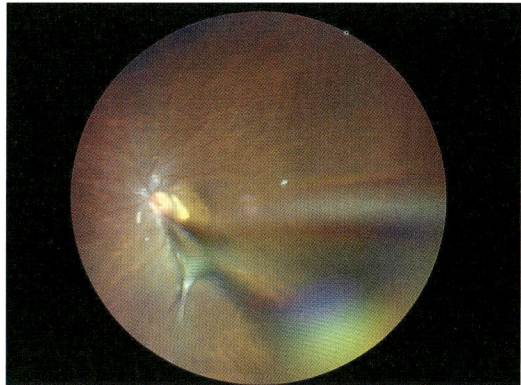

Fig. 22: Fundus photo of persistent hyperplastic primary vitreous (PHPV) associated with cataract.

and hereditary factors. Older children may struggle with distant vision or watch TV closely.
- *Prenatal/perinatal factors:* Factors such as drug use during pregnancy, prematurity, retinopathy of prematurity, or galactosemia should be explored, along with trauma details.
- *Systemic examination:* Systemic examination including facial dysmorphic features, skin, hair changes, skeletal abnormalities, cranial and facial signs, and other syndromic associations.
- Dilated ocular examination of siblings and both parents
- *Comprehensive eye examination:*
  - *Slit lamp examination:* Evaluate the morphology, density, and location of the cataract.
  - *Dilated fundus examination:* Rule out any posterior segment anomalies such as PHPV, retinal detachment, or optic nerve anomalies **(Fig. 22)**
  - *Red reflex test:* Any abnormality or asymmetry requires urgent evaluation.
- *Assessment of visual acuity:*
  - For preverbal children, use techniques such as preferential looking or fixation behavior assessment.
  - In older children, perform visual acuity testing with age-appropriate methods.
- *Amblyopia risk evaluation:*
  - Consider the size, density, and centrality of the cataract to assess the risk of amblyopia
  - Early intervention is critical in dense, central cataracts that affect visual development
  - *Ocular investigations:* Keratometry, axial length, B-scan ultrasonography, intraocular lens (IOL) power calculation
  - *Genetic and metabolic screening:* Essential laboratory tests include TORCH titers, venereal disease research laboratory (VDRL), serum calcium, and phosphorus levels, and urine tests for reducing substances. Any additional systemic evaluation should be coordinated with the pediatrician, and dysmorphic features may warrant consultation with a geneticist.

TIMING OF SURGERY

- *Bilateral cataract:* Early surgery (within the first 6 weeks of life) for dense, bilateral cataracts to minimize amblyopia.

- *Unilateral cataract:* Surgery is ideally performed between 4 and 6 weeks of age for dense cataracts.
- Delayed surgery can lead to irreversible amblyopia.

Key point: Strabismus and nystagmus associated with congenital cataracts indicate the presence of amblyopia, highlighting the sensory deprivation caused by the cataract. This highlights the importance of early surgical intervention.[5]

PREOPERATIVE EVALUATION

Examination under anesthesia is conducted to assess essential parameters for IOL power calculation.[6] Important parameters to assess are the horizontal corneal diameter (HCD), axial length, keratometry, detailed evaluation of the cataract and posterior segment **(Figs. 23 and 24)**.

SURGICAL TECHNIQUE (VIDEO 1)

- *Surgical approach:* A superior corneal or scleral incision is preferred along with two side ports positioned 180° apart to enable 360° movement.
- *Capsulorhexis:* Trypan blue dye is used to stain the anterior lens capsule. A 26G cystitome creates a nick in the anterior lens capsule, followed by completion of the anterior capsulorhexis with appropriate capsulorhexis forceps. The goal is to achieve a continuous curvilinear capsulorhexis, using a manual or Zepto-assisted technique. Also, the two-incision push–pull technique is useful in a few situations where there may be preexisting fibrosis of the anterior lens capsule.
- *Lens aspiration:* Aspiration of the lens matter which is usually soft can be done using the bimanual or Blumenthal technique. In cases of delayed presentation, where the nucleus is hard, phacoemulsification of the nucleus may be necessary.
- *Posterior capsule management:* Primary management of the posterior capsule is critical to prevent visual axis opacification (VAO). In children under 6 years, consider performing a posterior capsulotomy and anterior vitrectomy to reduce the risk of posterior capsule opacification (PCO) and the need for future YAG laser treatment.

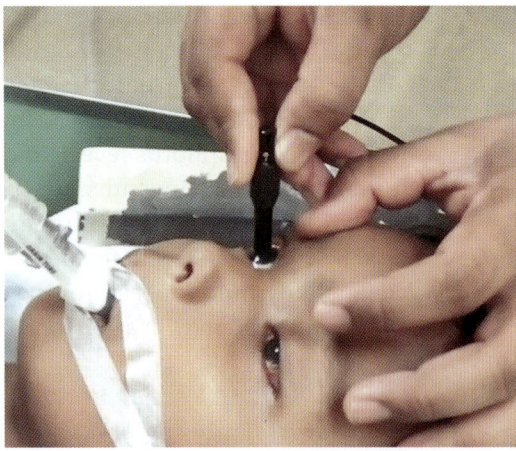

Fig. 23: A-scan biometry being done on a child under anesthesia.

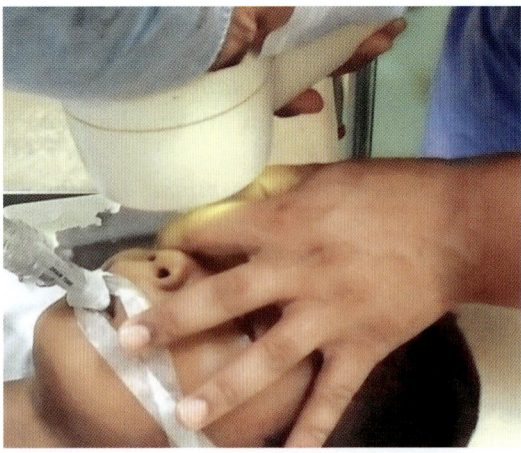

Fig. 24: Handheld keratometry being done on a child under anesthesia.

Pediatric Cataract

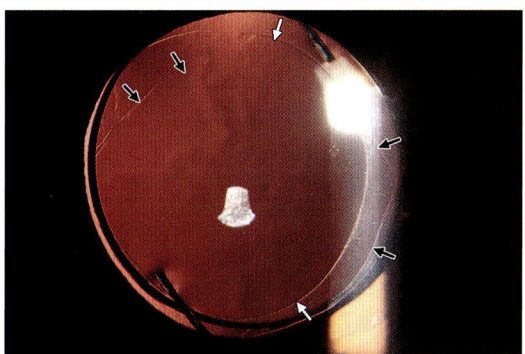

Fig. 25: Posterior optic capture performed with a 3 piece-IOL (white arrows depicting the anterior capsulorhexis margin and black arrows depicting the posterior capsulorhexis margin).

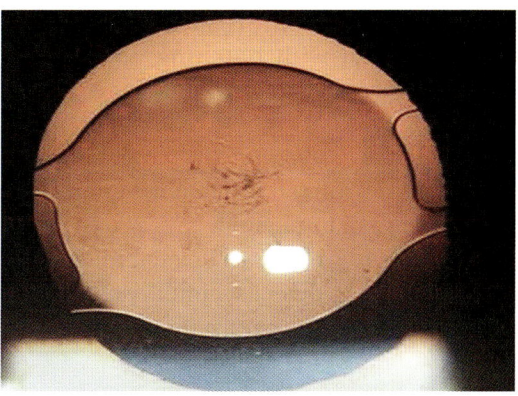

Fig. 26: Retrofixated iris-claw intraocular lens postimplantation in a case of Marfan's syndrome.

Posterior capsulotomy can be attained either with manual technique or using a vitrector.
- *IOL insertion techniques:* The IOL is inserted via a corneal/scleral entry wound, ensuring proper placement in the bag. Primary IOL implantation is generally recommended for children older than 2 years. For infants under 6 months, the decision is more individualized.[7]
- *Optic capture:* IOL optic can be captured behind the posterior capsule, this reduces the incidence of PCO and also prevents IOL decentration **(Fig. 25)**.
- *Special considerations:* For lens subluxation, intralenticular aspiration with retrofixated iris claw IOL and peripheral iridectomy is preferred. In traumatic cases, posterior capsulorhexis with optic capture is recommended **(Fig. 26)**.[8]
- *Suturing techniques:* Incisions should be sutured with 10-0 monofilament nylon due to risks of anterior chamber collapse and endophthalmitis, while side ports can be left sutureless if no leakage occurs.
- *Key point for IOL power calculation:* Use pediatric-specific formulas such as Holladay, Hoffer Q, or SRK/T. Consider undercorrecting by 20–30% due to future ocular growth.
- *Type of IOL:*
  - *Acrylic hydrophobic IOLs:* Preferred for pediatric cases due to their durability and lower risk of PCO. Square edge optics in the IOL also help in reducing the incidence of PCO.
  - *Monofocal IOLs:* Avoid multifocal lenses in pediatric patients to minimize visual disturbances.
  - If IOL implantation is deferred (e.g., in very young infants), use aphakic glasses or contact lenses postsurgery.
  - Retrofixated IOLs and scleral fixated/glued IOLs are useful in cases where there is poor capsular support.

POSTOPERATIVE MANAGEMENT

- *Medication protocol:* Postoperatively, patients are typically prescribed topical steroids (prednisolone acetate 1% eight times a day) with tapering over 4–6 weeks postoperatively, topical broad-spectrum antibiotics, and cycloplegics (preferably homatropine 2%). In infants, atropine 1% eye drops may be necessary.

- *Amblyopia therapy:* Aggressive treatment is essential with patching or pharmacological penalization of the better-seeing eye.
- *Refractive correction:* Use contact lenses or glasses for refractive correction if an IOL was not implanted.
- *Monitor for glaucoma:* Regular follow-ups are crucial to detect secondary glaucoma, especially in younger patients and those who underwent early surgery.
- *REAL follow-up at every visit:* R (Refraction and Visual acuity), E (eye pressure or IOP), A (Amblyopia and alignment of eyes), and L (Lens or IOL-related factors such as VAO)

COMPLICATIONS OF PEDIATRIC CATARACT SURGERY

- *Wound leak or shallow anterior chamber:* It can be prevented by appropriate wound suturing.
- *Severe anterior chamber inflammation:* It can be managed with higher frequency of topical steroids and intraoperative injection of subconjunctival dexamethasone.
- *Visual axis opacification*: VAO is the most common complication of cataract surgery in children and can lead to amblyopia. Strategies to prevent VAO include performing a posterior capsulorhexis and anterior vitrectomy. If opacification occurs, Nd laser capsulotomy can be attempted, although general anesthesia may be necessary for younger children, and surgical membranectomy might be required if laser treatment is ineffective.
- *Secondary glaucoma:* Children may develop secondary glaucoma following cataract surgery, especially those who are younger at the time of surgery or have microphthalmia. Open-angle glaucoma can develop months to years later, while angle-closure glaucoma can arise from anterior synechiae. Treatment may involve topical medications or additional surgical interventions, and lifelong monitoring for glaucoma is essential. It is thus essential not to implant IOLs in small eyes or eyes having anterior segment dysgenesis.
- *Retinal detachment:* Key risk factors include persistent fetal vasculature (PFV), high myopia, and multiple surgeries. Regular dilated fundus examinations are necessary for monitoring.
- *Endophthalmitis and suture-related infection*

PROGNOSIS

- Prognosis varies widely due to ocular or systemic comorbidities. A well-done surgery with good postoperative optical rehabilitation leads to good visual outcomes.
- The timing of surgery is crucial for visual development. Stimulus deprivation for an extended period of time can cause irreversible amblyopia.
- Unilateral cataracts have poorer outcomes than bilateral ones, requiring prompt surgical intervention, proper optical correction, and amblyopia treatment, necessitating disciplined commitment from both ophthalmologist and parents.

VIDEO LEGEND

Video 1: Demonstrating steps of pediatric lens aspiration, IOL implantation, primary posterior capsulotomy, and anterior vitrectomy

REFERENCES

1. Khokhar SK, Pillay G, Dhull C, Agarwal E, Mahabir M, Aggarwal P. Pediatric cataract. Indian J Ophthalmol. 2017;65:1340-9.
2. Medsinge A, Nischal KK. Pediatric cataract: challenges and future directions. Clin Ophthalmol. 2015;9:77-90.

3. Foster A, Gilbert C, Rahi J. Epidemiology of cataract in childhood: a global perspective. J Cataract Refract Surg. 1997;23(Suppl 1):601-4.
4. Trumler AA. Evaluation of pediatric cataracts and systemic disorders. Curr Opin Ophthalmol. 2011;22:365-79.
5. Khokhar SK, Pillay G, Agarwal E, Mahabir M. Innovations in pediatric cataract surgery. Indian J Ophthalmol. 2017;65:210-6.
6. Vasavada V, Shah SK, Vasavada VA, Vasavada AR, Trivedi RH, Srivastava S, et al. Comparison of IOL power calculation formulae for pediatric eyes. Eye (Lond). 2016;30:1242-50.
7. Khokhar S, Sharma R, Patil B, Sinha G, Nayak B, Kinkhabwala RA, et al. A safe technique for in-the-bag intraocular lens implantation in pediatric cataract surgery. Eur J Ophthalmol. 2015;25:57-9.
8. Muthukumar B, Chhablani PP, Salman A, Bhandari V, Kapoor R. Comparison of retropupillary fixated iris claw lens versus sclera fixated lens for correction of pediatric aphakia secondary to ectopia lentis. Oman J Ophthalmol. 2021;14(1):20-6.

Mastering the Art of Capsulorhexis: A Transition to Forceps Continuous Curvilinear Capsulorhexis

CHAPTER 14

Shivani P Pattnaik, Kumar Doctor

SECTION 1

THE HIDDEN POWER OF FORCEPS IN CCC: ARE YOU READY TO LEVEL UP?

Professor Howard Gimbel and Professor Thomas Neuhann introduced the world to the technique of continuous curvilinear capsulorhexis (CCC). CCC is a critical surgical step in cataract surgery that involves creating a smooth and circular opening in the anterior lens capsule. Traditionally, we are trained to use a cystotome for creating a CCC. This chapter will guide your transition to forceps-based CCC creation which is an important tool in cataract surgery.

Why Stick with Cystotome? The Benefits You Already Know

As students, most of us learn the CCC with the 26 gauge cystotome because it is cheap and easily available. There are several benefits of performing a cystotome CCC including:

- The instrument can go through a small 0.25 mm side port incision
- Cystotome is held close to the tip and there is much greater control than in a case of a microrhexis forceps
- As opposed to the solid steel/titanium forceps, one can modify the structure of a cystotome and fashion it to be as curved as needed for a case (the bevel and the shaft angulation).

The Shift: Why Bother Switching to Forceps?

Despite cystotome's versatility, there are cases where complications arise—how can mastering the forceps technique rescue you from trouble? Let us dive into scenarios where forceps CCC shines.

While using a cystotome, the capsule is pierced and torn against the underlying nucleus mass by gently pressing down with the cystotome and the direction of tear is then controlled either by tangential tear forces or by using centripetal rip forces. Unchecked pressure onto the anterior capsule can disturb the underlying cortex and also damage the flap of the created rhexis, tearing it.

With forceps the tearing edge of the capsule is held and lifted upward to create the tear and the nuclear support is not necessary; traction applied is bidimensional giving the surgeon a feel of the flap as compared to a unidimensional tug of war in the cystotome technique where the flap can give way with the smallest change in vector forces.

The lens has a tapered shape which slopes downward from center to periphery. If the anterior chamber is shallow or if the rhexis is made slightly larger, there is a high probability of a peripheral run-off. This is where forceps rhexis comes to the rescue. In the forceps rhexis, it is not difficult to control the rhexis tear, even if the anterior chamber is slightly shallow.

When are Forceps Your Best Friend?

- Hypermature cataracts where the capsular bag is weak, turgid with positive pressure and more convex than usual
- Create a posterior CCC
- Extend a small size rhexis after intraocular lens (IOL) implantation
- To pull a runaway rhexis inward using the Little's maneuver

Creating a Perfect CCC: Cystotome versus Forceps—Which Technique Reigns Supreme?

The creation of CCC begins by making a small incision in the center of the anterior capsule either with a cystotome or rhexis forceps.

Needling Your Way to Perfection

> **Key Surgical Tip: Managing the Initial Tear**
> The *initial tear* is crucial. If too long, it may extend beyond the equator and lead to complications. Ensure the incision is *smaller than the desired size*. Aim for a *1.5-mm radius* for a *5-mm rhexis*, as the tear will typically extend *2–3 mm beyond* the expected result.

While using a cystotome for CCC, one can use a bent 26-gauge needle to initiate an incision in the center of the anterior capsule. Purkinje images work as a guide to place the incision in the center or it is recommended to use a ring caliper **(Video 1)**.

Forceps in Focus: Controlled Rotations for Precision—Forceps in Action

In contrast, *forceps CCC* involves the use of specially designed forceps to pierce, grasp, and carefully rotate it in a controlled and circular motion. This technique may offer better control over the flap of CCC, allowing the surgeon to adjust the pressure applied to the capsule based on resistance felt through the instrument **(Video 2)**.

Physics of CCC: What Forces are at Play?

The lens capsule behaves similarly to cellophane: it tears easily at sharp angles but can provide adequate support for an artificial lens when stretched. When the capsule is stretched, elastic fibers store potential energy, which can cause an unintended tear even after the external force is removed. Surgeons must also consider zonular forces, which apply a centrifugal pull on the capsule, potentially diverting the tear peripherally. To counter this, a surgeon uses both *stretching forces* (parallel to zonular forces) with a cystotome and *shearing forces* (perpendicular to the capsule) with forceps **(Video 3)**.

What makes Forceps CCC standout? Precision, control, and feedback

Using forceps offers tactile feedback, allowing surgeons to feel the capsule's resistance, signaling the need for careful adjustments in force application. This contrasts with needle CCC, where the instrument lacks the same degree of feedback, increasing the likelihood of overextension **(Table 1)**.

SECTION 2

TRANSITIONING TO FORCEPS: WHAT YOU NEED TO KNOW BEFORE MAKING THE SWITCH?

Factors	Description
Visualization	Poor pupil dilation hinders the view of the anterior capsule, increasing the risk of incomplete capsulorhexis/rhexis run-off. Clear corneal visibility ensures accurate assessment of the capsule
Chamber maintenance	Escape Of viscoelastic, large incision/leaky wounds can lead to radial extension, compromising capsule integrity
Adequate viscoelastic	Fill up the chamber with viscoelastic only up to mild pupil dilation, overfilling can cause radial tears, avoid viscoelastic escape
Stain	Always stain the capsule with trypan blue for better visualization of capsule
Ring rhexis marker for cornea	Using a ring rhexis corneal marker for providing an outline for rhexis helps to guide path for a complete and well sized CCC

Mastering the Art of Capsulorhexis: A Transition to Forceps Continuous Curvilinear Capsulorhexis

TABLE 1: Key factors for safe and effective forceps capsulorhexis (CCC).

Feature	CCC with cystitome	CCC with forceps
Viscoelastic escape	Minimal to none	Higher due to larger incision, requiring more OVD refill, use of cohesive OVD is beneficial (soft shell technique)
Control over CCC	Moderate control (requires dexterity and experience)	High control, precise feedback from forceps movement
Initial tear creation	Puncture with cystotome to initiate the tear	Can directly grasp the capsule edge to start the tear or nick the capsule with the Utrata forceps itself
Tactile feedback	Less tactile feedback	Significant tactile feedback for controlled tearing
Instrument maneuverability	Good, especially in narrow or small chambers	Can be challenging if the anterior chamber is shallow
Use in complex cases	Preferred for small pupils or difficult cases	Ideal for cases where better control is needed, but requires larger incision
Procedure speed	Generally faster, simpler to initiate	Faster and can be completed in four quick sweeps

(CCC: continuous curvilinear capsulorhexis; OVD: ophthalmic viscosurgical device)

When transitioning to forceps CCC, beginning with simpler cases is critical. The following factors help to minimize complications and ensure optimal visualization of the capsule.

SECTION 3

GRADUALLY ADAPTING TO FORCEPS: CAN YOU PERFECT THE ENTRY AND GRIP?

Incorporating forceps into CCC requires gradual adaptation, and a key part of this is mastering how to enter the eye with capsulorhexis forceps and hold them correctly for optimal control.

How to Enter the Eye Like a Pro (Video 4)

- Use a *2.2–2.4-mm incision* for stability
- Enter with *closed forceps* parallel to the *iris*, gently grasp the *capsular edge*, and avoid pressure on the *lens* or *wound* to prevent *stress* or *viscoelastic escape*.
- *Incision alignment:* Ensure the corneal incision is wide enough to accommodate the forceps without excessive stretching, typically around 2.2–2.4 mm. This minimizes fluid egress and maintains anterior chamber stability.
- *Approach:* Enter the anterior chamber in a closed position to avoid damaging the corneal endothelium or disturbing intraocular structures. The forceps should be introduced with the tips aligned parallel to the iris plane horizontally to maintain a clear line of sight.
- *Minimal disturbance:* Once inside, turn the tip of the forceps to face the anterior capsule, then nick the anterior capsule. The chord length of the nick should be 1.5–1.75 mm. Avoid placing pressure on the lens or capsule to prevent disturbance of the cortical matter beneath and

CHAPTER 15

Tips and Tricks in Phacoemulsification

Ankita Mulchandani

INTRODUCTION

Phacoemulsification is the standard procedure for cataract surgery, originally introduced by Charles Kelman in 1967.[1] While several modifications have been made to the technique, the core principles remain unchanged. The procedure involves making a small, an approximately 2 mm, clear corneal incision along with two smaller side port incisions adjacent to it. Through the main incision, an ultrasonic probe is used to break up and remove the cataractous lens. The development of small incisions has transformed modern cataract surgery by providing self-sealing, astigmatically neutral wounds with a reduced risk of complications. This advancement has also enabled the use of foldable intraocular lenses (IOLs). This chapter will provide readers with fundamental tips and techniques to refine their phacoemulsification skills.

BEFORE STARTING ANY SURGERY

Verify patient information such as name, age, the correct eye, and IOL power to prevent any errors during surgery. Cross-check the eye to be operated on with both your records and the patient, and mark it using a pen or sticker to avoid wrong-site surgery. Ensure that the surgeon is comfortably positioned, with hands properly supported. A solid grasp of ergonomics helps to prevent work-related injuries and allows the surgeon to operate for extended periods without discomfort.

DURING THE SURGERY

Globe Exposure

After painting and draping, a speculum should be applied to hold the eyelids apart. The speculum should be applied wide enough to allow easy instrumentations, but at the same time, it should not be opened too wide to cause patient discomfort or postoperative ptosis or tight belt syndrome (occurs when the canthus starts pressing on the eye on excessive exposure with speculum). Make sure the eyelashes are not in the way of the surgical field and the eye is sufficiently exposed. Make sure that you are well focused and are able to visualize all the structures properly and the eye is in the center of your visual field.

- Do a *par focalization* (**Fig. 1**) before starting every case. Increase the magnification to the highest available level on your microscope and then do a fine focusing to see the iris plane or the anterior zonules clearly
- This plane gives you the best depth and focus (from the corneal plane to the posterior capsule) to operate at all magnifications during different steps of the surgery
- Adjust the magnification as suited to you, after focusing the microscope

- Check all patient details before starting your surgery.
- Be comfortable before starting
- Be well focused
- Parfocalize the microscope

WOUND CONSTRUCTION

- Mark the site of the incision at the desired position by creating a groove on the limbus **(Fig. 2)**. The main incision can be made triplanar by entering through this groove.
- Make the side port incisions 80–90° (2–3 clock hours) away from the main incision as per your comfort. Avoid depressing the posterior lip of the incision to prevent egress of fluid from the eye and thus prevent the chamber from collapsing.
- Fill the anterior chamber with ophthalmic viscosurgical device (OVD) and make the main incision by entering through the groove created previously.
- A *triplanar incision* is superior to the uniplanar or biplanar incision as it is more stable, does not leak when pressure is applied to the lower lip of the incision.
- The triplanar wound has a stronger architecture as it involves more corneal stroma.
- Triplanar wounds are self-sealing and watertight when made correctly. They close better than uniplanar or biplanar wounds thereby decreasing chances of postoperative leaky wounds and postoperative infections.

CAPSULORHEXIS

Use the first Purkinje image on the cornea as a guide and center the capsulorhexis around it.

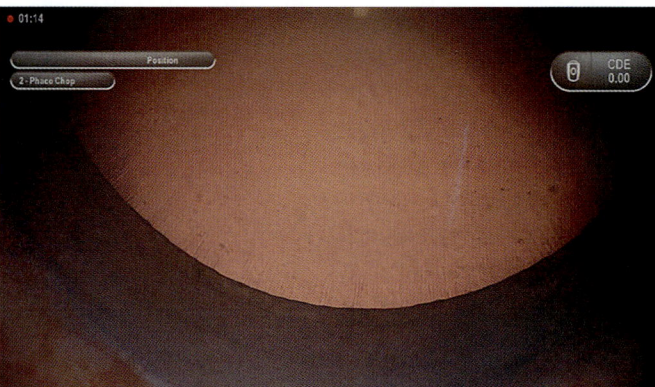

Fig. 1: Parfocalization.

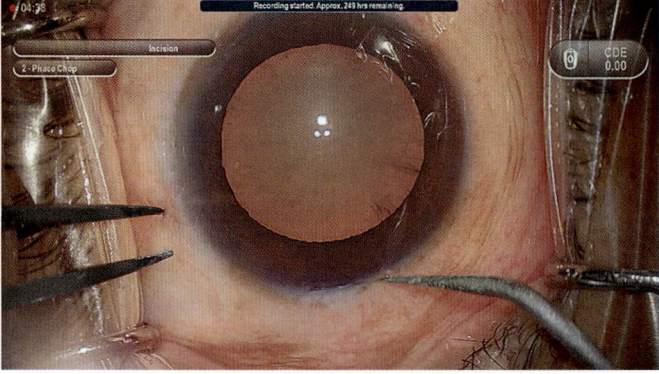

Fig. 2: Creating limbal groove.

This will help to ensure that the capsulorhexis is centered around the visual axis **(Fig. 3)**. To make a good continuous curvilinear capsulorhexis (CCC) you require a cystitome that is made properly.

Many a times, the side port incision tears because the tip of the cystitome is too long and needs to be pushed into the eye forcefully.

To Make a Good Cystitome (Refer to Video 1)

- Use a 26-G or 27-G needle
- Place the bevel side of the needle against the round handle of a barraquer needle holder and push the handle of the needle holder against the tip of the needle. This gives you the first bend on the bevel of the needle. The bend is small enough to safely enter through the side port without tearing it and at the same time it is sufficient enough to tear the anterior capsule.
- Use the jaws of the needle holder to create the second bend at the hub of the needle. This bend is >90° according to surgeon's comfort.

HYDROPROCEDURES

- Make sure to decompress the anterior chamber by removing some OVD before doing any hydroprocedures.
- Direct the 27G hydro cannula toward the equator as shown in **Figure 4** (in the space between the anterior capsule and cortex for hydrodissection and in the space between the epinucleus and endonucleus

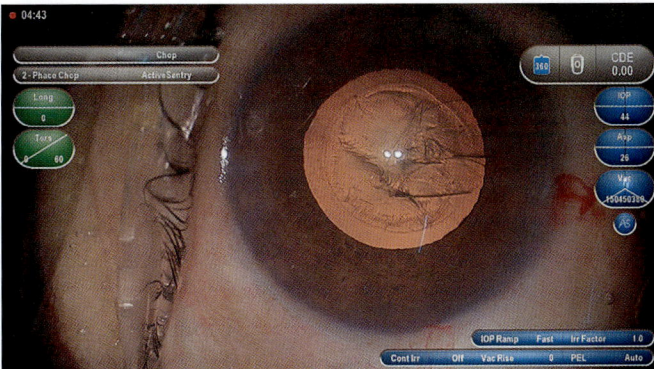

Fig. 3: Well-centered continuous curvilinear capsulorhexis (CCC).

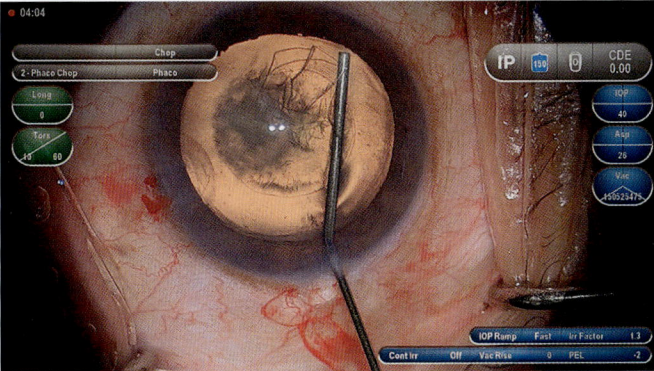

Fig. 4: Direction of hydro cannula.

for hydrodelineation) and inject a small jet of fluid.
- Make sure to tap the opposite pole of the nucleus to prevent entrapment of fluid and capsular blow-out!

DEMARCATING THE CONTINUOUS CURVILINEAR CAPSULORHEXIS

Many a times, we are not able to demarcate the CCC margins after hydroprocedures; especially when the anterior capsule is not stained. A good trick here is to remember the margins of the CCC and demarcate the area by aspirating the cortex and epinucleus from that area **(Fig. 5)**. This step also helps the surgeon to gauge the density of the nucleus.

- Make a triplanar incision
- Center the CCC around visual axis
- Do a good hydrodissection or delineation as required
- Tap on the opposite pole and release the entrapped fluid
- Stain the CCC if needed
- Demarcate the CCC before starting phaco to prevent CCC split with phaco probe

Standard Techniques of Nucleotomy

Divide and Conquer

Divide and conquer is the oldest described technique for phacoemulsification. Two deep central grooves (approximately two phaco tips deep) are made in the form of a plus sign of sufficient depth and the nucleus is mechanically broken.

Stop and Chop

A central deeper (about 1.5–2 tips deep) linear groove is made. The nucleus is divided into two heminuclei by mechanical cracking using a chopper in the nondominant hand and a phaco probe in the dominant hand.

Direct Chop

In this technique, the phaco tip is buried into the central most dense part of the nucleus and the nucleus is cracked in two halves. Each heminucleus is further cracked into multiple pieces.

Types of direct chopping techniques:
- Horizontal chop
- Vertical chop

In the Beginning or when Working with any New Machine

- *Start with a low flow rate:* This ensures that the turnover of events is slow and controlled and the turbulence in the chamber is maintained.
- *Higher bottle height:* Maintains chamber stability and prevents surge

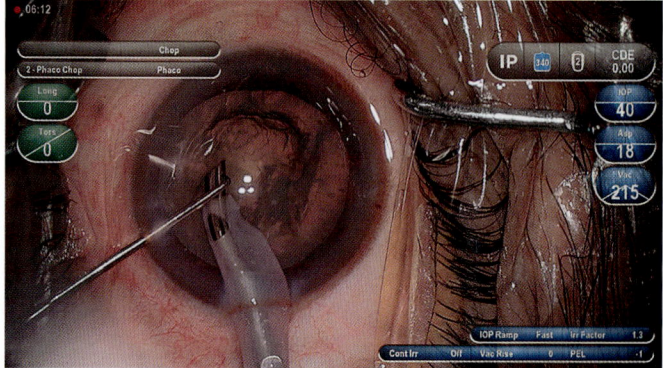

Fig. 5: Demarcation of continuous curvilinear capsulorhexis (CCC).

- *Lesser vacuum:* Use lesser vacuum initially and modify as you become comfortable and as per the grade of the nucleus.

Once you are comfortable with your machine, you can try to modify your settings and find out what works best for you.

> - Do not proceed without being comfortable
> - Avoid sudden decompression of chamber
> - Avoid forceful hydroprocedures
> - Do not push the nucleus while engaging it
> - Do not chop the nucleus by holding it superficially

To Begin Chopping (Refer to Video 2)

- First *engage the phaco tip* into the nuclear matter by using sufficient vacuum **(Fig. 6)**.
- After the phaco tip is occluded by the nucleus, use power to *bury the tip* into the most dense part of the nucleus and then come back to footswitch position two and hold the nucleus at a high vacuum.
- Once the tip has stabilized and has held the nucleus, *use the chopper* from the opposite end to chop the nucleus.
- Bury the chopper in the midperiphery of the nucleus and chop it toward the center and then laterally separate the two halves of the nucleus **(Fig. 7)**.
- *Rotate the heminucleus by 180°* and repeat the same procedure to divide the heminucelus into multiple small pieces **(Fig. 8)**. Smaller the pieces, lesser is the

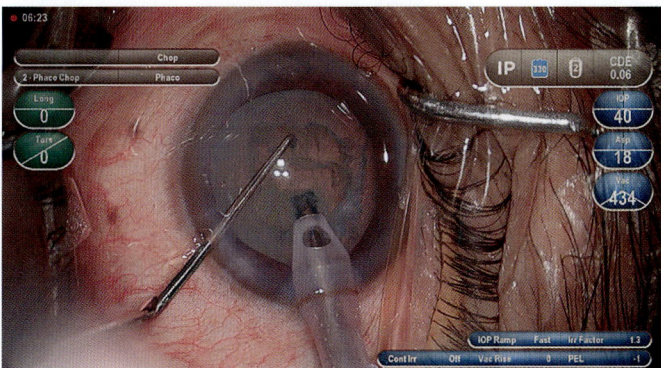

Fig. 6: Engaging the phaco tip in the nucleus.

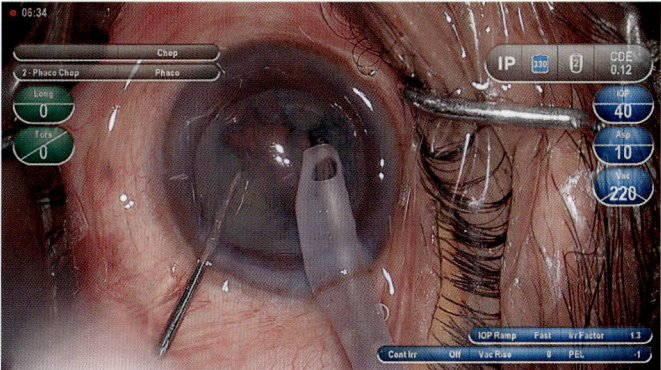

Fig. 7: Creating two heminuclei.

energy required to emulsify the piece. This translates into lesser inflammation postoperative and faster recovery!
- Use the chopper to feed the pieces into the phaco tip if required
- Decrease the vacuum while emulsifying the last piece

- Start with low flow rate, higher bottle height, lesser vacuum and modify as per the case
- Engage the phaco tip using vacuum
- Bury the tip and hold the nucleus
- Chop from mid periphery from opposite end
- Divide the heminuclei
- Rotate and repeat

CORTEX WASH

Before starting the cortex wash, inspect the instruments for any sharp or irregular edges which are a threat to the posterior capsule. One can choose a bimanual or coaxial I/A as per their convenience. Use tangential forces to aspirate the cortex **(Fig. 9)**. This decreases the stress on the zonules.

CAPSULAR POLISH (FIG. 10)

Polish the anterior and posterior capsule and remove all cortical remnants to prevent or delay the formation of posterior capsular

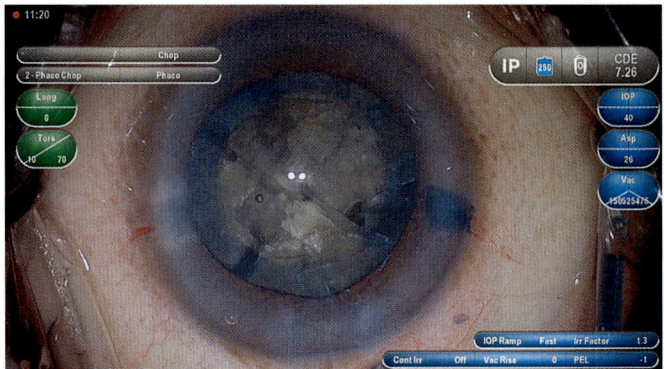

Fig. 8: Creating multiple small pieces of the nucleus.

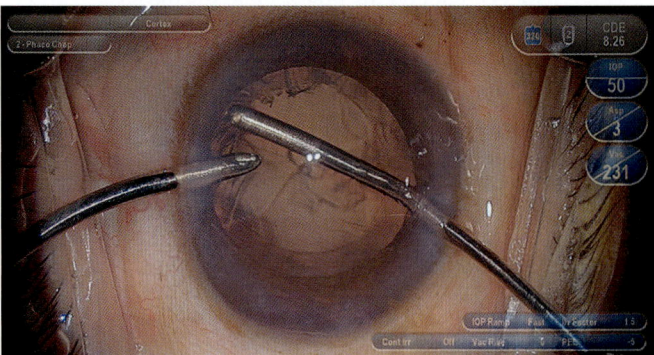

Fig. 9: Cortex wash.

opacification. Use low parameters to increase safety margin of the procedure.

INTRAOCULAR LENS INSERTION

One can consider IOL implantation under cover of OVD or do a hydroimplantation of IOL. What is important is that the anterior chamber should be maintained at all times while inserting the IOL. Assess and aim for a good and symmetrical IOL overlap **(Fig. 11)** to prevent tilting of IOL and maintaining the effective lens position.

VISCO WASH

One must completely remove the OVD from the anterior and posterior chambers before closing the eye.

FORMING THE CHAMBER AND HYDRATING THE WOUNDS

When wound construction is good, and the wounds are self-sealing, they can close on their own if one gently massages the wound and waits patiently. A minimal stromal hydration of the wounds can otherwise be

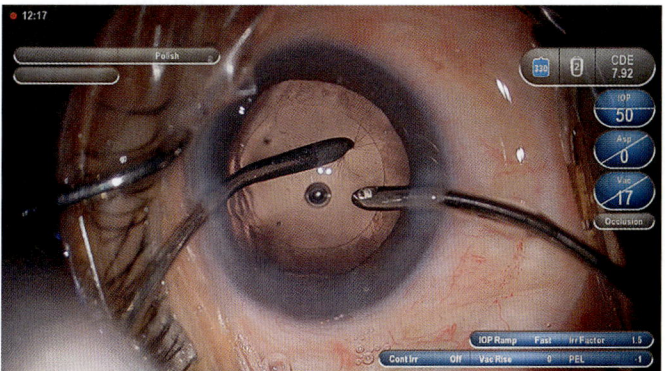

Fig. 10: Posterior capsular polish.

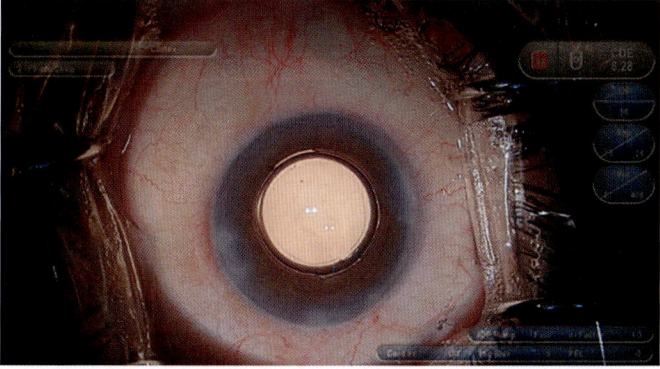

Fig. 11: Symmetrical intraocular lens (IOL) overlap.

done to form the chamber and ensure that there are no leaks. Remove the speculum under visualization.

- Strip the cortex tangentially
- Anterior and posterior capsular polish prevents posterior capsule opacification (PCO) formation
- Place IOL in the bag under cover of OVD or hydroimplantation
- Form the chamber with or without stromal hydration
- Call for help whenever needed

ACKNOWLEDGMENTS

It is with the greatest gratitude that I acknowledge the efforts of my parents who have supported me incessantly and unconditionally in my personal and professional journey.

A big thank you to my mentors who made me the surgeon I am today.

I am immensely thankful to Dr Mehul Shah, Dr Shreya Shah, and Dr Abhijeet Desai for their mentorship. Thank you for your patience, wisdom and encouragement. Your guidance has shaped my professional and personal journey in ways I never imagined!

I appreciate all the lessons and advice you have shared with me. Your mentorship has been a priceless gift. Thank you!

VIDEO LEGENDS

Video 1: How to make a cystitome
Video 2: Tips and tricks in phacoemulsification

REFERENCE

1. Davis G. The Evolution of Cataract Surgery. Mo Med. 2016;113(1):58-62.

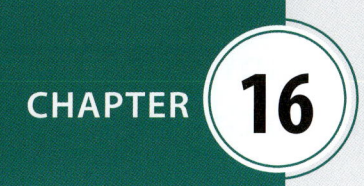

Argentinian Flag Sign Management

Anuj Kodnani

A mature cataract with extreme positive lenticular pressure caused an Argentinian flag sign. To safely remove the nucleus, the surgeon completed one side of the rhexis, enlarged the incision, and gently extracted the nucleus without additional anterior chamber manipulations. A PMMA lens was then implanted in the sulcus, and the incision was closed.

Kindly scan the QR code below to access the online Videos.

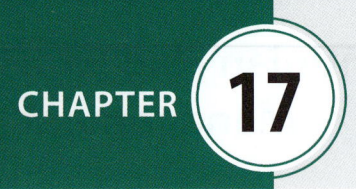

CHAPTER 17

2.5-mm Blunt Tip Chopper to the Rescue

Anuj Kodnani

In a complex case involving a white cataract with a hard nucleus and liquid cortex, the use of a 2.5-mm ball tip chopper proved highly effective. It allowed precise horizontal chopping, successfully breaking the tough nucleus into smaller segments, which eased the phacoemulsification process. During surgery, a tear in the anterior capsule occurred while extracting a sharp nuclear fragment from the capsular bag. The tear was managed and made continuous with capsulorhexis forceps. After phacoemulsification, an intraocular lens was implanted. The patient showed excellent visual recovery, emphasizing the success of the 2.5-mm ball tip chopper in handling difficult cataract cases.

Kindly scan the QR code below to access the online Videos.

CHAPTER 18

CM-T Flex IOL and XNIT

Madanagopalan VG, Nivean M

XNIT TECHNIQUE FOR SCLERAL FIXATION OF IOLs

When there is absent capsular support, the surgeon has to rely on the iris or on the sclera to fix the intraocular lens (IOL). While iris claw IOLs are versatile options, sclera-fixated IOLs (SFIOLs) have proven their safety and efficacy over a long time. Sutureless techniques are preferred these days for sclera fixation of IOLs. The XNIT technique utilizes three-piece IOLs with a 26-G needle to help with haptic exteriorization.

Docking the haptic to the needle happens outside the eye and this is the major advantage offered by this technique. When compared to previous methods such as the handshake technique that involves significant movements within the eye, novice surgeons find the XNIT technique easier to master. To ensure proper centration and to avoid tilt, it is necessary to make symmetric haptic tunnels parallel to the limbus at 3 and 9 o'clock meridians. A silicone stopper can be fashioned from any sterile material and this helps to keep the leading haptic exteriorized as the trailing haptic is being manipulated and tucked into the haptic tunnel. The video demonstrates the important steps and provides nuggets to simplify the process for young surgeons.

CM-T FLEX IOL

Fixation of an IOL to the sclera allows the IOL to be in a more anatomically suitable position. In fixing IOLs to the sclera, many techniques have been tried over the decades. Sutured IOLs were preferred initially. These IOLs had a specially designed hole in the haptics to thread the suture material. Later on, sutureless IOL techniques came into vogue. When performing sutureless SFIOL surgery, surgeons use three piece IOLs. A learning curve is required to exteriorize the haptics and then tuck them into pre-formed partial thickness scleral tunnels. Occasionally, when performing these maneuvres, issues such as decentration, optic tilt and haptic breakage are encountered.

The CM-T flex IOL is a novel IOL that employs a T-shaped haptic design. It allows for a simple pull and release technique that automatically ensures centration and stabilization without need for complex maneuvres. This IOL design offers all the advantages associated with a SFIOL while make the surgery as simple as an iris claw IOL surgery. The video details the nuances of this IOL and decodes the surgery in a simplified manner.

Kindly scan the QR code below to access the online Videos.

CM-T Flex IOL

XNIT

CHAPTER 19: Decoding Secondary Glaucomas

Rinal Pandit

INTRODUCTION

Now that we have a foundational understanding of the primary triad of glaucoma—high intraocular pressure (IOP), optic disc changes, and visual field defects, let us learn about various secondary glaucomas with the help of an image equation.

COMMON SECONDARY OPEN-ANGLE GLAUCOMAS

PIGMENT DISPERSION GLAUCOMA

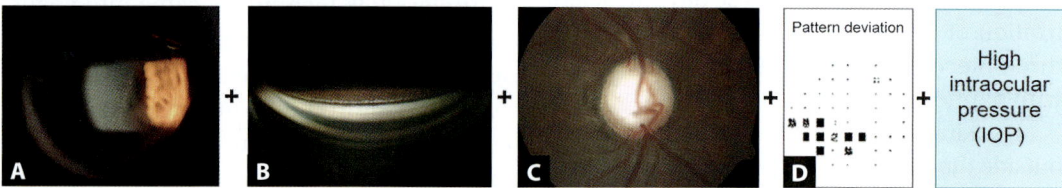

Figs. 1A to D: (A) Krukenberg spindles; (B) Uniform hyperpigmented trabecular meshwork (TM); (C) Disc damage; (D) Visual field (VF) defect.

PSEUDOEXFOLIATION GLAUCOMA

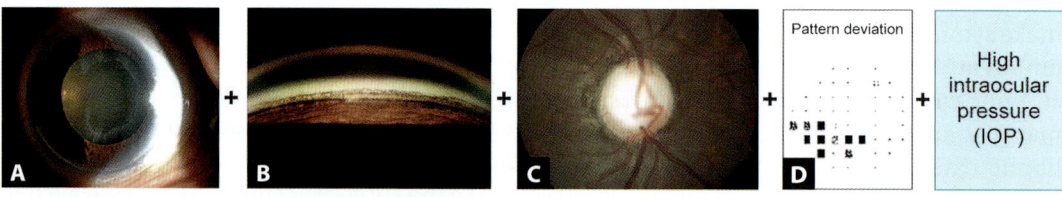

Figs. 2A to D: (A) Pseudoexfoliation (PXF) deposits on anterior lens capsule; (B) Hyperpigmented trabecular meshwork (Patchy pigmentation) with PXF deposits; (C) Disc damage; (D) Visual field (VF) defect.

ANGLE RECESSION GLAUCOMA

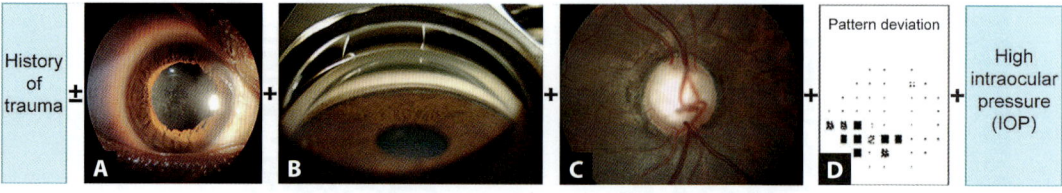

Figs. 3A to D: (A) Iris sphincter tears; (B) Widening of ciliary body band + hyperpigmented TM + Loss if iris processes; (C) Disc damage; (D) Visual field (VF) defect.

STEROID-INDUCED GLAUCOMA

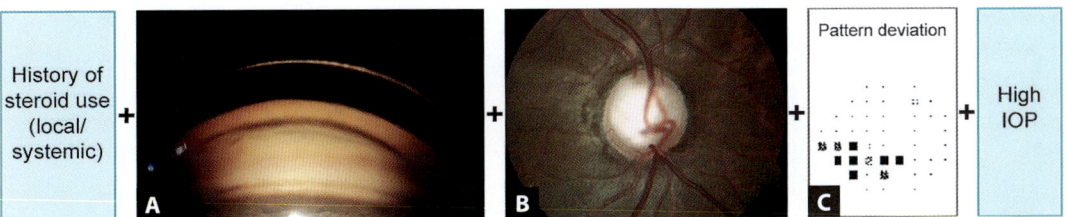

Figs. 4A to C: (A) Open angles; (B) Disc damage; (C) Visual field (VF) defect.

GLAUCOMA SECONDARY TO RAISED EPISCLERAL VENOUS PRESSURE

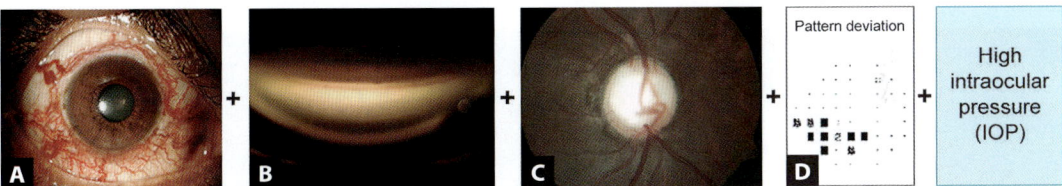

Figs. 5A to D: (A) Dilated and tortuous episcleral vessels; (B) Blood in Schlemm's canal; (C) Disc damage; (D) Visual field (VF) defect.

SILICONE OIL-INDUCED (OPEN ANGLE) GLAUCOMA

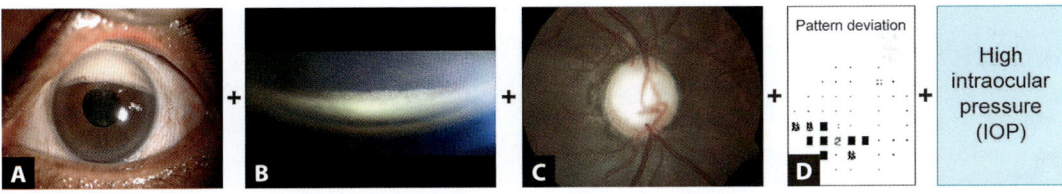

Figs. 6A to D: (A) Emulsified silicone oil in situ; (B) Emulsified oil particle deposits in angle; (C) Disc damage; (D) Visual field (VF) defect.

JUVENILE OPEN-ANGLE GLAUCOMA

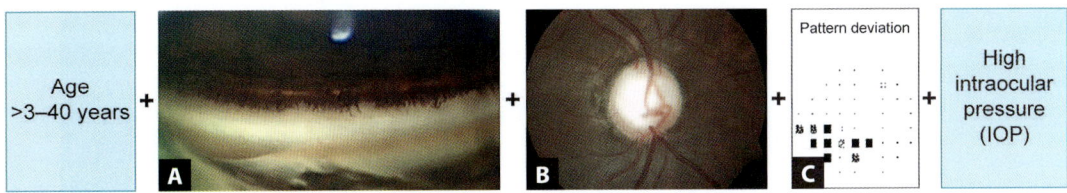

Figs. 7A to C: (A) Open angles with prominent iris processes ± High iris insertion; (B) Disc damage; (C) Visual field (VF) defect.

LENS-INDUCED (OPEN ANGLE) GLAUCOMA: PHACOLYTIC GLAUCOMA

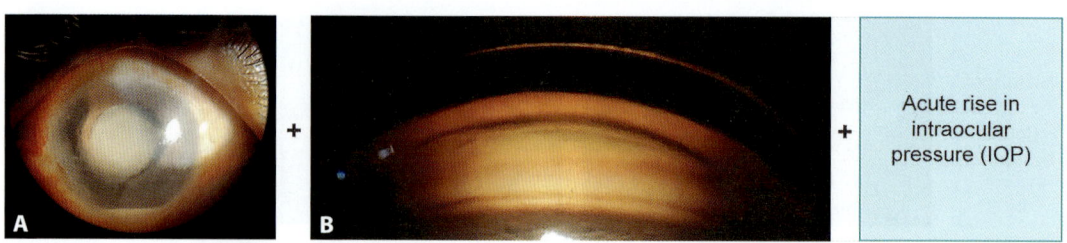

Figs. 8A and B: (A) Leaking hypermature cataract; (B) Open angles.

HEMOLYTIC/GHOST CELL GLAUCOMA

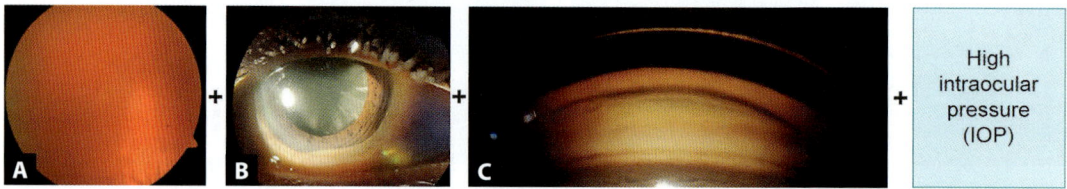

Figs. 9A to C: (A) Long-standing vitreous hemorrhage; (B) Tan hyphema; (C) Open angles.

POSNER–SCHLOSSMAN SYNDROME

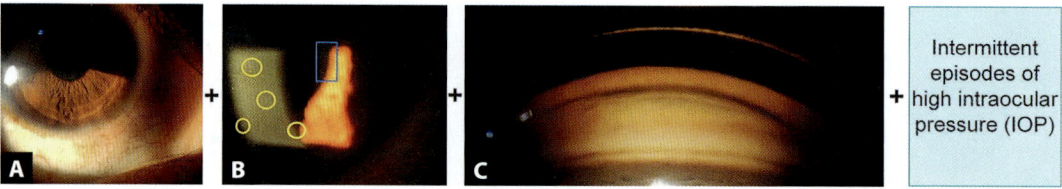

Figs. 10A to C: (A) Minimal ciliary congestion; (B) Fine keratic precipitates + minimal anterior chamber cells; (C) Open angles.

CHAPTER 20

Secondary Angle-closure Glaucomas

Rinal Pandit

NEOVASCULAR GLAUCOMA

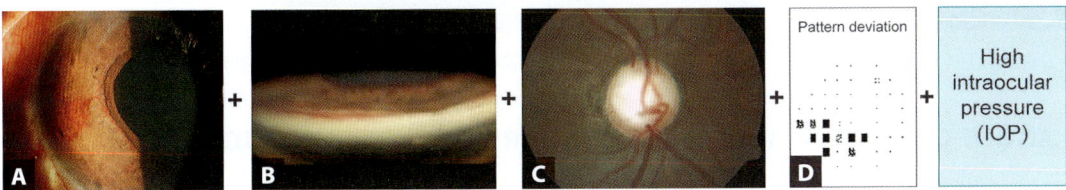

Figs. 1A to D: (A) Neovascularization of iris; (B) Neovascularization of angle; (C) Disc damage; (D) Visual field (VF) defect.

MALIGNANT GLAUCOMA

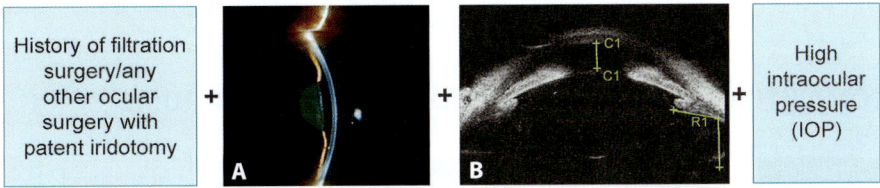

Figs. 2A and B: (A) Uniformly shallow anterior chamber (AC); (B) Forward displacement of iridolenticular diaphragm and forward rotation of ciliary body on Ultrasound Biomicroscopy (UBM).

ANGLE-CLOSURE GLAUCOMA SECONDARY TO MULTIPLE IRIS AND CILIARY BODY CYSTS

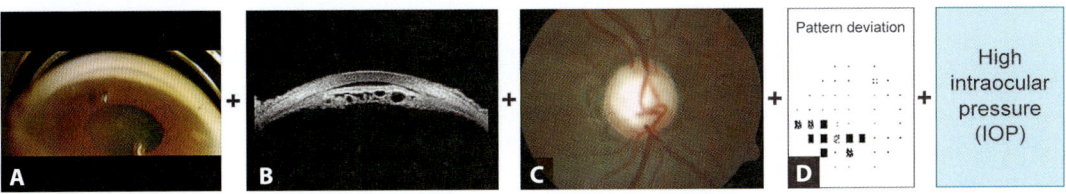

Figs. 3A to D: (A) Closed/occludable angles; (B) Multiple ciliary body cysts on Ultrasound Biomicroscopy (UBM); (C) Disc damage; (D) Visual field (VF) defect.

PHACOMORPHIC GLAUCOMA

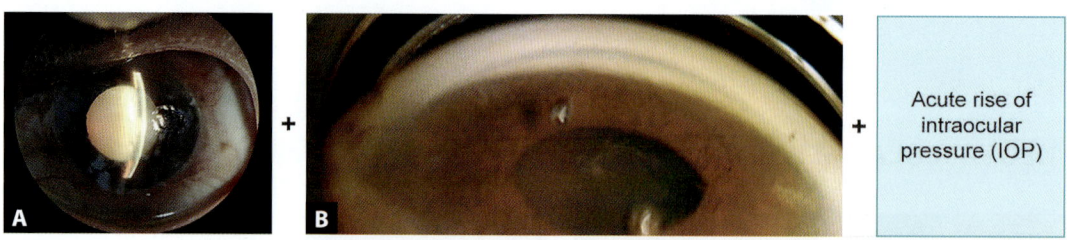

Figs. 4A and B: (A) Total intumescent cataract; (B) Closed angle.

ANGLE-CLOSURE GLAUCOMA SECONDARY TO UVEAL EFFUSION

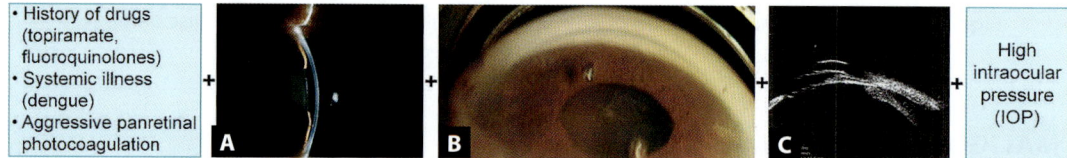

Figs. 5A to C: (A) Uniformly shallow anterior chamber (AC); (B) Closed angles; (C) Supraciliary effusion on Ultrasound Biomicroscopy (UBM).

GLAUCOMA IN ICE (IRIDOCORNEAL ENDOTHELIAL) SYNDROME

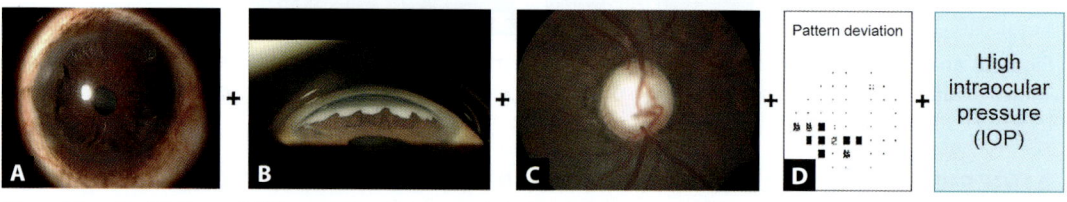

Figs. 6A to D: (A) Essential iris atrophy, ±iris stretch holes, beaten metal appearance of corneal endothelium; (B) Broad-based peripheral anterior synechiae (PAS); (C) Disc damage; (D) Visual field (VF) defect.

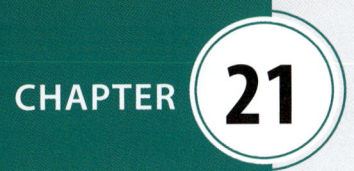

Insights into Intraocular Pressure and Glaucoma Dynamics

Nitika Beri

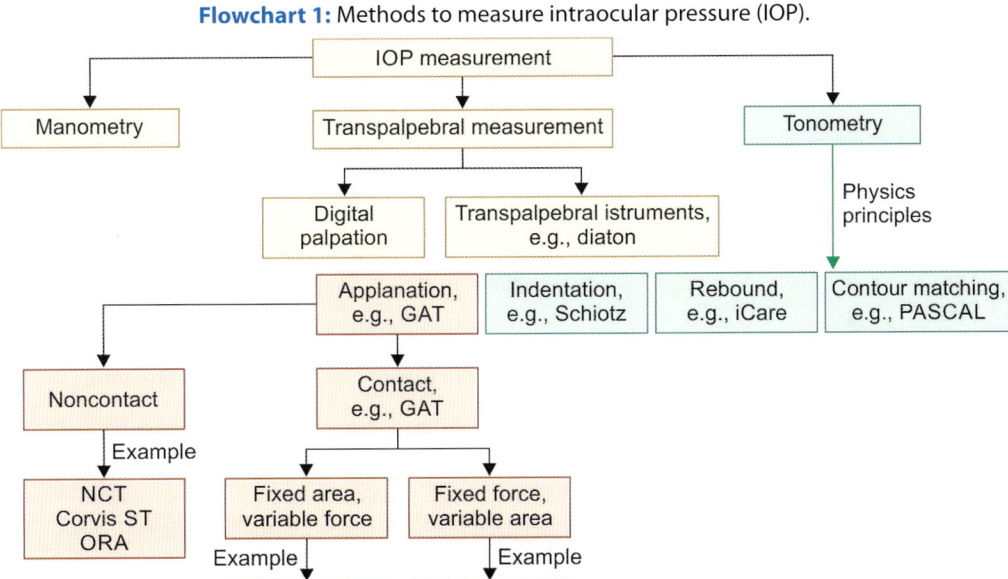

Flowchart 1: Methods to measure intraocular pressure (IOP).

(Corvis ST: corneal visualization Scheimpflug technology; GAT: Goldmann applanation tonometer; NCT: noncontact tonometer; ORA: ocular response analyzer)

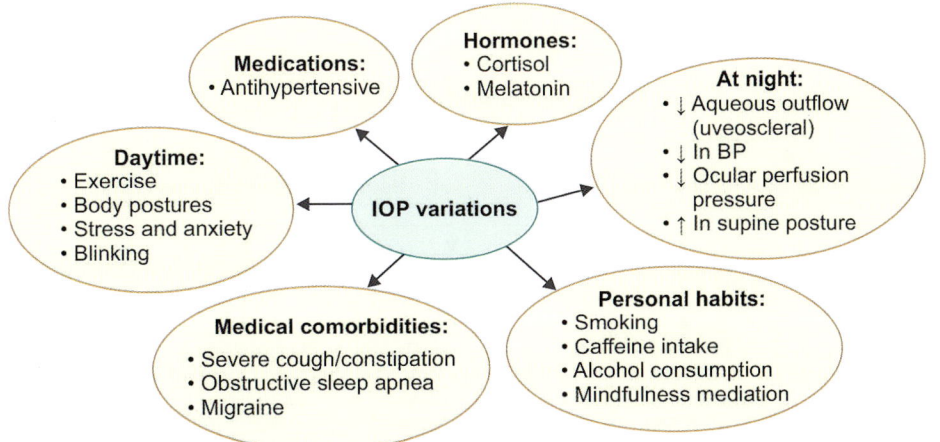

Fig. 1: IOP variations in daily life (physiology). (BP: blood pressure; IOP: intraocular pressure)

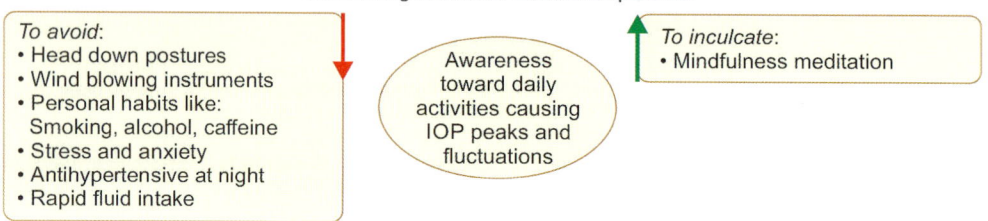

Fig. 2: Ocular perfusion pressure and glaucoma. (IOP: intraocular pressure)

Counseling sessions: Glaucoma patients

To avoid:
- Head down postures
- Wind blowing instruments
- Personal habits like: Smoking, alcohol, caffeine
- Stress and anxiety
- Antihypertensive at night
- Rapid fluid intake

Awareness toward daily activities causing IOP peaks and fluctuations

To inculcate:
- Mindfulness meditation

Fig. 3: Daily activities causing IOP peaks and fluctuations. (IOP: intraocular pressure)

- Check for refractive error
- Check for broken glass of prism
- Confirm last calibration
- Explain the procedure to the patient
- Avoid touching the eyelashes
- Avoid excessive pressure on the upper eyelid with your hand
- Keep the drum at mark of 1 (= 10 mm Hg) to start
- If expecting high IOP (e.g., 40 mm Hg)–can keep drum at higher mark like 20 mm Hg to start
- Avoid prolonged time of contact and be gentle– corneal abrasion
- Remember to put antibiotic eyedrop in the end

Fig. 4: Clinical tips for GAT. (GAT: Goldmann applanation tonometer; IOP: intraocular pressure)

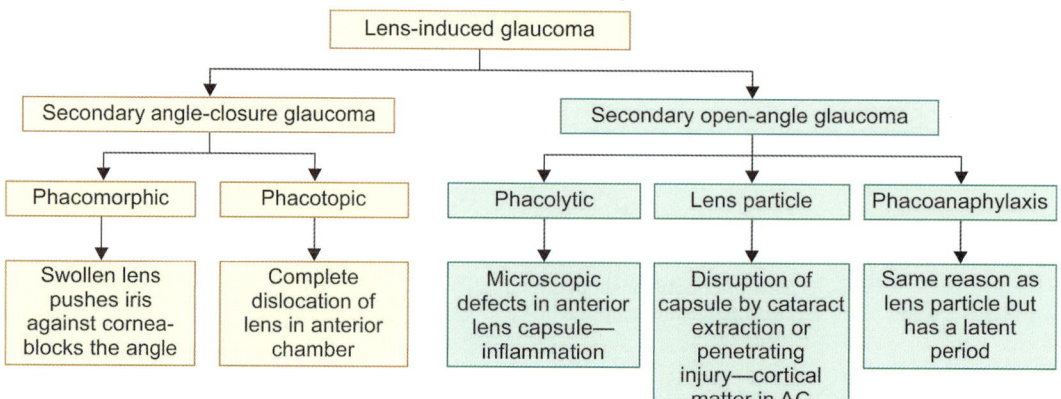

Flowchart 2: Lens-induced glaucoma.

CHAPTER 22

Recent Advances in Medical Management

Rinal Pandit

Omidenepag Isopropyl 0.002% (Omlonti/Eyebelis eye drop)

Fast facts

Mechanism of action
Relatively selective prostaglandin EP2 receptor agonist, which increases aqueous humor drainage through the conventional (or trabecular) and uveoscleral outflow pathways.

Indication
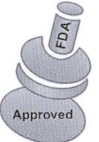
FDA approved in 2022 for use in primary open angle glaucoma and ocular hypertension patients.

Efficacy
Mean IOP reduction is 5–7 mm Hg.

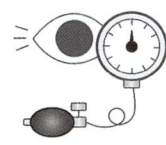

Dosage
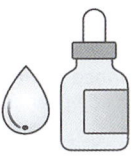
One drop in the affected eye(s) once daily in the evening.

Side effect profile
Conjunctival hyperemia, photophobia, blurred vision, dry eye, instillation site pain, ocular hyperemia, punctate keratitis.

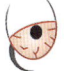 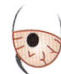

Unique feature
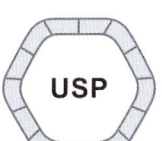
Claimed to have minimal to no incidence of Prostaglandin-associated periorbitopathy (PAP).

Claimed to be effective in non-responders to conventional PG analogues.

Latanoprostene Bunod 0.024% (Vyzulta eye drop)

Fast facts

Mechanism of action
In addition to acting as a prostaglandin analogue increasing uveoscleral outflow, it is expected to release nitric oxide, which in turn reduces IOP by relaxing the trabecular meshwork and Schlemm's canal improving trabecular outflow.

Indication
FDA approved in 2017 for use in primary open angle glaucoma and ocular hypertension patients.

Efficacy
- IOP reduction: 32% from baseline.
- Additional 1.2 mm Hg IOP reduction as compared to latanoprost alone.

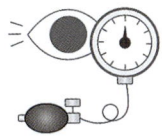

Dosage
One drop in the affected eye(s) once daily in the evening.

Side effect profile
- Similar to PG analogue.
- Conjunctival hyperemia, instillation site pain, irritation, hyperpigmentation of iris, changes in eyelashes (increase in length, thickness), uveitis, reactivation of herpetic keratitis, cystoid macular edema.

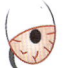 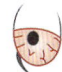

Clinical trials
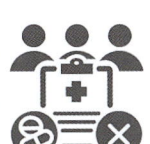
APOLLO and LUNAR: Compared to timolol noninferiority to timolol 0.5% at all time points and superior diurnal IOP reduction compared to timolol 0.5%.
VOYAGER: Compared to latanoprost lowered mean diurnal IOP by 1.23 mm Hg more than latanoprost 0.005% at 1 month.

Fast facts
DURYSTA
(Bimatoprost 10 μg implant)

#1
FDA approved intracameral biodegradable Bimatoprost sustained release implant.

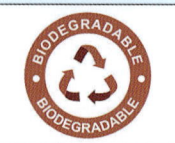

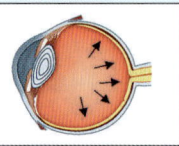

#2
Approved for use in open angle glaucoma and ocular hypertension patients.

#3
Injected via preloaded injector into the anterior chamber in the superotemporal region under topical anesthesia.

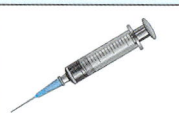

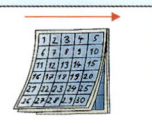

#4
Sustained release of drug up to 6 months.

#5
Offers up to 32% IOP reduction.

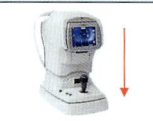

#6
Ocular surface friendly improves compliance.

#7
Costs approximately $2000/dose.

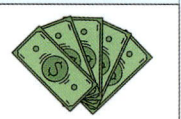

Fast facts
iDOSE TR
(Travoprost intracameral implant 75 μg)

#1
FDA approved intracameral bio-compatible sustained-release Travoprost titanium implant.

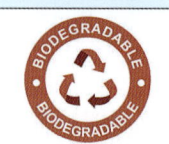

#2
Approved for use in open angle glaucoma and ocular hypertension patients.

#3
Injected via preloaded injector through the trabecular meshwork and anchored into scleral tissue under direct gonioscopic view.

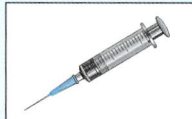

#4
Designed to continuously release the medication for at least 1 year.

#5
IOP reductions from baseline to 3 months ranging between 6.6 mm Hg and 8.4 mm Hg.

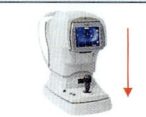

#6
Ocular surface friendly improves compliance.

#7
Costs approximately $13,950/dose (implant).

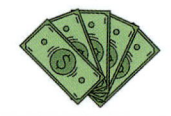

CHAPTER 23

Disorders of Vitreous

Kushal S Delhiwala

ANATOMY OF VITREOUS

The vitreous is a transparent gel-like spheroidal structure which occupies approximately 80% volume of the eyeball. It is divided into central core vitreous and the peripheral cortical vitreous and is primarily made up of consisting of collagen, hyaluronic acid, water, and hyalocytes.[1-3] The anterior vitreous, in contact with the posterior lens capsule, constitutes Wieger's ligament, while central vitreous is traversed by Cloquet canal, which represents remnant of hyaloid artery course. The vitreous is firmly attached to the posterior lens capsule, the vitreous base near the ora serrata, retinal blood vessels, the optic nerve, and the fovea.[4]

DISORDERS OF VITREOUS

These can be categorized into:
- Developmental abnormalities
- Hereditary vitreoretinopathies with optically empty vitreous
- Diseases secondary to primary diseases of adjacent ocular sites

Developmental Abnormalities

- *Persistent tunica vasculosa lentis remnants* **(Video 1)**
- *Mittendorf dot*: An anterior remnant, adherent to the posterior lens capsule.
- *Bergmeister papilla:* A prepapillary remnant at the margin of the optic nerve head **(Figs. 1A and B)**.[2]
- *Prepapillary vascular loops:* Normal retinal vessels grow into Bergmeister papilla before returning to the retina. These are predominantly arterial.
- *Persistent fetal vasculature (PFV):*
  - It results from failure to primary vascular vitreous to regress. It is usually unilateral and without any associated systemic findings.
  - *Anterior PFV:* It presents as leukocoria due to white fibrovascular tissue adherent to posterior to the lens.

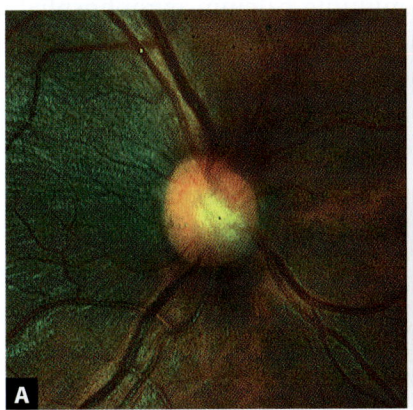
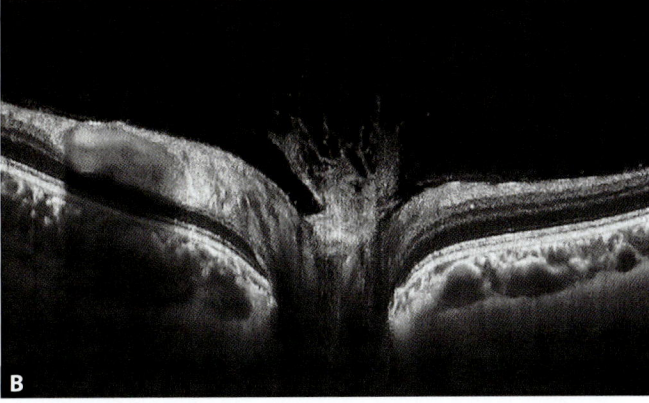

Figs. 1A and B: (A) Fundus image showing Bergmeister papilla; (B) Optical coherence tomography (OCT) scan of Bergmeister papilla.

These may be associated with microphthalmos, elongated ciliary processes, cataract, and secondary angle-closure glaucoma.
- *Posterior PFV:* This may have an isolated presentation or may be associated with anterior PFV. There is a presence of fibrovascular tissue stalk extending from optic nerve head, which courses anteriorly toward the retrolental area and also involving the anterior retina with formation of retinal fold.[5]

Hereditary Vitreoretinopathies with Optically Empty Vitreous

These group of abnormalities show liquefaction of vitreous with thin cortical vitreous leftover and avascular membranes adherent to retina. These are autosomal dominant conditions and may present with myopia, glaucoma, and cataract.

These vitreoretinopathies include:[1]
- *Wagner syndrome:* This is not associated with systemic abnormalities.
- *Stickler syndrome:* This is associated with development of retinal detachment along with orofacial and skeletal abnormalities.

Disorders Secondary to Primary Diseases of Adjacent Ocular Sites[3]

These usually present in the form of vitreous opacities and include the following:
- *Vitreous degeneration and detachment (Fig. 2 and Video 2):*
  - With senile changes, collagen fibers in vitreous get coalesced, leading to loss of transparent property of vitreous.
  - These clusters can be perceived by patients a floaters, which can get further increased following vitreous detachment.
  - Separation of vitreous from optic nerve head creates ring-shaped condensation known as Weiss ring.
  - These floaters gradually reduce with progressive vitreous liquefaction.
- *Vitreous hemorrhage (Video 3):*
  - These can result from multiple etiologies such as proliferative vascular retinopathies, trauma, avulsion of retinal blood vessel following posterior vitreous detachment, and systemic conditions such as bleeding disorders and Terson syndrome **(Figs. 3A and B)**.
  - In mild form, patients may experience symptoms of floaters, while severe vitreous hemorrhage may lead to significant reduction in visual acuity and may require vitrectomy surgery to clear the hemorrhage.
  - In case of severe vitreous hemorrhage, B-scan ultrasonography can provide a clue for possible underlying etiology.
  - Sometimes even examination of the fellow eye can provide a clue with regards to possibility of unilateral or bilateral condition of the disease.
- *Asteroid hyalosis (Fig. 4A):*
  - It is characterized by accumulation of multiple calcium pyrophosphate crystals within vitreous gel *(Fig. 4B)*.
  - These appear as numerous yellowish-white vitreous opacities and move with ocular movements.

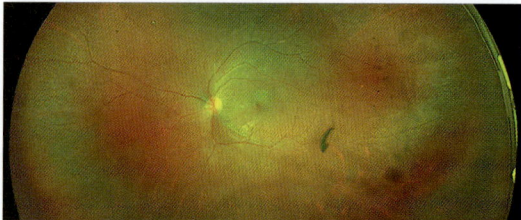

Fig. 2: Fundus image depicting vitreous degeneration.

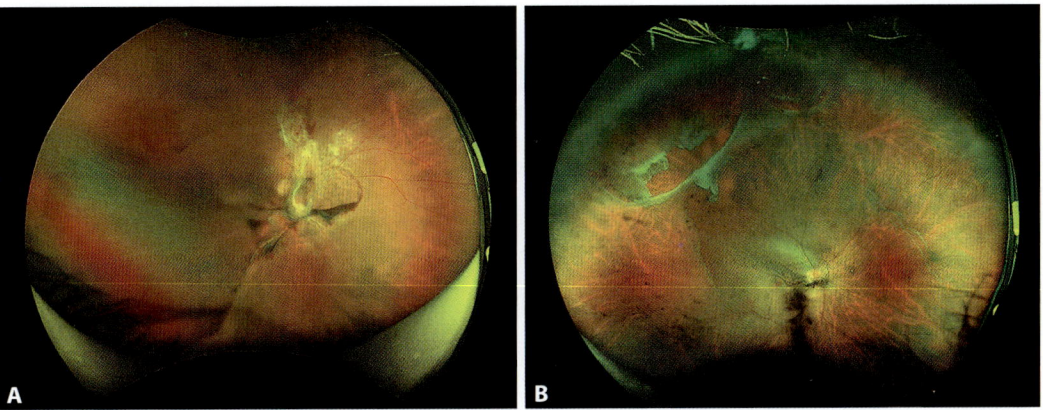

Figs. 3A and B: (A) Fundus image of vitreous hemorrhage in proliferative diabetic retinopathy (PDR); (B) Fundus image of vitreous hemorrhage associated with a retinal tear.

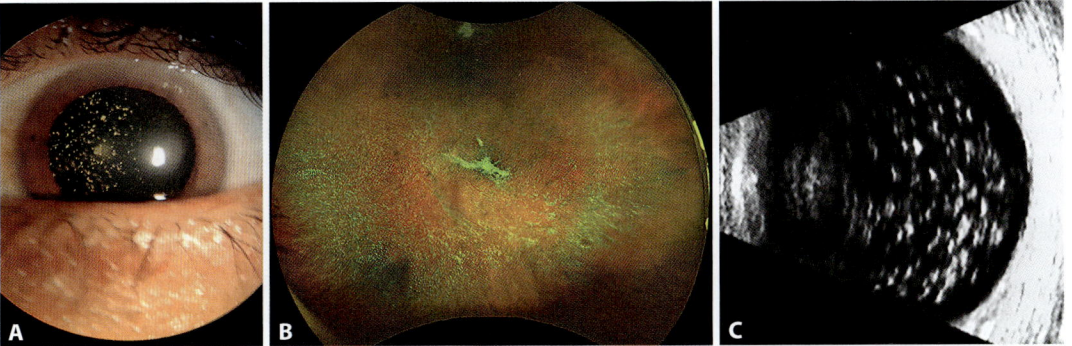

Figs. 4A to C: (A): Slit-lamp image of asteroid hyalosis; (B) Fundus image of asteroid hyalosis; (C) B-scan ultrasound image of asteroid hyalosis.

- These are found to be unilateral in approximately 3/4th cases and are usually asymptomatic.
- B-scan ultrasonography of asteroid hyalosis characteristically shows clear zone between the dot echoes and the retina **(Fig. 4C)**.
- Asteroid hyalosis can sometimes obscure the details of coexisting retinal pathology and hence may require investigations such fluorescein angiography and optical coherence tomography to evaluate them.

- *Synchysis scintillans:*
  - This condition can result as consequence of an old vitreous hemorrhage and are composed of cholesterol crystals.
  - This may mimic asteroid hyalosis however crystals tend to settle inferiorly in this condition while crystals in asteroid hyalosis stay suspended in resting position of eye.
- *Amyloidosis:*
  - It is characterized by deposition of extracellular fibrillary protein

in vitreous and is seen in familial amyloidosis.
- Vitreous opacities may be unilateral or bilateral and may get adherent to posterior lens capsule.

▪ *Vitreous cyst* **(Fig. 5)**:
- These are either congenital or secondary to trauma and inflammation.
- They may also be seen in association with hereditary conditions such as retinitis pigmentosa.
- These are found to be freely floating and are usually asymptomatic.

▪ *Vitritis* **(Videos 4 and 5)(Fig. 6)**:
- Inflammatory cells and mediators released following intraocular inflammation, can get accumulated within vitreous leading to development of visually affecting vitreous opacities.
- These are commonly seen in intermediate uveitis, pan uveitis, and endophthalmitis and may present along with retinal vasculitis and retinitis.
- These are usually responsive to anti-inflammatory treatment and nonresolving opacities may need vitrectomy for visual recovery.
- Intravitreal injection of triamcinolone acetonide given for various retinal pathologies can mimic vitritis due to yellowish-white appearance of triamcinolone crystals **(Fig. 7)**.
- Similarly retained lens matter in vitreous following posterior capsular rent during cataract surgery an also mimic vitritis **(Fig. 8)**.

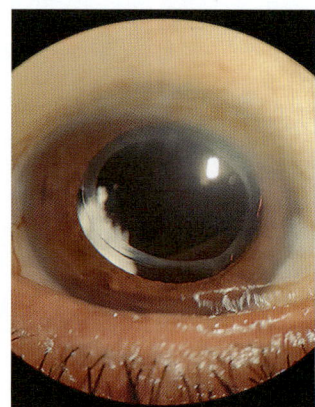

Fig. 7: Slit-lamp image of intravitreal triamcinolone acetonide (IVTA).

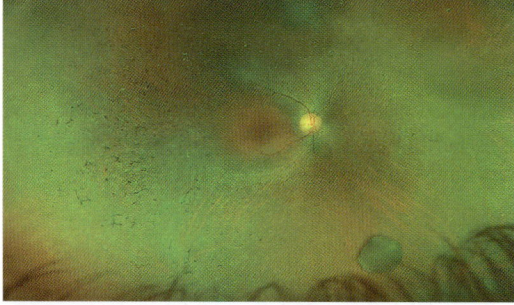

Fig. 5: Fundus image showing a vitreous cyst.

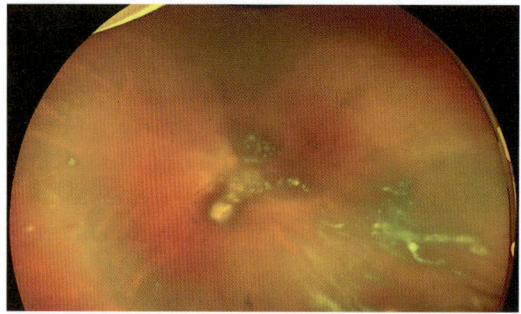

Fig. 6: Fundus image demonstrating vitritis.

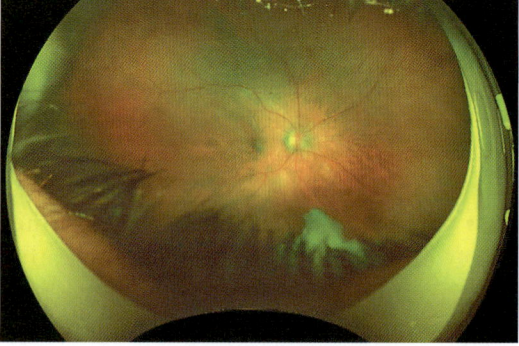

Fig. 8: Fundus image revealing lens matter in the vitreous cavity.

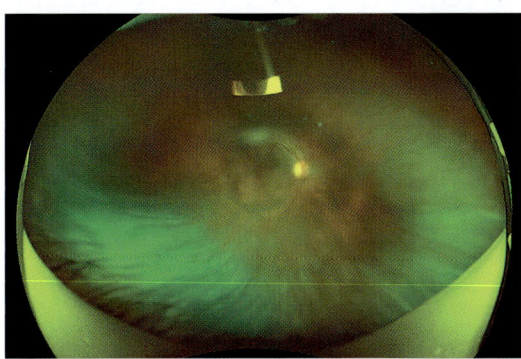

Fig. 9: Fundus image illustrating vitreoretinal lymphoma with an "aurora borealis" appearance.

- *Primary vitreoretinal lymphoma:*[1]
  - It is non-Hodgkin's diffuse large B-cell lymphoma which may appear initially within the eye and eventually may lead to central nervous system (CNS) involvement on most of the patients.
  - It is characterized by presence of large vitreous cells, which may show "string of pearls" pattern or can appear as multiple, aligned vitreous fibrils described as "aurora borealis" pattern.
  - This is considered to be a uveitis masquerade and should be considered as one of the major differential diagnoses in uveitis patients showing suboptimal or no response to conventional corticosteroid treatment.
  - In such cases, vitreous biopsy can prove to be confirmatory. This requires to stop all steroidal treatments 2–3 weeks before taking biopsy as steroids lead to lysis of lymphoma cells and thereby reducing the yield **(Fig. 9)**.

VIDEO LEGENDS

Video 1: Mittendorf dot with Cloquet canal remnant.
Video 2: Vitreous degeneration.
Video 3: Vitreous hemorrhage.
Video 4: Intravitreal triamcinolone acetonide (IVTA).
Video 5: Vitritis.

REFERENCES

1. Sadda SR (2022). Ryan's retina, 7th edition. Elsevier.
2. Ye Q, Zhang C, Gao F, Min, H (2020). Vitreous Diseases. In: Min H (Eds). Stereo Atlas of Vitreoretinal Diseases. Springer, Singapore.
3. Salmon JF (2024). Kanski's clinical ophthalmology (10th edition). Elsevier.
4. Worst JGF, Los LI. Cisternal Anatomy of the Vitreous. Kugler; 1995.
5. Goldberg MF. Persistent fetal vasculature (PFV): an integrated interpretation of signs and symptoms associated with persistent hyperplastic primary vitreous (PHPV). LIV Edward Jackson Memorial Lecture. Am J Ophthalmol. 1997;124(5):587-626.

CHAPTER 24

Retinopathy of Prematurity

Puja Maitra, Aditya Maitray, Manan Balvant Mistry

PATHOGENESIS[1]

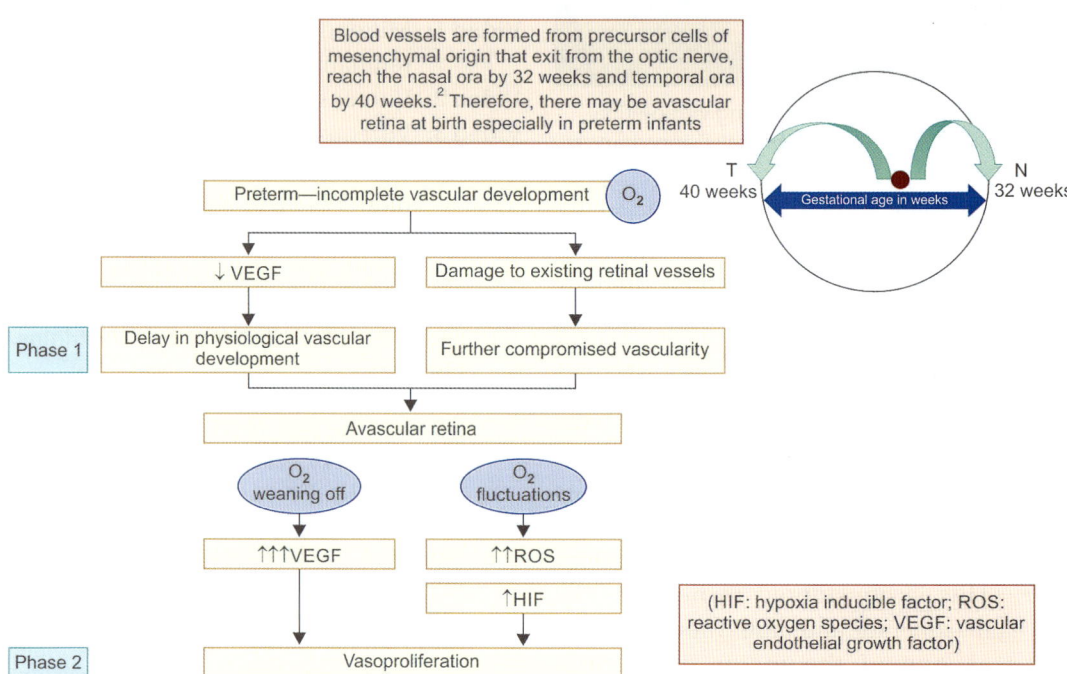

Retinopathy of Prematurity

SCREENING

Whom to screen?
<2,000 g
<34 weeks
34–36 weeks of gestation with risk factors

RBSK 2017, NNF 020

When to screen?
*First screening →
4 weeks of birth
Gestational age <28 weeks or birthweight
<1,200 g → 3 weeks*

How to screen?
- Dilate using ROP drops (2.5 mL of tropicamide phenylephrine combination diluted with 2.5 mL tear substitute). All extra eye drops to be wiped off to prevent systemic absorption through skin)
- Withhold feeding for at least 40 minutes
- Swaddle the baby (as in image)
- Topical anesthesia 0.5% proparacaine instilled
- Alfonso speculum used to keep lids apart
- Indirect ophthalmoscopy with 28D (or 20D) used to at least see posterior pole, nasal and temporal periphery and a vectis is used to rotate globe and for scleral indentation
- Topical antibiotics instilled at the end

How to document?

Handwritten detailed records	Photodocumentation using retcam, retcam shuttle, NeoForus, Smartphone based fundus cameras

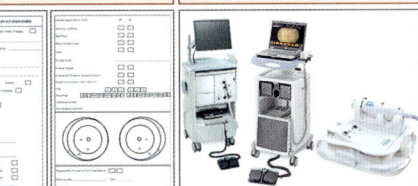

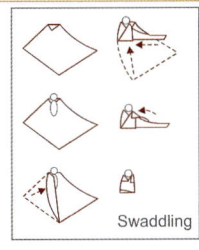
Swaddling

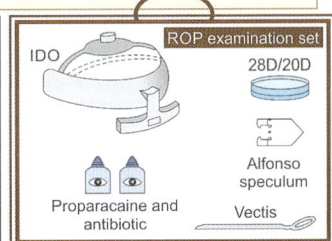
IDO — ROP examination set — 28D/20D
Proparacaine and antibiotic — Alfonso speculum — Vectis

ZONES AND STAGES[3-5]

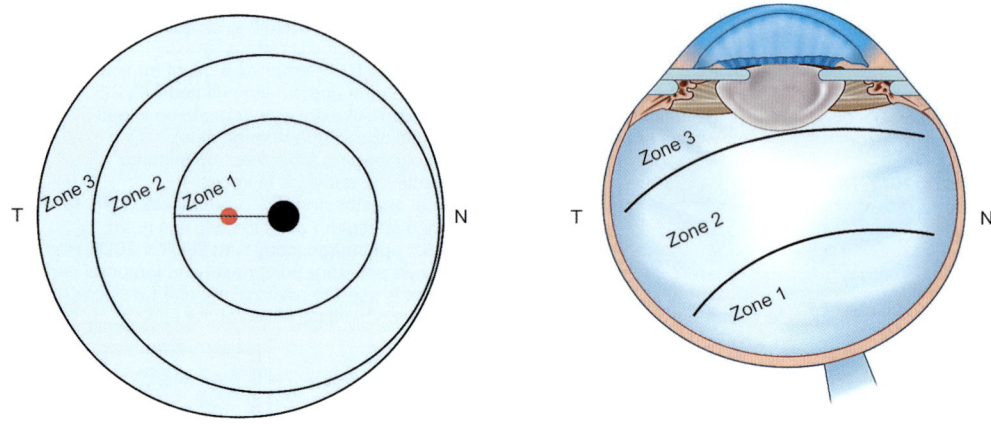

A rough estimate of zone 1 is when we examine with 28D lens. If the disc is at one edge of the field, we are roughly able to see the temporal or nasal half of zone 1

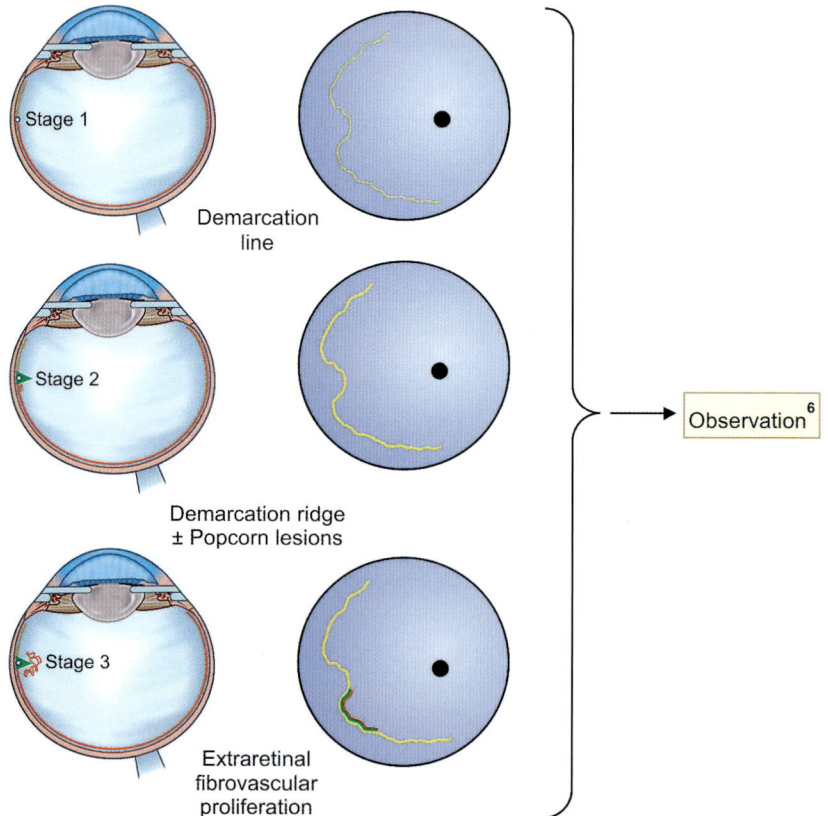

Stage 1 — Demarcation line

Stage 2 — Demarcation ridge ± Popcorn lesions

Stage 3 — Extraretinal fibrovascular proliferation

Observation[6]

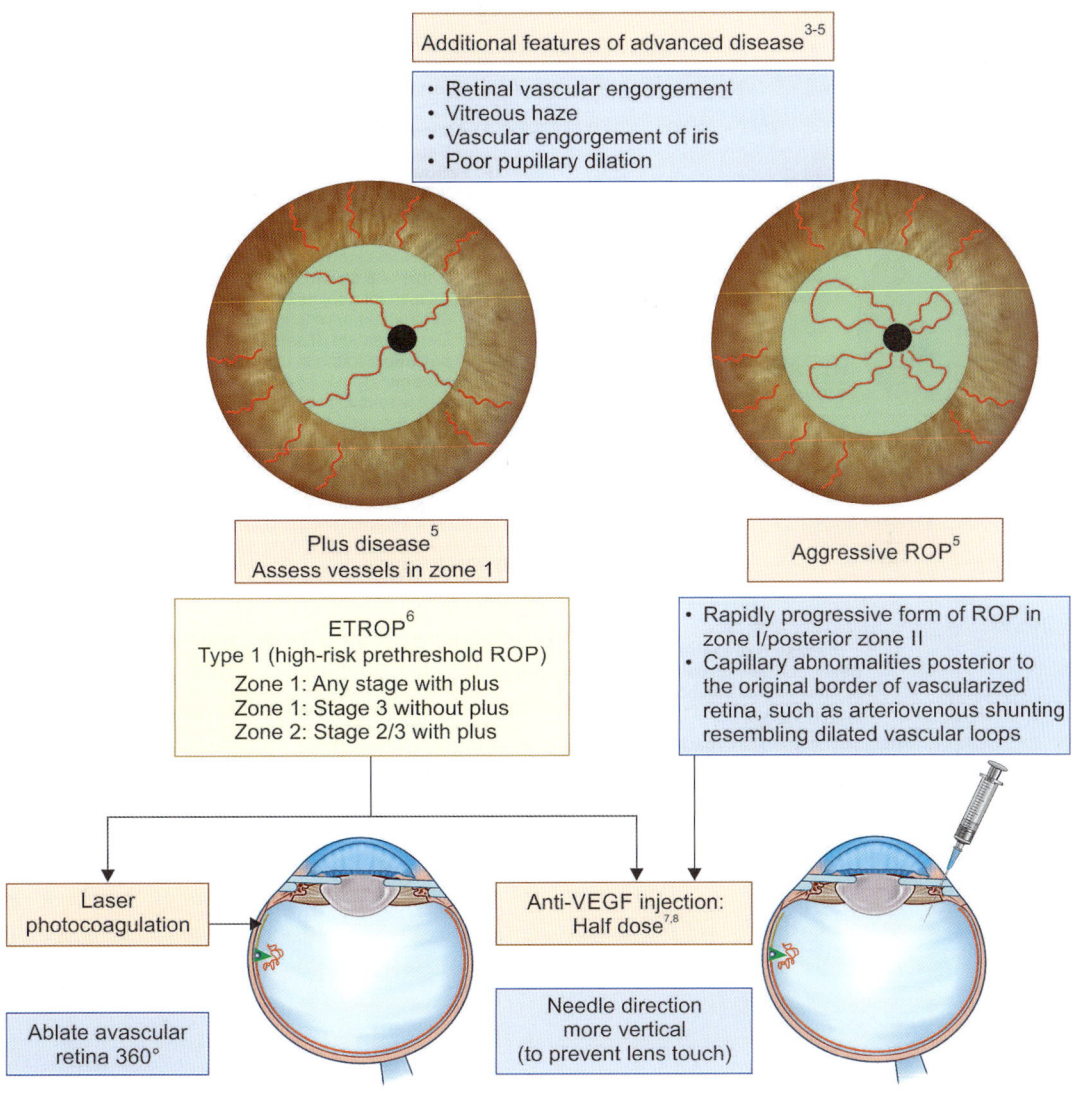

Retinopathy of Prematurity

Near confluent nonoverlapping burns

- Start with worse eye
- Start posteriorly close to ridge
- Watch for bradycardia/desaturation during the procedure

Red laser	Green laser
810 nm	532 nm
Deeper penetration—better for hazy media but causes more pain	Lesser pain Can cause cataract in eyes with TVL

SAFER ROP injection technique[9]

S: Short Needle
- ✔ 32-gauge 4.0 mm TSK SteriJect needle

A: Antiseptic/Antibiotic
- ✔ Betadine 5% or 10% both before and after treatment

F: Follow-Up
- ✔ 2–7 days post-injection to examine for injection complications

E: Extra Attention to Detail
- ✔ Maintain clean environment (gloves, masks, single-use caliper, and eyelid speculum)
- ✔ Assess for conjunctivitis and nasolacrimal duct obstruction prior to injection
- ✔ Determination of safe injection site 0.75–1.0 mm posterior to limbus using the ora nonogram

R: Recheck
- ✔ 1–2 weeks following injection and until mature vascularization is complete
- ✔ Use fluorescein angiogram for all treated patients between 60 and 65 weeks postmenstrual age if not vascularized
- ✔ Laser avascular areas if necessary

Monitoring disease activity after treatment

Disease regression
Better pupillary dilatation
Decrease in plus component
Vessel progression up to ora

After initial regression, reactivation of stage 2/3 after injection must be treated with laser to any avascular retina

Disease progression
Development of traction requires surgery

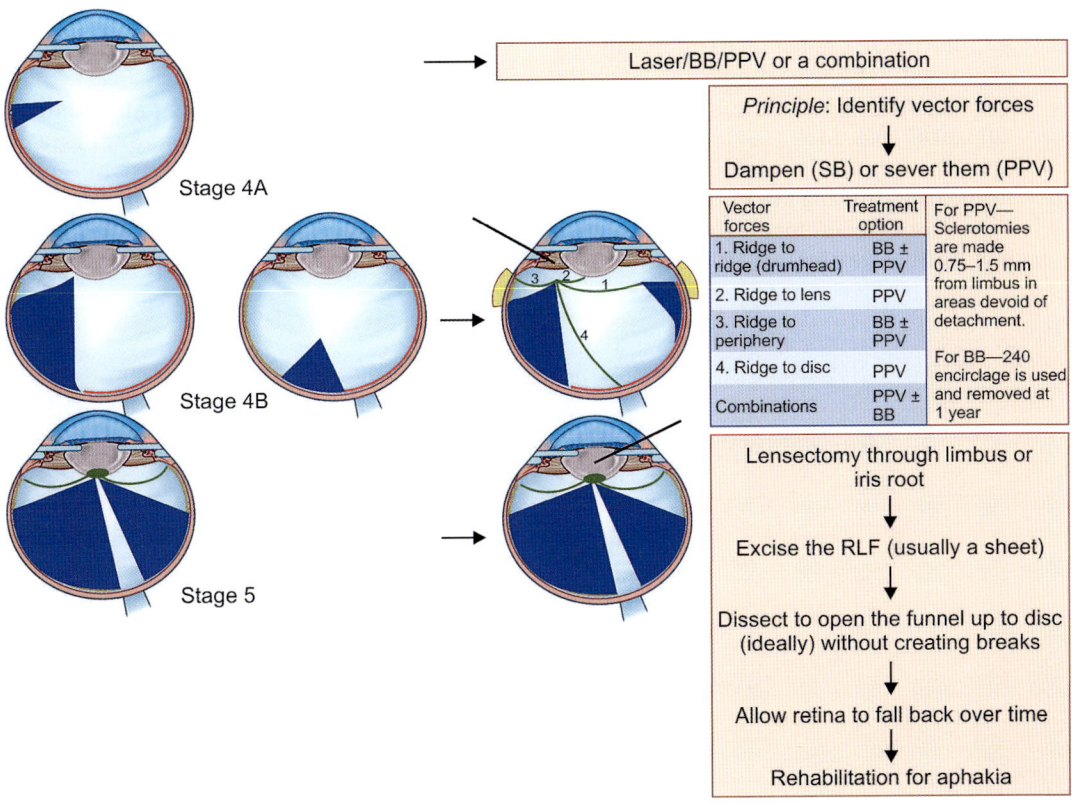

REFERENCES

1. Hughes S, Yang H, Chan-Ling T. Vascularization of the human fetal retina: Roles of vasculogenesis and angiogenesis. Invest Ophthalmol Vis Sci. 2000;41:1217-28.
2. Hartnett E. The pathophysiology of retinopathy of prematurity. In: Wu WC, Lam WC (Eds). A Quick Guide to Pediatric Retina. Singapore: Springer Nature Singapore Pte Ltd; 2021. pp. 3-9.
3. International Classification of Retinopathy of Prematurity Committee for Classification of Late Stages of ROP. An international classification of retinopathy of prematurity: II. The classification of retinal detachment. Arch Ophthalmol. 1987;105:906-12.
4. Committee for the Classification of Retinopathy of Prematurity. The International Classification of Retinopathy of Prematurity revisited. Arch Ophthalmol. 2005;123(7):991-9.
5. Chiang MF, Quinn GE, Fielder AR, Ostmo SR, Paul Chan RV, Berrocal A, et al. International Classification of Retinopathy of Prematurity, Third Edition. Ophthalmology. 2021;128(10):e51-e68.
6. Early Treatment For Retinopathy Of Prematurity Cooperative Group. Revised indications for the treatment of retinopathy of prematurity: results of the early treatment for retinopathy of prematurity randomized trial. Arch Ophthalmol. 2003;121(12):1684-94.

7. Mintz-Hittner HA, Kennedy KA, Chuang AZ; BEAT-ROP Cooperative Group. Efficacy of intravitreal bevacizumab for stage 3+ retinopathy of prematurity. N Engl J Med. 2011;364(7):603-15.
8. Stahl A, Lepore D, Fielder A, Fleck B, Reynolds JD, Chiang MF, et al. Ranibizumab versus laser therapy for the treatment of very low birthweight infants with retinopathy of prematurity (RAINBOW): an open-label randomised controlled trial. Lancet. 2019;394(10208):1551-9.
9. Beck KD, Rahman EZ, Ells A, Mireskandari K, Berrocal AM, Harper CA. SAFER-ROP: Updated Protocol for Anti-VEGF Injections for Retinopathy of Prematurity. Ophthal Surg Lasers Imag Retina. 2020;51(7):402-6.

CHAPTER 25

Diabetic Eye Disease

Aman Khanna, Gaurav M Kohli, Tanya Jain, Pratik Shenoy, Pallavi Goel

INTRODUCTION

Diabetic retinopathy (DR) is a microangiopathy associated with diabetes mellitus. It is a significant vision-threatening condition and a leading cause of preventable blindness worldwide.

The overall prevalence of DR in India (considering both known diabetes and undiagnosed diabetes) is approximately 12.5% with no reported difference between the rural and urban population.

The prevalence of vision-threatening diabetic retinopathy (VTDR) is 4% which implies that one-third of patients with DR develop vision loss due to the disease.

Even though the prevalence of DR in India is reported to be lower than the global prevalence, the disease burden of VTDR cases in India remains comparable to the rest of the world.

PATHOGENESIS OF DIABETIC RETINOPATHY

The pathogenesis of retinopathy involves an interplay of three pivotal factors, namely: of (a) oxidative/osmotic stress, (b) inflammation, and (c) vascular dysfunction.[1-5]

Chronic hyperglycemia can trigger the development of DR through glycation end products, polyol pathway activation, and phosphokinase C (PKC). Elevated blood glucose levels lead to the formation of advanced glycation end products (AGEs), which induce oxidative stress. This oxidative stress damages retinal cells and disrupts the retinal microvasculature **(Flowchart 1)**.[6]

In the retina, excess glucose is processed via the polyol pathway, where aldose reductase converts glucose into sorbitol. The accumulation of sorbitol is responsible for osmotic stress-related cellular damage.

Hyperglycemia has also been reported to activate PKC, which is critical in vascular dysfunction. Activation of PKC results in increased vascular leakage, abnormal blood flow, and disruption of the blood-retinal barrier.

Apart from the aforementioned metabolic disarray which initiates the retinopathy, the presence of inflammation remains the

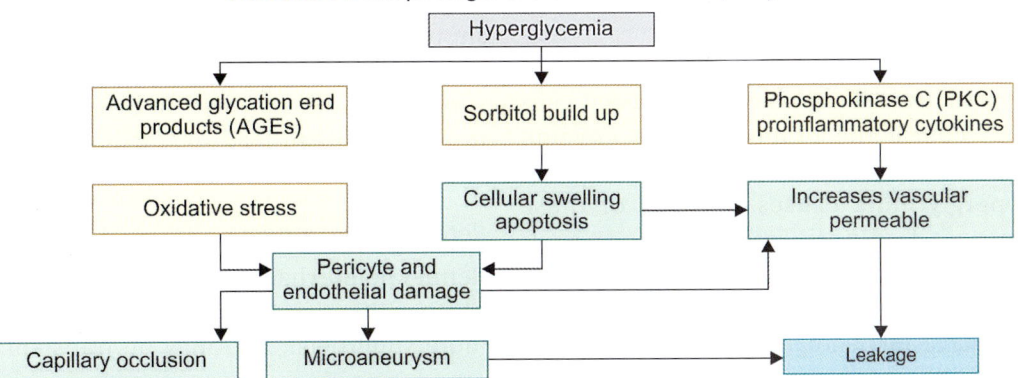

Flowchart 1: The pathogenesis of diabetic retinopathy.

central component for the development of vascular leakage after angiopathy sets in. Hyperglycemia triggers the release of proinflammatory cytokines [e.g., tumor necrosis factor-alpha (TNF-α) and nterleukin-6 (IL-6)] and chemokines, leading to leukocyte adhesion to retinal endothelial cells, further exacerbating vascular injury and capillary occlusion, responsible for retinal ischemia.

In response to retinal ischemia, hypoxia-inducible factors (HIFs) are activated, leading to increased expression of vascular endothelial growth factor (VEGF), a potent angiogenic factor. VEGF promotes abnormal blood vessel growth and increases vascular permeability, contributing to diabetic macular edema (DME), and proliferative changes.

> Clinical nuggets:
> - The hallmark of DR is the breakdown of the blood-retinal barrier and microvascular dysfunction. Damage to the endothelial cells and loss of pericytes lead to capillary leakage, edema, and the formation of microaneurysms.
> - Capillary occlusion results in areas of retinal ischemia, promoting the release of vascular endothelial growth factor (VEGF), which drives abnormal neovascularization, leading to proliferative diabetic retinopathy (PDR).

PATHOLOGICAL CHANGES IN DIABETIC RETINOPATHY

Microscopic Changes

Microvascular Damage

Pericyte loss: Pericytes are specialized cells with contractile properties that envelop the endothelial cells of capillaries. In DR, hyperglycemia causes the loss of these pericytes, leading to weakened blood vessels and increased vascular permeability. Cellular damage is first noted in the pericytes which are crucial for maintaining capillary structure and function. Pericyte lost is the earliest histological change in diabetic angiopathy.

Endothelial dysfunction: High blood glucose levels damage endothelial cells, impairing the functioning of the retinal capillaries, leading to the breakdown of the blood-retinal barrier, resulting in leakage of plasma proteins, lipids, and fluids into the retina.[7,8]

Capillary Occlusion

Basement membrane thickening and the accumulation of advanced glycation end products leads to capillary blockages. The occlusion of capillaries results in areas of retinal ischemia, which promotes the release of proangiogenic factors; VEGF.

Macroscopic Changes

Microaneurysms

The earliest clinical signs of DR are the formation of microaneurysms which are small outpouchings of blood vessels. These occur due to the weakening of capillary walls due to loss of pericytes and increased intravascular pressure.

Neovascularization

In proliferative diabetic retinopathy (PDR), ischemia stimulates the release of VEGF, which drives the formation of fragile, abnormal new blood vessels at the junction of ischemic, and nonischemic retina. These fragile vessels grow into the vitreous and rupture, leading to vitreous hemorrhage. The neovessels can grow over the retinal surface, and the contraction of this fibrotic proliferation can lead to tractional retinal detachments.

Retinal Hemorrhages

Retinal hemorrhages are "dot/blot-shaped" (deep within the retina) or "flamed-shaped" more superficial, and may be transient in appearance. These appear due to capillary ruptures.

Hard Exudates

As capillaries leak plasma components, hard exudates (lipid deposits) form. This disrupts retinal function and contributes to the progression of vision loss, particularly when it affects the macular region.

Intraretinal Microvascular Abnormalities

The microvascular loops originate in the distended preexisting capillaries, which act as vascular shunts. Some consider intraretinal microvascular abnormality (IRMA) as the Harbinger of neovascular growth.

Venous Beading/Looping

This is a sign of retinal ischemia and occurs adjacent to an area of decreased perfusion. It is one of the significant indicators of progression toward PDR.

Macular Edema

Diabetic macular edema results from the accumulation of fluid in the macula due to leakage of retinal capillaries secondary to pericyte loss. This causes thickening of the retina and leads to central vision impairment.

RHEOLOGICAL CHANGES IN DIABETIC RETINOPATHY

Increased Blood Viscosity

Hyperglycemia increases the viscosity of blood. This impairs blood flow through the retinal capillaries, exacerbating ischemia and increasing the likelihood of vessel occlusion.

Hypercoagulability

Hypercoagulability is a hallmark of diabetes. This is due to elevated levels of clotting factors, reduced fibrinolysis, and increased platelet activity. These changes promote microthrombosis in the retinal vasculature.

Leukostasis

Hyperglycemia leads to leukocyte adhesion to the retinal endothelium (leukostasis). This abnormal adhesion is mediated by increased expression of adhesion molecules like intercellular adhesion molecule-1 (ICAM-1). Leukocytes obstruct blood flow and release inflammatory mediators that exacerbate endothelial damage and capillary leakage.

Platelet Dysfunction

Diabetes is associated with increased platelet aggregation and activation, which contributes to capillary thrombosis. Activated platelets promote clot formation and obstruct blood flow, promoting increasing retinal ischemia.

Altered Plasma Fibrinogen Levels

Elevated levels of fibrinogen, a blood clotting protein, are commonly observed in diabetic patients. Increased fibrinogen contributes to higher blood viscosity and enhances the risk of thrombosis in retinal vessels.

RISK FACTORS

The development and progression of DR are influenced by both modifiable and nonmodifiable risk factors. Modifiable risk factors include glycemic status, hypertension, and lifestyle habits. The nonmodifiable factors such as genetics, duration of diabetes, and age are important in identifying high-risk individuals who may benefit from more frequent monitoring and early interventions.

Modifiable Risk Factors

Poor Glycemic Control

Elevated blood sugar levels are the most significant modifiable risk factor contributing to the development and progression of DR. Hemoglobin A1c (HbA1c) levels, which reflect average blood sugar levels over 2–3 months can used to assess glucose control.

Good glycemic control (target HbA1c <7%) reduces the risk and progression of DR.

Hypertension
Hypertension accelerates retinal microvascular damage, exacerbating the progression of DR. An effective blood pressure control can slow the progression of DR, especially in patients with type 2 diabetes.

Dyslipidemia
Elevated cholesterol and triglyceride levels have been associated with more severe forms of DR, including the presence of hard exudates in the retina. Managing dyslipidemia through diet, exercise, or medications like statins can reduce this risk.

Smoking
Smoking increases the risk of DR by contributing to oxidative stress, endothelial dysfunction, and increased vascular damage. Smoking cessation can significantly lower the risk of developing or worsening DR.

Obesity
Truncal/centripetal obesity is associated with poor glycemic control, hypertension, and dyslipidemia—all of which contribute to the development and progression of DR. Weight loss through diet and exercise can reduce these associated risks.

Nonmodifiable Risk Factors

Duration of Diabetes
The longer a person has diabetes, the higher their risk for developing DR.[9]

Age
Older age is associated with a higher risk of DR. This is due to the cumulative effect of long-term diabetes and age-related vascular changes that affect the retinal microvasculature.

Type of Diabetes
Type 1 diabetes patients are at a higher risk for developing severe forms of DR due to the early onset of the disease, often during childhood or adolescence. In children and adolescents with type 1 diabetes, the onset of puberty is associated with an increased risk of developing DR. Hormonal changes during this time may contribute to the progression of microvascular complications. However, patients with type 2 diabetes often have a delayed diagnosis, which means some degree of retinopathy is already present by the time diabetes is recognized.

Genetic Predisposition
A family history of diabetes and retinopathy can influence the likelihood of developing DR, independent of glycemic control.

Ethnicity
African Americans, Hispanics/Latinos, and South Asians have a higher risk of developing DR compared to other populations.

> Clinical nuggets:
> Who are at a risk of developing diabetic retinopathy?
> - Patients with uncontrolled diabetics: HbA1c >6.5%, random blood sugar (RBS) >200 mg/dL, gestational diabetes
> - Patients with obesity
> - Patients with type 1 diabetes mellitus (DM)

CLINICAL DIAGNOSIS OF DIABETIC RETINOPATHY

Diabetic retinopathy is often asymptomatic in its early stages, but as the disease progresses, it leads to various clinical signs and symptoms. It is important to recognize these, as early detection and treatment can prevent significant vision loss. The clinical manifestation of DR can be grouped under two headings, primary vascular changes and secondary retinal changes. The vascular changes are seen as red lesions, these include microaneurysms, vascular looping/beading, IRMA, and new vessels. The retinal changes can be either as red lesions **(Figs. 1A and B)** due to retinal hemorrhages or yellow lesions **(Figs. 2A to C)** due to outpouring and accumulation of lipoproteins (hard exudates) or white due to superficial retinal ischemia and axoplasmic status involving the nerve fiber layer (soft exudates). When the adobe changes are localized to the macular area, it is called "maculopathy" whereas when these changes are localized to outside the macular, we refer to as background retinopathy.

Based on the conglomeration of clinical signs we can classify retinopathy into two main stages: Nonproliferative diabetic retinopathy (NPDR) and PDR **(Fig. 3)**.

CLINICAL STAGES OF DIABETIC RETINOPATHY

Nonproliferative Diabetic Retinopathy

Early Stage (Mild-to-Moderate NPDR) (Figs. 4A and B)

Microaneurysms: The earliest clinical sign of NPDR. These appear as tiny red dots on the retina during fundoscopic examination.

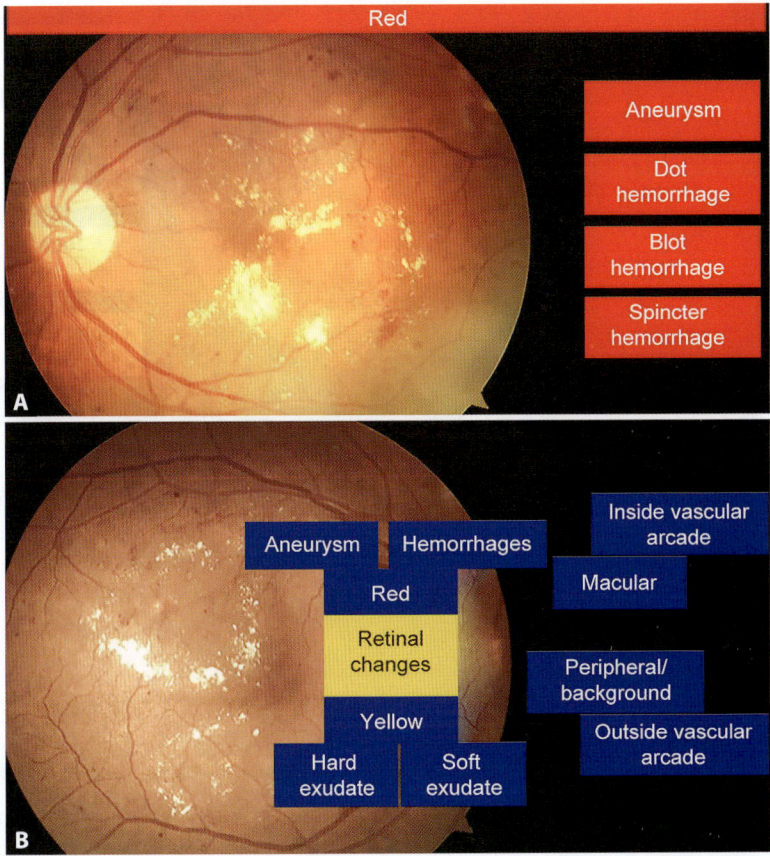

Figs. 1A and B: The fundus photograph shows (A) vascular lesions and (B) retinal lesions.

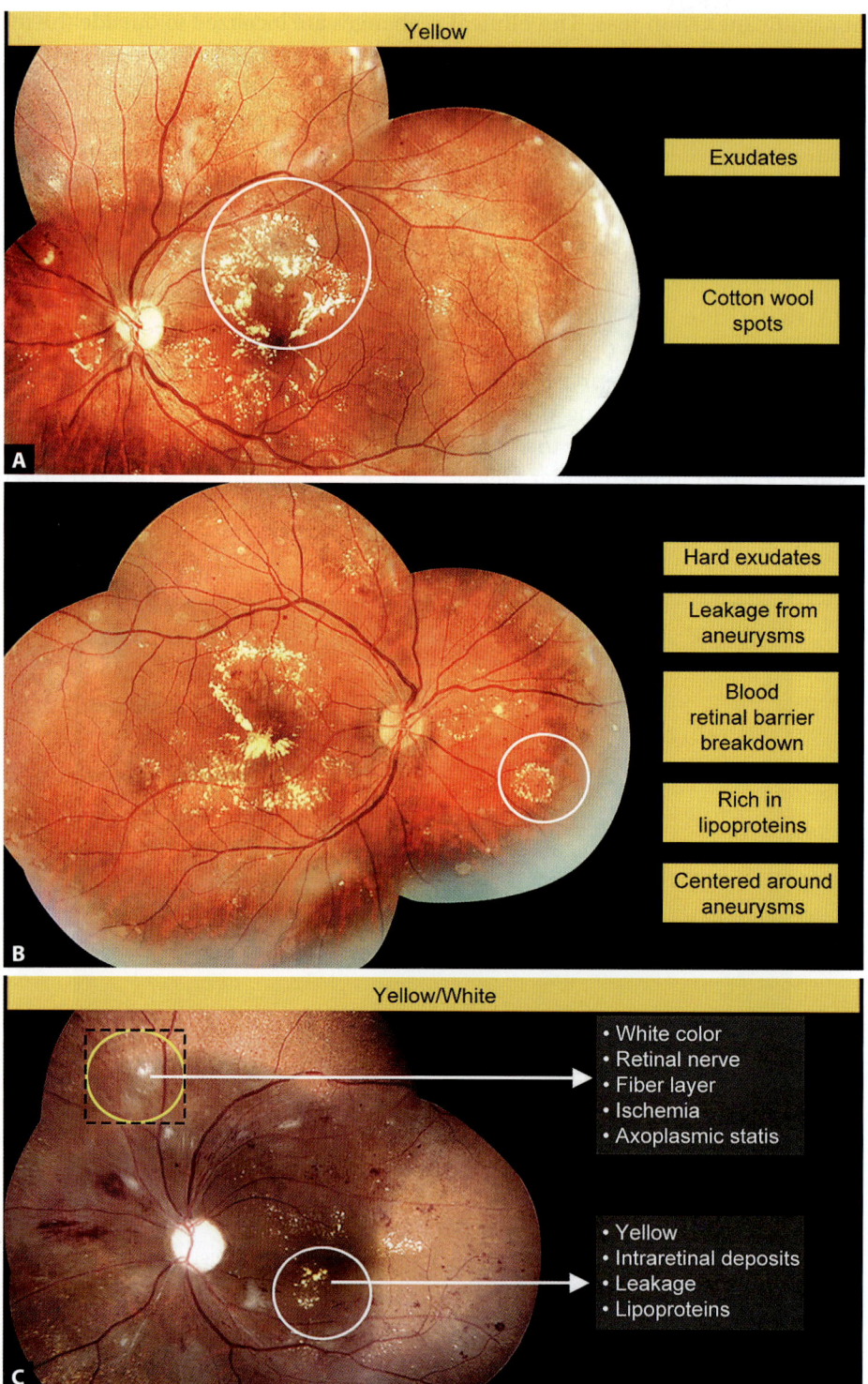

Figs. 2A to C: The fundus photographs showing yellow lesions on retina.

Diabetic Eye Disease

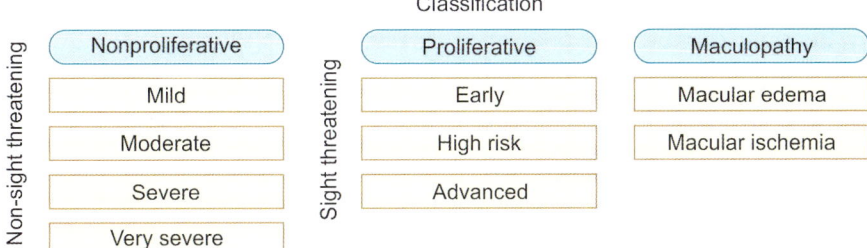

Fig. 3: Clinically diabetic retinopathy can be classified based on sight threatening and non-sight threatening. Observation can be considered for non-sight threatening cases. The sight threatening retinopathy group often warrants intervention inform of laser or anti-VEGF drugs.

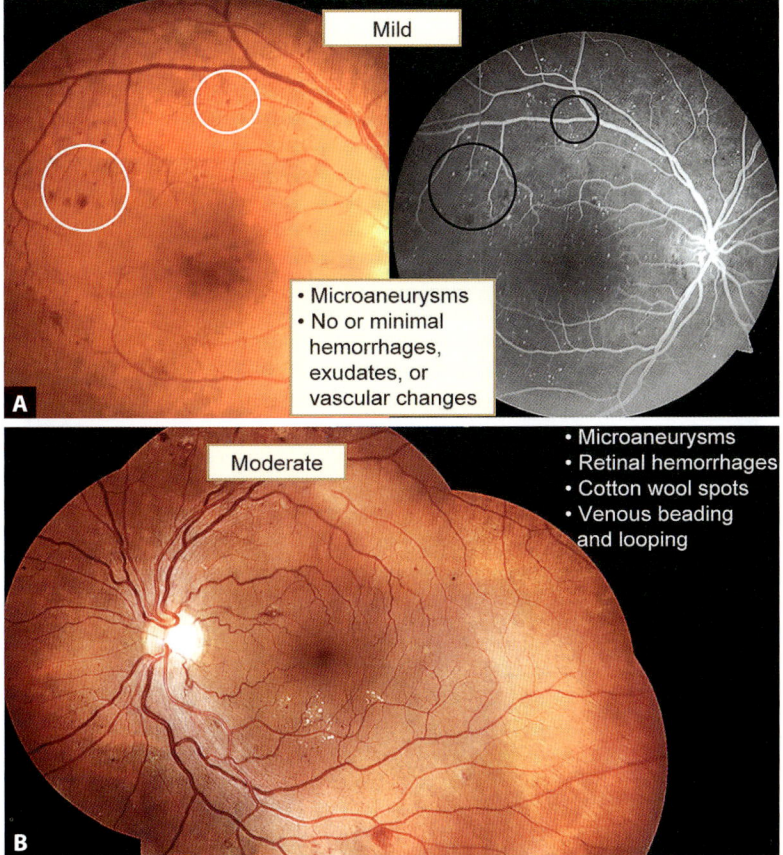

Figs. 4A and B: The fundus photographs showing (A) mild nonproliferative diabetic retinopathy and (B) moderate nonproliferative diabetic retinopathy.

Retinal hemorrhages: As NPDR progresses, small hemorrhages occur in the retina, appearing as red dots or blots.

Hard exudates: They appear as yellow-white spots, often surrounding areas of edema.

Retinal edema: Leakage of fluid from capillaries can cause swelling of the retina, particularly in the macular region. This leads to macular edema, which can affect central vision.

Venous beading and dilatation: The retinal veins may become dilated and take on a beaded appearance, indicating increased retinal ischemia and vascular damage.

Late Stage (Severe NPDR) (Figs. 5A and B)

Cotton wool spots are fluffy white patches on the retina that result from nerve fiber layer infarctions caused by retinal ischemia.

Intraretinal microvascular abnormalities: IRMAs are hallmarks of severe NPDR. These are abnormal, dilated retinal capillaries that form as a result of chronic retinal ischemia. IRMAs can be differentiated from neovascularization elsewhere (NVE) clinically. The IRMAs do not cross the major vessels while NVE can be seen anywhere on the retina. The fundus fluorescein angiography (FFA) helps in further differentiation of both as IRMAs do not leak in late phases as against NVEs that show intense leakage on the late phase of FFA.

Proliferative Diabetic Retinopathy

Clinical Signs

Neovascularization: The hallmark of PDR is the development of new, fragile blood vessels that grow on the surface of the retina or the optic disc. These vessels are prone to rupture, leading to bleeding into the retina and the vitreous.

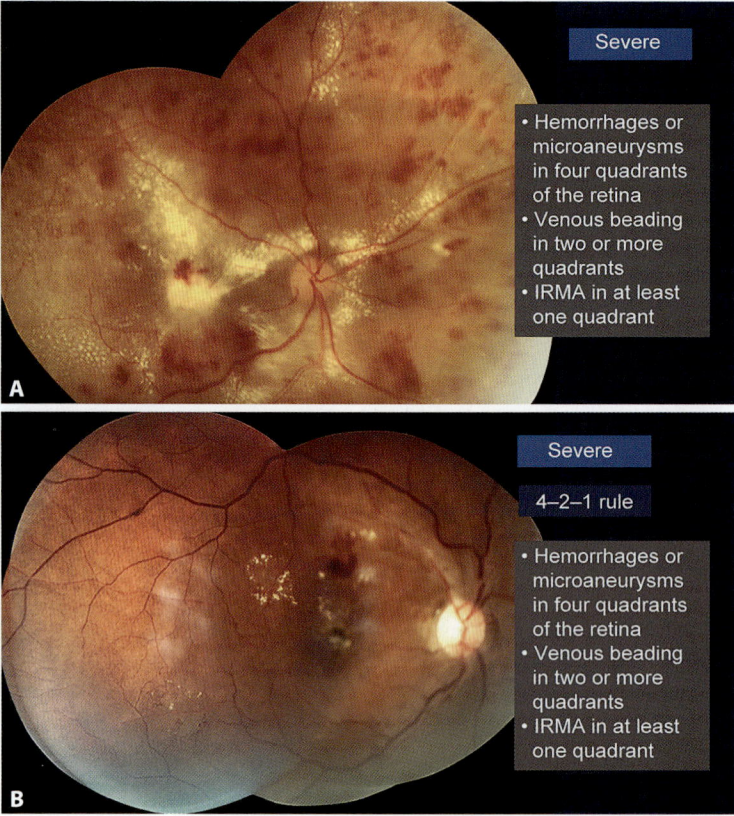

Figs. 5A and B: Two forms of severe NPDR. (A) Retinal hemorrhages in all four quadrants. (B) A case of severe NPDR, that shows the presence of IRMA along the inferotemporal vascular arcade, IRMAS are not picked up, the presence of few exudates and hemorrhages over the macula can create a false impression of moderate NPDR.

When the neovascularization is present on/within 1-disc diameter (1DD) of the disc, it is called as neovascularization of disc (NVD) and if the neovascularization is 1DD away from disc, it is addressed as NVE **(Figs. 6A to G)**.

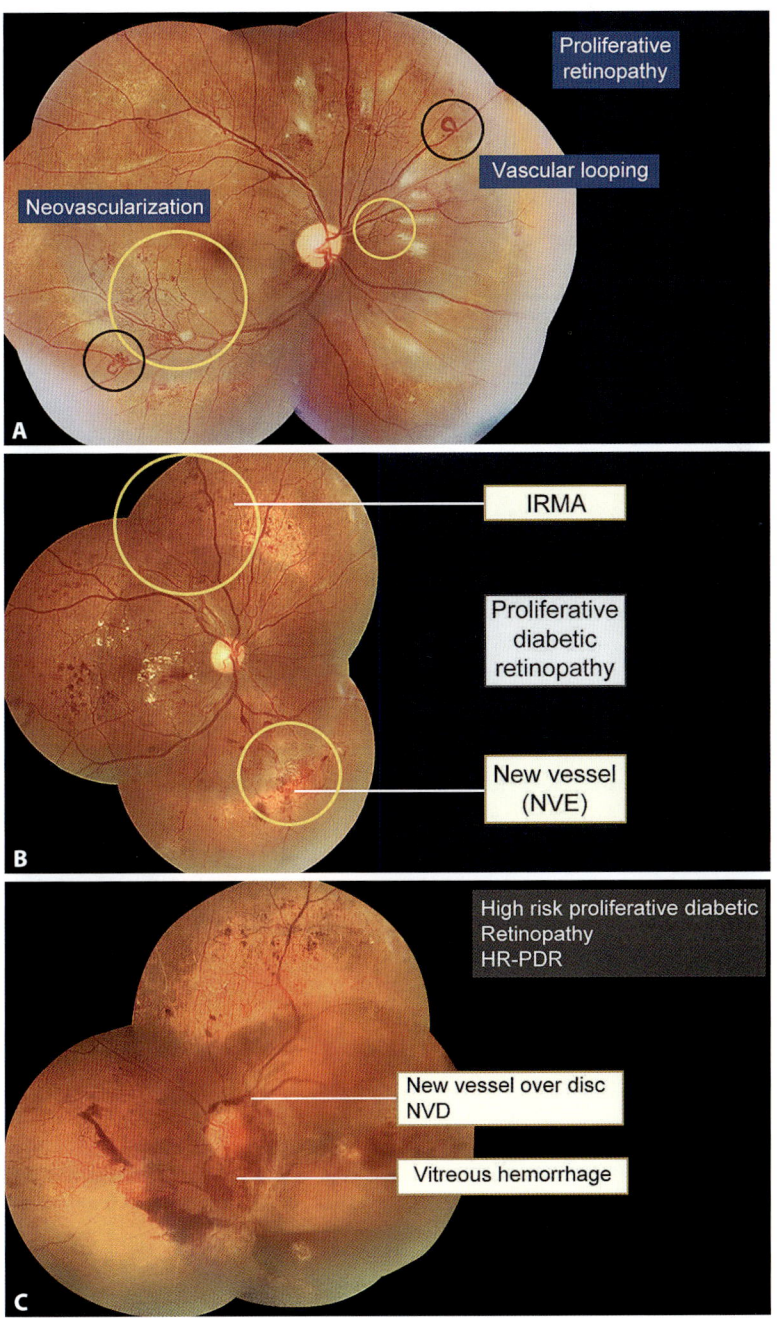

Figs. 6A to C

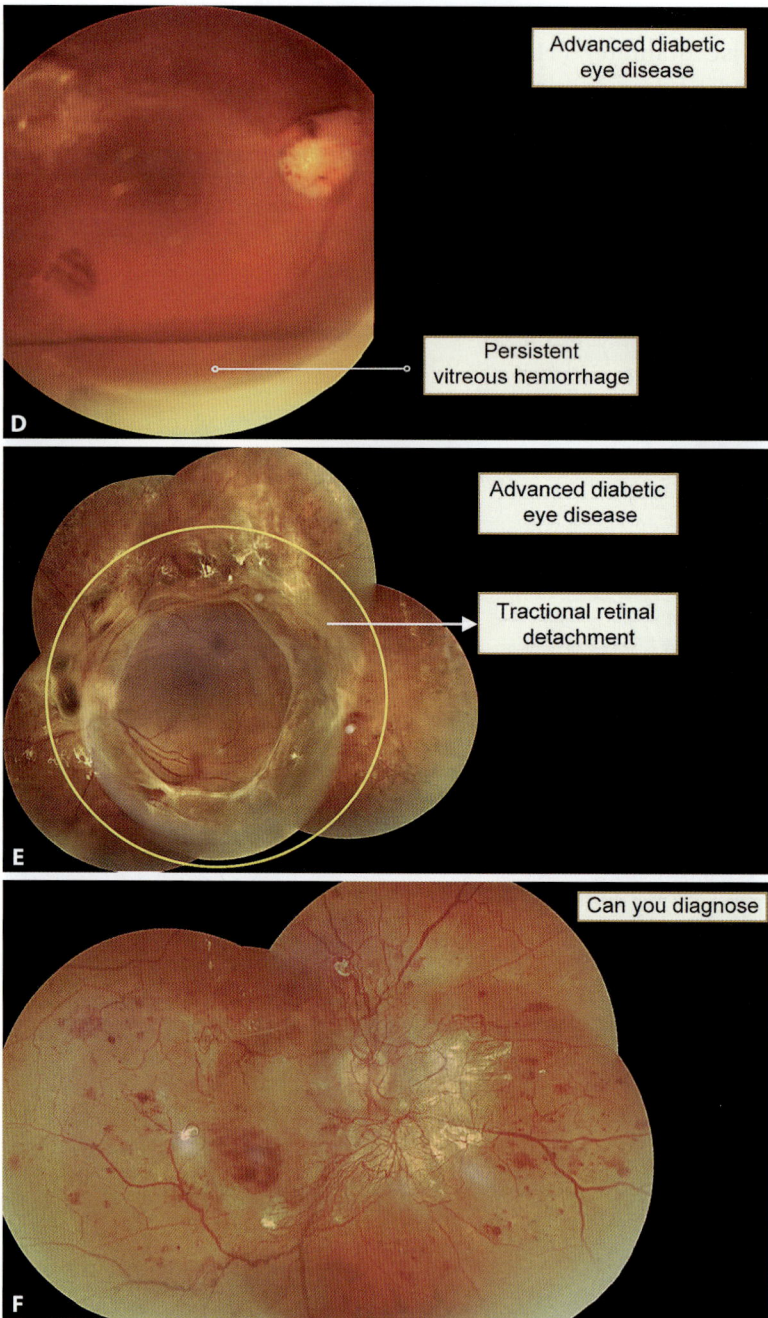

Figs. 6D to F

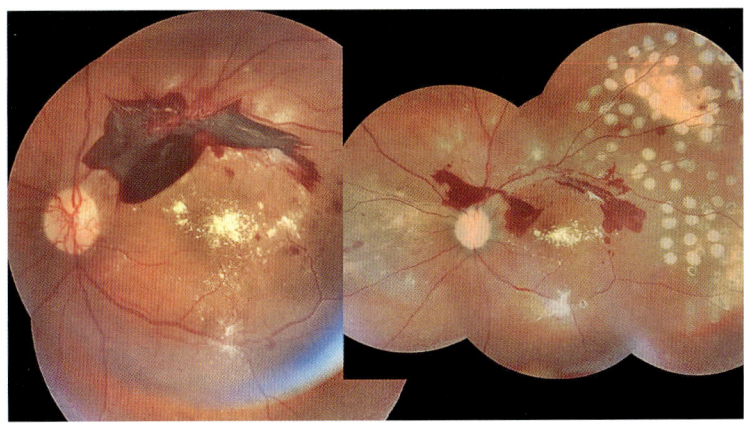

Fig. 6G

Figs. 6A to G: (A and B) A case of early PDR, with early neovascularization along the inferior temporal vascular arcade (A) and the inferonasal vascular arcade (B). (C) A case of high-risk PDR (HRPDR) with neovascularization of the disc (NVD) >1/3 disc area and associated preretinal hemorrhage; (D) A case of HRPDR, which has evolved into advanced diabetic eye disease (ADED) with multiple episodes of vitreous hemorrhage/persistent vitreous hemorrhage. (E) A case of tractional detachment threatening he macula with annular fibrovascular proliferation. (F) A case of high-risk PDR as there is prominent NVD >1/3 of disc area.

Vitreous hemorrhage: Neovascularization has fragile vessels which can rupture and cause vitreous hemorrhage resulting in sudden and significant loss of vision or floaters. This often occurs in advanced PDR, more commonly seen in patients with poor glycemic control.

Fibrovascular proliferation: As the new blood vessels grow, they may be accompanied by fibrous tissue formation, which can cause retinal traction and increase the risk of retinal detachment.

Tractional retinal detachment: Fibrous tissue from neovascularization can pull on the retina, leading to tractional retinal detachment, causing severe and permanent vision loss and may require surgical intervention.

Neovascular glaucoma (NVG): These abnormal blood vessels grow in the anterior chamber angle of the eye, blocking the drainage of aqueous fluid and leading to increased intraocular pressure and NVG. This can cause permanent vision loss. NVG is the secondary presentation of the long-standing ischemic condition of retina due to chronic DR changes leading to production of VEGF and causing neovascularization of the iris (NVI) formation that ultimately leads to development of NVG.

SYMPTOMS OF DIABETIC RETINOPATHY

While many patients may not experience symptoms in the early stages of DR, the following symptoms may develop as the condition progresses.

Blurred Vision

This is one of the earliest symptoms and may be due to macular edema or hemorrhages affecting the central vision. Near vision is affected more. The patient may experience metamorphopsia. This is often due to macular edema or retinal distortion from neovascularization and fibrosis.

Floaters

Patients may experience floaters in their vision, which is caused by blood floating in the vitreous, often from bleeding neovascular vessels in PDR.

Sudden Painless Vision Loss

Sudden and dramatic vision loss may occur due to vitreous hemorrhage or macula involving tractional/combined retinal detachment.

Night Vision Problems

Night vision difficulties may occur as a result of generalized retinal damage, particularly in areas affected by ischemia. Heavy panretinal photocoagulation can also lead to peripheral visual field loss and affect accommodation causing night vision problems.

Reduced Color Vision

Mainly due to photoreceptor damages secondary to macular ischemia or long-standing DME.

ETDRS CLASSIFICATION OF DIABETIC RETINOPATHY

The Early Treatment Diabetic Retinopathy Study (ETDRS) classification is one of the most widely used systems for grading the severity of DR. It provides a detailed framework to classify the stages of DR and guide treatment based on fundus examination. This system categorizes DR into NPDR and PDR, and it emphasizes the importance of macular edema as a key risk for vision loss.

The ETDRS classification is based on the severity of specific retinal findings, such as microaneurysms, hemorrhages, exudates, venous abnormalities, and neovascularization **(Table 1)**.

The ETDRS classification also emphasizes DME, which can occur at any stage of DR

TABLE 1: A simplified version of ETDRS classification is mentioned.

Stages of DR	Clinical signs
Mild NPDR	• Microaneurysms • No or minimal hemorrhages, exudates, or vascular changes
Moderate NPDR	• Microaneurysms • Retinal hemorrhages • Cotton wool spots • Venous beading and looping
Severe NPDR "4-2-1 rule"	• Hemorrhages or microaneurysms in four quadrants of the retina • Venous beading in two or more quadrants • IRMA in at least one quadrant
Very severe NPDR	• Two or more of the "4-2-1" criteria are indicative of NPDR
Early PDR	• Presence of neovascularization that is not causing significant complications yet. • NVD measuring 1/4 to 1/3 of the disc area or NVE
High risk character (HRC)—PDR	NVD measuring > 1/4 to 1/3 of the disc area or NVE associated with vitreous hemorrhage or preretinal hemorrhage
Advanced PDR	• Extensive vitreous hemorrhage • Fibrovascular proliferation causing TRD • Neovascular glaucoma (NVG)

(DR: diabetic retinopathy; ETDRS: Early Treatment Diabetic Retinopathy Study; IRMA: intraretinal microvascular abnormality; NPDR: nonproliferative diabetic retinopathy; NVD: neovascularization of disc; NVE: neovascularization elsewhere; PDR: proliferative diabetic retinopathy; TRD: tractional retinal detachment) and is a major cause of vision loss in diabetic patients. DME is defined by retinal thickening or hard exudates in the macular area. It is classified as:

Clinically Significant Macular Edema

Definition: Retinal thickening or hard exudates found within 500 µm (on-third of disc diameter) from the center of the macula, or thickening spanning over an area larger than a disc size within a disc diameter from the macula.

Clinically significant macular edema (CSME) has a high risk of central vision loss if untreated.

Clinical Work-up and Imaging Tools

Fundus photo: Color fundus photos help in documentation and follow ups of patients with DR. It is a helpful tool in grading DR and explaining the patient's disease progression.

Fundus Fluorescein Angiography

- It is an invasive tool that helps in the diagnosis of PDR due to the presence of intense leakage from the neovascularization at the disc (NVD) or elsewhere (NVE) in the late phases. NPDR can show localized leakages from MAs in the late phases.
- It is useful for the diagnosis of macular ischemia in cases of unexplained vision loss without clinical findings.

Diabetic maculopathy on FFA is classified as below:
- *Focal maculopathy*: Localized areas of leakage from microaneurysms and retinal capillaries, leading to hard exudates and retinal thickening.
- *Diffuse maculopathy:* Widespread capillary leakage causing diffuse retinal thickening, often affecting the entire macular region.
- *Ischemic maculopathy:* Caused by capillary occlusion in the macula, reducing blood supply and resulting in permanent vision loss.
- Assists in detecting areas of capillary nonperfusion (CNP) in cases of persistent or nonresolving DME.
- FFA also helps in planning targeted laser photocoagulation to leaky microaneurysms and areas of CNPs.

Optical coherence tomography (OCT): This noninvasive imaging technique provides cross-sectional images of the retina, showing areas of retinal thickening or edema, which may not be visible on a fundoscopic examination (**Box 1**).

Regular OCT imaging is essential for the timely detection and management of DME, ultimately helping to preserve vision in patients with diabetes.

Optical coherence tomography is a helpful tool in monitoring the treatment responses to intravitreal injections during follow-ups.

Optical coherence tomography angiography (OCTA): It is a helpful noninvasive diagnostic tool in DR. As most of the patients with DM have associated diabetic nephropathy, OCTA comes in handy for such cases where deranged renal function tests do not permit FFA.

- *To look for macular ischemia*: Distorted foveal avascular zone (FAZ) in superficial

---

BOX 1: Classification of diabetic macular edema (DME) based on optical coherence tomography (OCT).

OCT features:
- Diffuse retinal thickening
- Cystoid macular edema
- Posterior hyaloid traction
- Subretinal fluid/serous retinal detachment
- Tractional retinal detachment

capillary plexus (SCP), deep capillary plexus (DCP) slabs with associated reduced vessel density.
- *Helps to diagnose NVD/NVE*: By looking at vascular networks and flow signals in vitreoretinal interface (VRI) slab.
- Helps in grading macular edema and monitoring its response to treatment.
- PLEX Elite OCTA can help in capturing peripheral capillary nonperfusion areas as well.

Blood investigations in cases diagnosed with diabetic retinopathy: The most commonly advised blood work-up in patients with DR to look for a baseline control are as follows—
- *Complete blood count (CBC):* To look for Hb in particular as anemia is associated with DR progression.[10]
- Fasting and postprandial blood sugar
- *HbA1c:* A key indicator of control of disease. HbA1c levels exceeding 6.5% are associated with the progression of DR.
- *Renal function test (RFT):* To look for renal function
- *Lipid profile:* Treating hypercholesterolemia has been shown to reduce the need for intravitreal injections, especially in patients with hard exudates.[11]

Along with blood investigations, checking urine microalbumin helps in detecting albuminuria which has a significant relation to progressive of stages of DR in diabetics.

MANAGEMENT OF DIABETIC RETINOPATHY

To understand the treatment for DR, it is imperative to understand the clinical spectrum of the disease. DR represents a form of retinal microvascular injury following prolonged periods of hyperglycemia. At one end of the disease spectrum, the vascular insult and endothelial damage can lead to vascular leakage, exudation of intravascular fluids, development of macular edema, and exudation at the macula, a disease continuum similar to what we see in vascular inflammation. When these changes are predominantly in the macular area, it is labeled as diabetic maculopathy or DME, i.e., retinal thickening/exudates within one disk diameter of the center of the macula.

On the other end of the spectrum, diabetic angiopathy can lead to the closure of capillaries with a subsequent decrease in retinal perfusion. This can lead to retinal ischemia and release of VEGF with subsequent neovascularization of the optic disc and/or the retina. The rupture of the aberrant newly formed vessels can lead to the development of retinal hemorrhage with/without vitreous hemorrhage. This form of disease is labeled as PDR. Both DME as well as PDR can occur independently or in combination.

The treatment for DR needs to be approached on three levels of prevention: (1) Primary (prevent retinopathy from developing), (2) secondary (detect retinopathy early), and (3) tertiary (timely management of DME and PDR). We cannot prevent diabetes, but we can prevent retinopathy from developing if we are able to maintain good glycemic levels in the initial years of the disease.

The Diabetes Control and Complications Trial (DCCT) has shown that intensive glycemic control in the initial years after being diagnosed with diabetes is protective for the development of DR as compared to reestablishment of good glycemic control after a profound period of poor control, which does not immediately benefit the progression of retinopathy. It is because of this, that continued worsening/paradoxical worsening of DR may be observed, despite stabilized blood glycemia. This has been linked to the effect of metabolic memory.

Intensive treatment in the initial decade of being diagnosed with diabetes has shown to have a protective effect on the development of retinopathy. It is because of metabolic memory that the present HbA1c value is not the most important; rather, the HbA1c value 2–3 years has the highest impact.

In its early stages, DR is typically asymptomatic, and patients may not observe any changes in their vision. As a result, they might not seek treatment promptly. Secondary prevention is centered around screening strategies to detect early, treat early and prevent progression to a stage of VTDR. Individuals with type 1 diabetes should start annual screenings for DR 5 years after diagnosis. Those with type 2 diabetes need an immediate screening upon diagnosis, followed by yearly screenings.

The spectrum of VTDR include DME, severe preproliferative, and PDR. VTDR can initially be asymptomatic, with no impact on vision. Early screening is essential to detect VTDR promptly and deliver treatments to preserve or restore eyesight.

Metabolic control is the first line of management for both prevention and stopping the progression of retinopathy. The term metabolic control should not be limited to achieving only glycemia control but should be extended to encompass regulation of dyslipidemia, correction of anemia, and normalization of blood pressure. Ophthalmologists often underemphasize the importance of improving glycemic control, blood pressure, and lipid levels since systemic management is primarily overseen by internal medicine specialists.

Collectively, these measures help in achieving a rheological homeostasis, pertinent for stabilization of retinopathy.

Because high blood glucose level is the most modifiable risk factor, maintaining HbA1c levels between 6 and 7% is imperative. Caution and care must be exercised when choosing the oral hypoglycemics for achieving glycemic control. In particular, there is evidence suggesting that certain groups of newer generation oral hypoglycemic agents possibly worsen DME. These include peroxisome proliferator-activated receptor-γ (PPAR-γ) agonists and semaglutide [glucagon-like peptide-1 (GLP-1) receptor agonist] shows to worsen retinopathy and macular edema. Additionally, sodium-glucose cotransporter-2 (SGLT-2) inhibitors have been associated with a higher incidence of retinal vein occlusion, particularly in older patients and those with advanced kidney disease.

Tertiary prevention is aimed at cure and palliation, salvaging residual function, and preventing complications of the disease. A point of confusion can often arise for young doctors, as to whom to treat and when to treat. Not all cases of DR require treatment, only eyes presenting with sight threatening retinopathy require an active intervention.

The term of sight threatening retinopathy is reserved for cases with macular edema or with presence of neovascularization. These patients usually present with gradually progressive decrease in vision due to macular edema or may complain of acute onset, painless, diminishing vision with floaters due to development of vitreous hemorrhage in cases with proliferative retinopathy. Clinical examination augmented with OCT examination can help in establishing diagnosis of macular edema. FFA/B-scan can help in diagnosis of PDR associated with/without vitreous hemorrhage.

Strategies to Treat Diabetic Retinopathy

In clinical practice, a DR patient can present to you under five possible scenarios:

1. Asymptomatic with no maculopathy and no PDR
2. Asymptomatic with PDR and no maculopathy
3. Symptomatic with maculopathy but no PDR
4. Symptomatic with no maculopathy and only PDR
5. Symptomatic with maculopathy as well as PDR

For all asymptomatic cases with no evidence of PDR on clinical examination, metabolic control remains pivotal. Active intervention is required usually for symptomatic cases with macular edema and patients detected with PDR **(Table 2)**.

While patients with macular edema require intravitreal steroids/anti-VEGF with or without focal laser/grid laser for resolution of edema, those with PDR require green laser panretinal photocoagulation of the ischemic retina.

In DME, the macula becomes thickened due to an accumulation of extracellular fluid caused by hyperpermeable retinal capillaries. Patients with DME exhibit elevated vitreous concentrations of VEGF, ICAM-1, interleukin-6 (IL-6), monocyte chemoattractant protein-1, and other inflammatory cytokines. Anti-VEGF agents function by inhibiting VEGF's ability to increase vascular permeability. Corticosteroids, on the other hand, suppress *VEGF* gene expression, modulate the expression of various VEGF receptors, and exert additional non-VEGF-related effects. These include reducing leukocyte recruitment, lowering ICAM-1 production, and inhibiting collagenase activation, thereby decreasing the permeability of retinal microvasculature.

- *Laser therapy for diabetic retinopathy/ maculopathy* **(Table 3)**
  - Focal
  - Panretinal photocoagulation
- Intravitreal injections for DR (anti-VEGF/ steroid) **(Table 4)**
  - Anti-VEGF (drug/brand name/ dosage)
  - Steroids (Ozurdex/IVTA)

Intravitreal Injections (Table 5)

Anti-vascular endothelial growth factor:
- *Mechanism of action*: The VEGFs secreted by the retinal pigment epithelium (RPE) cells, endothelial cell, and muller cells in response to retinal ischemia. These growth factors are responsible for the sequelae of retinal and preretinal

TABLE 2: Screening and follow-up guidelines for people with and without diabetic retinopathy.	
Stage of DR	**Follow-up**
No diabetic retinopathy (DR)	Every 12 years
Mild nonproliferative diabetic retinopathy (NPDR)	Every year
Moderate NPDR	Every 6 months
Severe NPDR	Every 3 months
Proliferative DR	Every 3 months
No diabetic macular edema (DME)	Every year
Non-center-involving diabetic macular edema (non-Ci-DME)	Every 3 months
Center-involved DME (Ci-DME)	Every 1–2 months + intravitreal anti-vascular endothelial growth factor (anti-VEGF) injections

TABLE 3: Indications and types of laser treatment for DR.

	Focal laser	Panretinal photocoagulation
Area treated	Macula: • Leaking microaneurysms • Retinal thickening • Avascular areas	Peripheral retina Usually done in 2–3 sittings
Indications	Diabetic macular edema	Retinal neovascularization due to proliferative diabetic retinopathy

TABLE 4: Various types of intravitreal anti-VEGF agents with its dosage.

Molecule	Brand name	Dosage
Bevacizumab	Avastin	1.25 mg/0.05 mL
Ranibizumab	Lucentis/Accentrix	0.5 mg/0.05 mL
Aflibercept	Eylea	2 mg/0.05 mL
Brolucizumab	Pagenax	6 mg/0.05 mL
Faricimab	Vabysmo	6 mg/0.05 mL

TABLE 5: Various types of intravitreal steroid injections.

Molecule	Brand name	Dosage
Dexamethasone	Ozurdex implant	0.7 mg
Triamcinolone acetonide	Aurocort/Kenalog	40 mg/mL

neovascularization and vascular leakage due to alternation in blood retinal barrier. The use of humanized monoclonal antibodies directed against VEGF (anti-VEGF) molecule can block the effects of VEGF. These antibodies can block the angiogenic and proinflammatory effects and are helpful in resolution of macular edema and regression of new formed vessels.[12]

- *Dosage:* Anti-VEGF injections are administered as monthly loading doses initially (for the first 3 months) followed by the treatment and extended regimen or pro re nata (PRN).
- *Side effects:* The injection-related complications include endophthalmitis, retinal detachment, and vitreous hemorrhage.
- *Contraindications:* A recent history of a stroke or cardiovascular event (<6 months)

Intravitreal steroids
Mechanism of action: Steroids act on multiple vascular and inflammatory pathways responsible for DME.[13,14]
- Inhibit VEGF
- Decrease cytokines and growth factors
- Decrease leukotriene synthesis
- Decrease prostaglandin synthesis

The corticosteroids stabilize the blood-retinal barrier and regulate the endothelial tight junctions decreasing the DME.
- *Ozurdex:* It is a biodegradable sustained release dexamethasone implant which is injected into the eye.
- *Triamcinolone acetonide:* They are crystalline deposits which slowly dissolve in the vitreous cavity over a period of time.

Side effects: The most common side effects of steroid injections are cataract formation and glaucoma. The injection-related complications include endophthalmitis, retinal detachment, and vitreous hemorrhage.

Surgery for diabetic retinopathy
- Indications:
  - Nonresolving vitreous hemorrhage
  - Tractional retinal detachment
  - Tractional macular edema
- *Surgical steps*: Steps of vitreoretinal surgery for diabetic eye disease:
  - *Preoperative*:
    - Good metabolic control is a very important prerequisite before surgery. The stoppage of blood thinners a few days prior to a diabetic vitrectomy remains contentious as some surgeons prefer stopping it while the others do not.[15]
    - The presence of a cataract in phakic patients hinders viewing during surgery. Hence, a cataract surgery with intraocular lens implantation can be combined with vitreoretinal surgery. A few surgeons advocate performing the cataract surgery 3–5 days before the vitreoretinal surgery to prevent corneal edema during the intraoperative period.[16]
    - An anti-VEGF injection 3–5 days before a vitrectomy has been demonstrated to reduce the intraoperative bleeding and use of endodiathermy.
  - *Intraoperative steps*:
    - *Ports:* A 3 port pars plana vitrectomy (PPV) is performed using 23/25/27-gauge instruments. A chandelier illumination system can be used to aid in bimanual dissection in eyes with advanced diabetic diseases with extensive proliferation.
    - *Core vitrectomy:* The central vitreous core is vitrectomized to clear the media in cases of vitreous hemorrhage and to gain access to the retinal surface for membrane dissection.
    - *Membrane dissection*: Fibrovascular proliferations/tractional detachments are dissected to relieve the traction using the vitrectomy cutter/vitrectomy scissors/forceps. Dissection of these membranes can lead to bleeding due to their vascular component. An endodiathermy is used to cauterize these bleeders. It is important to relieve all the tractions to ensure retinal reattachment in cases of tractional retinal detachment.

    Membrane dissection can be achieved by two main techniques:
    1. *Segmentation:* The large proliferations are segmented into smaller islands by dissecting between the segments.
    2. *Delamination:* The fibrovascular stalks connecting the membrane to the retinal surface are dissected.
    - *Endolaser:* A 360° panretinal photocoagulation is performed using endolaser to decrease the ischemic load on the retina. Retinal breaks (if any) should be also treated intraoperatively using endolaser.
    - *Tamponade:* Postsurgery, the infusion fluid-filled vitreous cavity can be left as it is if there are no active bleeders/retinal breaks. However, in most cases, an

endotamponade agent is used. The various types of tamponade agents used are as follows:
- *Air:* Air acts as a temporary tamponading agent whose effect lasts for 3–5 days till its absorption.
- *Gas:* Sulphur hexafluoride (SF6) and perfluoropropane (C3F8) are the gasses commonly used as tamponading agents. Their effect lasts for 2–3 weeks (SF6) and 6–8 weeks (C3F8).
- *Silicon oil:* Silicon oil (polydimethylsiloxane) acts as a long-acting tamponade and remains inside the vitreous cavity till removed.

REFERENCES

1. Caldwell RB, Bartoli M, Behzadian MA, El-Remessy AE, Al-Shabrawey M, Platt DH, et al. Vascular endothelial growth factor and diabetic retinopathy: role of oxidative stress. Curr Drug Targets. 2005;6(4):511-24.
2. Zatz R, Brenner BM. Pathogenesis of diabetic microangiopathy. The hemodynamic view. Am J Med. 1986;80:443-53.
3. Yamagishi S, Nakamura K, Imaizumi T. Advanced glycation end products (AGEs) and diabetic vascular complications. Curr Diabetes Rev. 2005;1(1):93-106.
4. Ciulla TA, Amador AG, Zinman B. Diabetic Retinopathy and Diabetic Macular Edema. Diabetes Care. 2003;26:2653-64.
5. Koya D, King GL. Protein Kinase C Activation and the Development of Diabetic Complications. Diabetes. 1998;47:859-66.
6. Antonetti DA, Klein R, Gardner TW. Diabetic retinopathy. N Engl J Med. 2012;366(13):1227-39.
7. Medscape. (2006). Diabetic Retinopathy. [online] Available from https://emedicine.medscape.com/article/1225122-overview?form=fpf [Last accessed March, 2025].
8. Suganami E, Ohasi H. Leptin stimulates ischemia-induced retinal neovascularization. Diabetes. 2004;53(9):2443-8.
9. Klein R, Klein BE, Moss SE, Cruickshanks KJ. The Wisconsin Epidemiologic Study of diabetic retinopathy. XIV. Ten-year incidence and progression of diabetic retinopathy. Arch Ophthalmol. 1994;112(9):1217-28.
10. Li Y, Yu Y, VanderBeek BL. Anaemia and the risk of progression from non-proliferative diabetic retinopathy to vision threatening diabetic retinopathy. Eye (Lond). 2020;34(5):934-41.
11. Pranata R, Vania R, Victor AA. Statin reduces the incidence of diabetic retinopathy and its need for intervention: A systematic review and meta-analysis. Eur J Ophthalmol. 2021;31(3):1216-24.
12. Stitt AW, Curtis TM, Chen M, Medina RJ, McKay GJ, Jenkins A, et al. The progress in understanding and treatment of diabetic retinopathy. Prog Retin Eye Res. 2016;51:156-86.
13. Wilson CA, Berkowitz BA, Sato Y, Ando N, Handa JT, de Juan E Jr. Treatment with intravitreal steroid reduces blood-retinal barrier breakdown due to retinal photocoagulation. Arch Ophthalmol. 1992;110:1155-9.
14. Hood PP, Cotter TP, Costello JF, Sampson AP. Effect of intravenous corticosteroid on ex vivo leukotriene generation by blood leukocytes of normal and asthmatic patients Thorax. 1999;54:1075-82.
15. Brown JS, Mahmoud TH. Anticoagulation and clinically significant postoperative vitreous hemorrhage in diabetic vitrectomy. Retina. 2011;31(10):1983-7.
16. Lahey JM, Francis RR, Kearney JJ. Combining phacoemulsification with pars plana vitrectomy in patients with proliferative diabetic retinopathy: a series of 223 cases. Ophthalmology. 2003;110(7):1335-9.

CHAPTER 26

Current Approaches in the Diagnosis and Management of Sub-internal Limiting Membrane Hemorrhage

Dhaivat Shah

INTRODUCTION

Sub-internal limiting membrane (sub-ILM) hemorrhage is a relatively rare condition, commonly caused by Valsalva retinopathy, blood dyscrasias, Terson syndrome, retinal macroaneurysm rupture, shaken baby syndrome, or ocular trauma, which can result in significant visual impairment.[1] The management of this condition should ideally be personalized, considering the location, duration, and any accompanying damage caused by the bleeding. While various treatment approaches have been documented, no established guidelines exist in the current literature.[2] In this article, we will explore the diagnostic criteria and management principles for sub-ILM hemorrhages in modern-day clinical practice.

ETIOPATHOGENESIS

The ILM is a rigid, nonelastic layer on the inner retinal surface, formed by astrocytes and Müller cell end feet.[3] It is tightly adherent to the underlying retinal nerve fiber layer (RNFL), making separation difficult. Sub-ILM hemorrhages commonly occur at the macula due to weaker ILM attachments in this area. These hemorrhages are associated with sudden pressure fluctuations, most commonly seen in Valsalva retinopathy caused by actions such as vomiting, coughing, or straining.

DIAGNOSTIC CRITERIA

Diagnosing sub-ILM hemorrhage **(Fig. 1)** can be challenging during clinical fundus examination, as it can be difficult to distinguish from preretinal or subretinal hemorrhages. However, several clues may assist in the diagnosis:

- *Clinical observation:* Sub-ILM hemorrhage usually exhibits a glistening white reflex from the overlying ILM, a yellow line at its margin, and relative immobility.
- *Color fundus photography:* A thick yellow line outlines the hemorrhage, corresponding to a greenish line in multicolor imaging (e.g., Spectralis and Heidelberg Engineering), indicating elevation.
- *Optical coherence tomography (OCT):* OCT scans reveal a dome-shaped elevation with sharply defined edges and varying reflectivity—either hyperreflective or hyporeflective—depending on the coagulation state of the red blood cells (RBCs) within the hemorrhage **(Fig. 2)**.[4] It is crucial to perform the OCT line scan

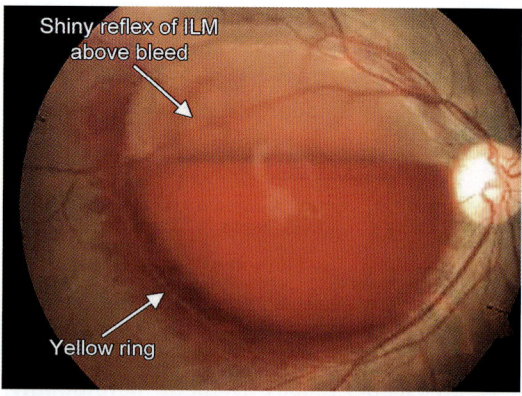

Fig. 1: Fundus image illustrating a sub-internal limiting membrane (sub-ILM) hemorrhage, characterized by a glistening white reflex from the overlying ILM and a yellow ring at the margins.

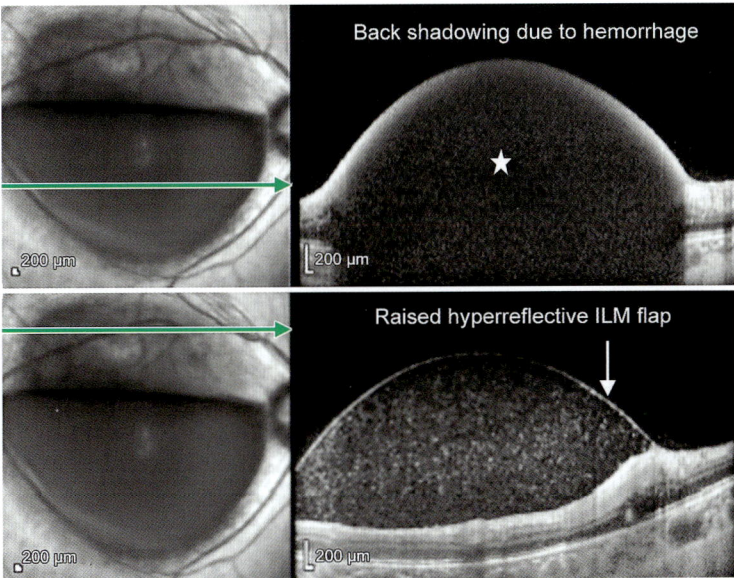

Fig. 2: OCT scans depict a dome-shaped elevation with sharply defined edges. The reflectivity varies, showing alternating hyporeflective and hyperreflective areas. (ILM: internal limiting membrane; OCT: optical coherence tomography)

through both the blood-accumulated area (hyperreflective) and the adjacent area devoid of blood (hyporeflective). In regions with hyperreflectivity, distinguishing between sub-ILM and subhyaloid hemorrhage can be challenging. However, in the hyporeflective zone which is usually superior owing to gravity, a thick hyperreflective line is typically observed, indicating the presence of a raised ILM flap.

A characteristic OCT feature of a sub-ILM bleed in a few cases is the presence of large hyperreflective foci at the outer nuclear layer (ONL), extending into the inner retinal layers **(Fig. 3)**. These are hypothesized to be distended Müller cells caused by tension on the ILM after a bleeding event.[5] Müller cells, which span the retina and support neuronal function, may swell due to hypoxia or ischemia. This is linked to disrupted potassium channels

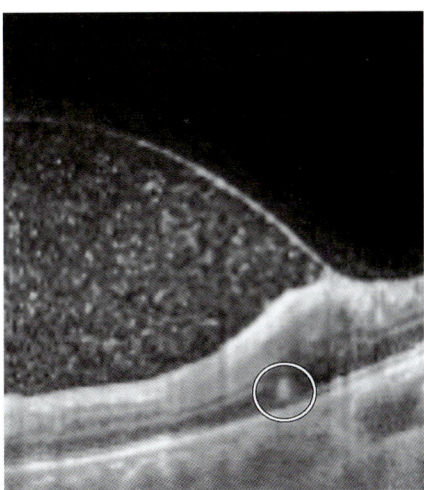

Fig. 3: Optical coherence tomography (OCT) scan showcasing the FAT MÜLLER SIGN—large hyperreflective foci at the outer nuclear layer (ONL), extending into the inner retinal layers within a sub-ILM bleed.

and abnormal water influx, causing cellular edema, leading to dilated Müller cells, which we term as "FAT MÜLLER

TABLE 1: Comparison between preretinal (subhyaloid) hemorrhages and sub-ILM hemorrhages.

Feature	Subhyaloid hemorrhage	Sub-ILM hemorrhage
Mobility	More mobile	Less mobile
Settling behavior	Settles over time with head position	Does not settle as readily
OCT imaging	Shows two distinct membranes: 1. Hyperreflective band above the hemorrhage—ILM 2. Patchy membrane with low reflectivity (posterior hyaloid)	Shows dome shape elevation with sharp edges: • Hyper- or hyporeflective areas based on RBC coagulation • Thick hyperreflective line in areas devoid of blood indicating raised ILM flap

(ILM: internal limiting membrane; OCT: optical coherence tomography)

SIGN." This swelling is believed to be a key indicator of sub-ILM hemorrhage.

- *Histopathology:* The most definitive method for distinguishing between the two is intraoperative staining of the preretinal membrane, followed by excision and histopathological examination.

Table 1 summarizing the differences between preretinal (subhyaloid) hemorrhages and sub-ILM hemorrhages.

MANAGEMENT

The literature provides various management strategies for sub-ILM hemorrhage, but no specific guidelines are established. The main approaches include:

- *Observation:*
  - *Pros:* Spontaneous absorption is possible, especially for hemorrhages <1 disc diameter, typically resolving within 2 weeks.[6]
  - *Cons:* Larger hemorrhages may take months to clear. If there are no signs of resolution after 1 month, treatment is necessary to prevent potential toxic retinal damage from prolonged hemoglobin exposure **(Fig. 4).**
- *Laser puncture of ILM* **(Fig. 5)**:
  - *Pros:* Neodymium-doped yttrium aluminum garnet (Nd:YAG) laser can effectively clear hemorrhages, especially if performed within 2–3 weeks of onset.[7]
  - *Cons:* Risks include retinal hole formation and retinal detachment. Care must be taken to ensure the bleed's lower margin does not involve the fovea or papillomacular bundle, and media clarity is essential.
- *Pneumopexy ± intravitreal injection of tPA:*
  - *Pros:* Intravitreal gas injection, combined with prone positioning, can effectively displace subfoveal hemorrhages. tPA promotes fibrinolysis, aiding in blood breakdown.[8]
  - *Cons:* The timing of tPA administration is crucial; a delay of 2–3 hours may be necessary for optimal efficacy, especially in sub-ILM cases. There is also a need for careful monitoring of the gas bubble position.
- *Vitrectomy with ILM peeling* **(Fig. 6)**:
  - *Pros:* This is the definitive treatment for sub-ILM hemorrhage, often resulting in significant and immediate visual improvement. The ILM can be sent for histological analysis if needed.
  - *Cons:* Common complications include increased intraocular pressure, cataract

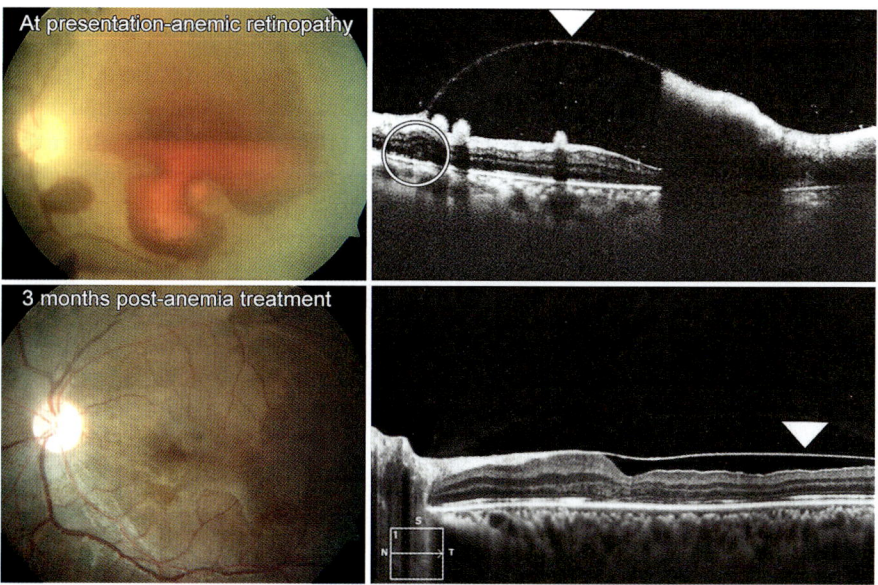

Fig. 4: Combined OCT and fundus images showing sub-ILM hemorrhage associated with anemic retinopathy at presentation, alongside the resolution observed 3 months after anemia treatment. (ILM: internal limiting membrane; OCT: optical coherence tomography)

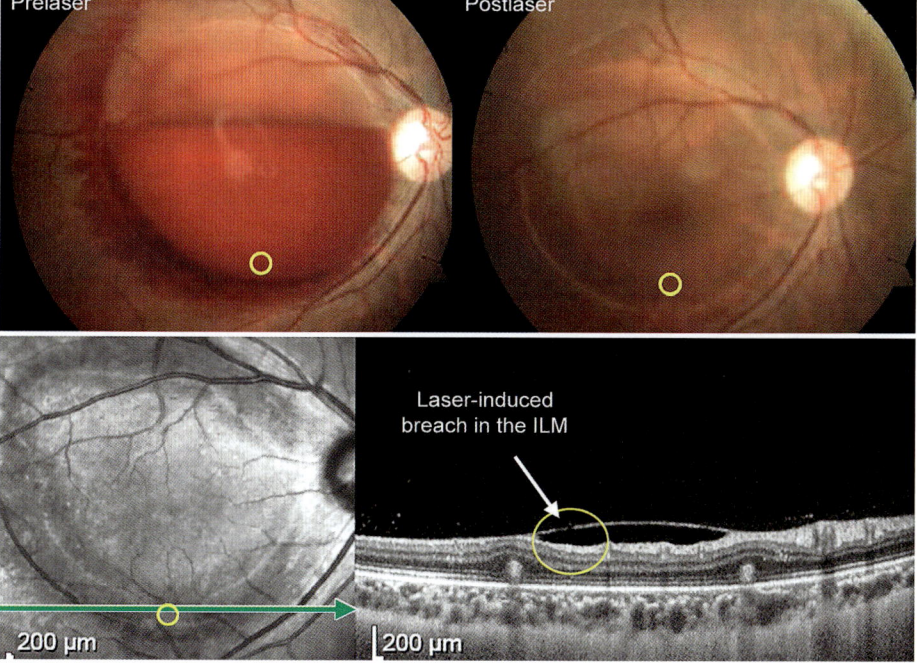

Fig. 5: Collage displaying a fundus photo of sub-ILM hemorrhage before and after laser puncture of the ILM. Accompanying OCT image demonstrates the laser-induced breach in the ILM. (ILM: internal limiting membrane; OCT: optical coherence tomography)

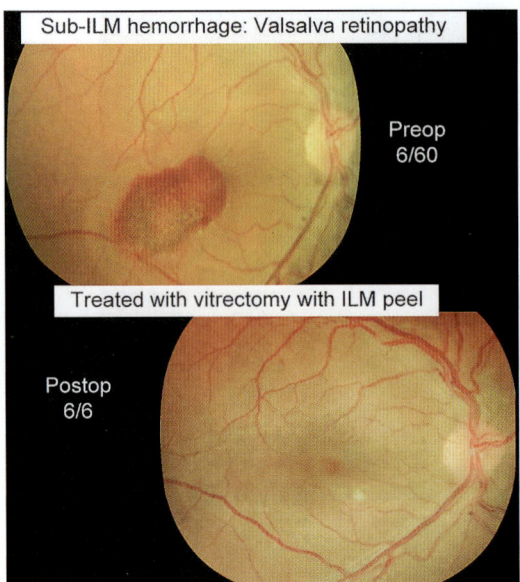

Fig. 6: Fundus photographs of sub-ILM hemorrhage before and after vitrectomy with ILM peeling. (ILM: internal limiting membrane)

formation, and retinal detachment, though these are rare when performed by experienced hands.

CONCLUSION

Sub-ILM hemorrhage is frequently misdiagnosed during routine clinical examinations. However, specific imaging clues can assist ophthalmologists in accurately identifying the condition. Notable indicators include the yellow outline observed in fundus photography, the dome-shaped elevated hyperreflective line on OCT, and the stretched hyperreflective foci in the ONL. The size and location of the hemorrhage are critical factors that influence the timing and type of management required. Additionally, thorough patient counseling is essential, particularly for those with large macular bleeds, as it sets realistic expectations regarding potential outcomes.

ACKNOWLEDGMENTS

I sincerely thank my teachers at Sankara Netralaya, Kolkata and Chennai my colleagues at Choithram Netralaya, Indore and the optometry staff for their invaluable support. Most importantly, I am grateful to my patients for their trust, which inspires my work.

REFERENCES

1. De Maeyer K, Van Ginderdeuren R, Postelmans L, Stalmans P, Van Calster J. Sub-inner limiting membrane haemorrhage: causes and treatment with vitrectomy. Br J Ophthalmol. 2007;91(7):869-72.
2. Semeraro F, Morescalchi F, Duse S, Gambicorti E, Russo A, Costagliola C. Current Trends about Inner Limiting Membrane Peeling in Surgery for Epiretinal Membranes. J Ophthalmol. 2015;2015:671905.
3. Reichenbach A, Bringmann A. New functions of Müller cells. Glia. 2013;61(5):651-78.
4. Suzuki AC, Miranda RS, Zacharias LC, Monteiro ML, Takahashi WY. Novel Outer Retinal Optical Coherence Tomography Hyperreflective Abnormality Associated With Sub-Internal Limiting Membrane Hemorrhage. Retina. 2015;35(8):1713-4.
5. Guidry C. The role of Müller cells in fibrocontractive retinal disorders. Prog Retin Eye Res. 2005;24:75-86.
6. Azzi TT, Zacharias LC, Pimentel SL. Spontaneous absorption of extensive subinternal limiting membrane hemorrhage in shaken baby syndrome. Case Rep Ophthalmol Med. 2014;2014:360829.
7. Raymond LA. Neodymium:YAG laser treatment for hemorrhages under the internal limiting membrane and posterior hyaloid face in the macula. Ophthalmology. 1995;102(3):406-11.
8. Chou YK, Huang YM, Lin PK. Sub-internal limiting membrane hemorrhage treated with intravitreal tissue plasminogen activator followed by octafluoropropane gas injection. Taiwan J Ophthalmol. 2015;5(4):198-201.

Optical Coherence Tomography Biomarkers in Diabetic Macular Edema

Isha Acharya, Himanshu Prakash

INTRODUCTION

Structural optical coherence tomography (OCT) is a key tool in diagnosing and monitoring diabetic macular edema (DME) **(Box 1)**.

Image resolution and field of vision have been significantly increased since time-domain OCT (TD-OCT—400 A-scans/second) was replaced by spectral-domain OCT (SD-OCT—20,000–40,000 A-scans/second).[1]

Spectral domain OCT provides high-resolution images that reveal critical retinal structures like the retinal pigment epithelium (RPE), inner segment/outer segment (IS/OS) junction, and external limiting membrane (ELM) that predict visual outcomes. Analyzing these structures and other morphological characteristics on OCT can yield useful biomarkers which can help in tracking disease progression and guiding treatment decisions for better vision preservation.

With the advent of ultrahigh-speed swept-source OCT (SS-OCT—100,000–400,000 A-scans/second),[1] which offers superior spatial resolution, a larger field of view and deeper penetration, it is now possible to examine choroidal structures in detail and identify potential choroidal biomarkers for predicting DME. The enhanced depth imaging (EDI) mode of SD-OCT can also visualize choroidal layers in greater depth than the conventional mode.

TO IDENTIFY MILD DIABETIC RETINOPATHY AND EARLY DIABETIC MACULAR EDEMA

By identifying diabetic retinopathy (DR) at an early stage, we can counsel the patient regarding the importance of regular follow-ups and strict systemic control **(Figs. 1 and 2)**.

Location of Diabetic Macular Edema

According to the 2018 guidelines from the International Council of Ophthalmology (ICO),[2] DME has been classified into two categories based on fundus examination:
1. Center-involved diabetic macular edema (CI-DME) **(Fig. 3)**
2. Non-center involved diabetic macular edema (non-CI-DME) **(Fig. 4)**

CI-DME	NON-CI-DME
Retinal thickening in the macula that involves the central subfield zone (1 mm in diameter)	Retinal thickening in the macula that does not involve the central subfield zone (1 mm in diameter)

Optical coherence tomography facilitates confirming the location of DME based on which treatment can be directed.

PATTERNS AND/OR CLASSIFICATION OF DIABETIC MACULAR EDEMA

Several classification systems have been described in the literature based on OCT

BOX 1: Why optical coherence tomography in diagnosing diabetic macular edema (DME)?

- To identify early diabetic retinopathy (DR) and DME
- Location of DME
- Patterns and/or classification of DME
- Assessing visual prognosis and chronicity

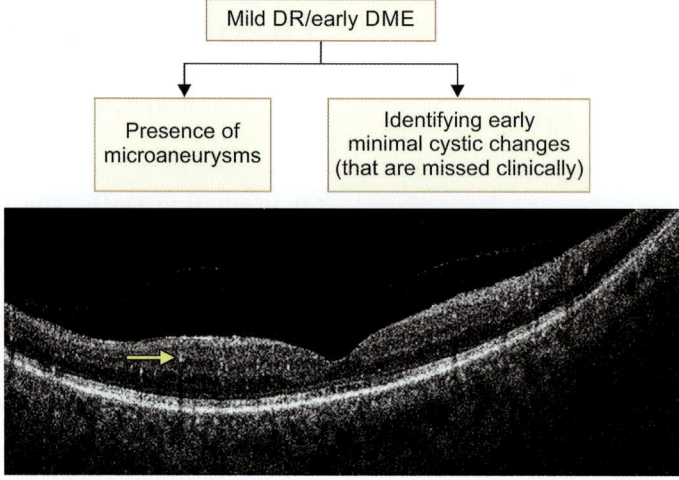

Fig. 1: Mild diabetic retinopathy with occurrence of multiple microaneurysms (yellow arrow). (DME: diabetic macular edema; DR: diabetic retinopathy)

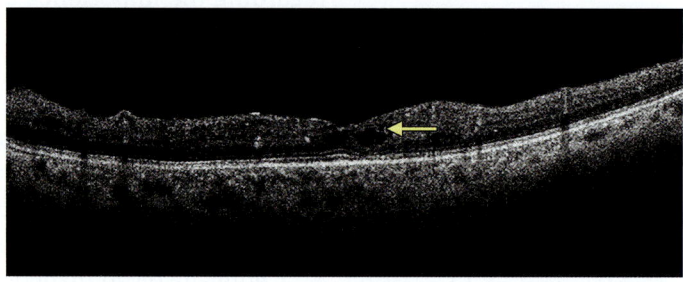

Fig. 2: Minimal cystic changes at the macula signifying early diabetic macular edema (DME).

morphology[3] (some of which have been discussed in **Table 1**)

One of the widely accepted classifications was given by Kim et al.[3] in 2006 on TD-OCT:
- Diffuse retinal thickening **(Fig. 5)**
- Cystoid macular edema **(Fig. 6)**
- Serous retinal detachment **(Fig. 7)**
- Posterior hyaloid traction **(Figs. 8A and B)**
- Tractional retinal detachment

Based on these classification systems, DME can be simply categorized into:

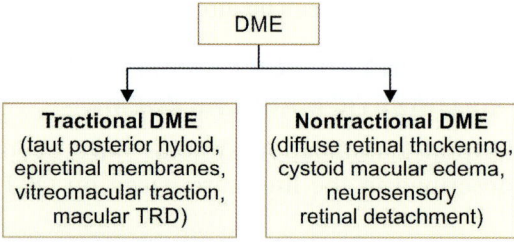

ASSESSING VISUAL PROGNOSIS AND CHRONICITY

The evaluation of retinal and choroidal OCT biomarkers is pivotal in determining the chronicity and severity of DME, and in predicting visual prognosis. These OCT biomarkers ensure precise treatment strategies and help in setting achievable expectations for patients.

Table 2 provides a comprehensive summary of these important retinal OCT biomarkers.

Central subfield thickness (CST) is defined as the circular region of 1 mm in diameter centered around the foveola, with a measurable thickness on OCT software. It is an unreliable visual prognostic marker. Visual acuity particularly depends upon the

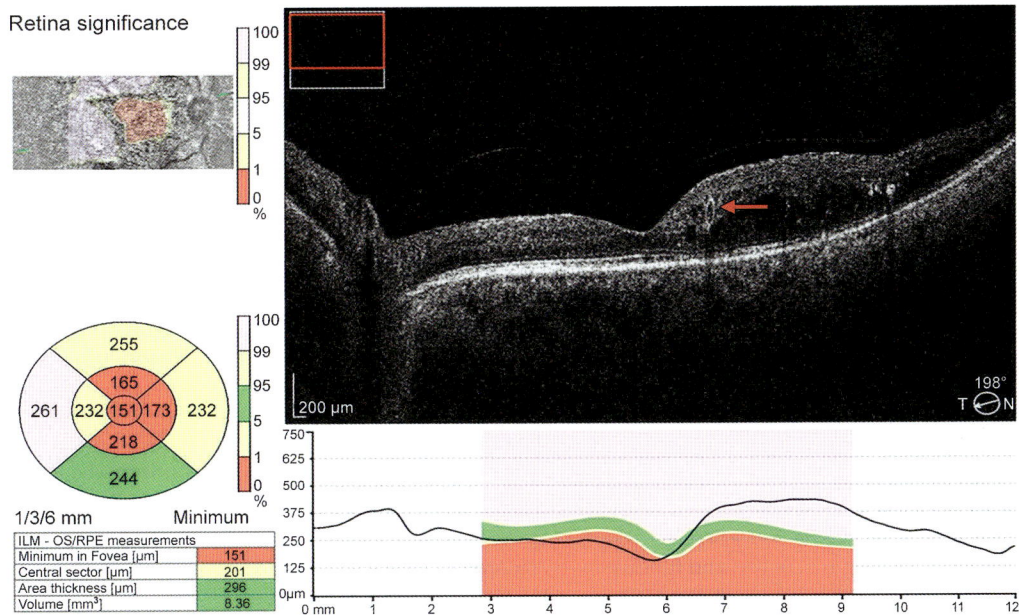

Fig. 3: Spectral-domain optical coherence tomography (SD-OCT) image of right eye showing non-center involved diabetic macular edema (non-CI-DME) sparing the central 1 mm ETDRS circle. Microaneurysm (red arrow) is noted with hyperreflective oval walls and hyporeflective lumen.

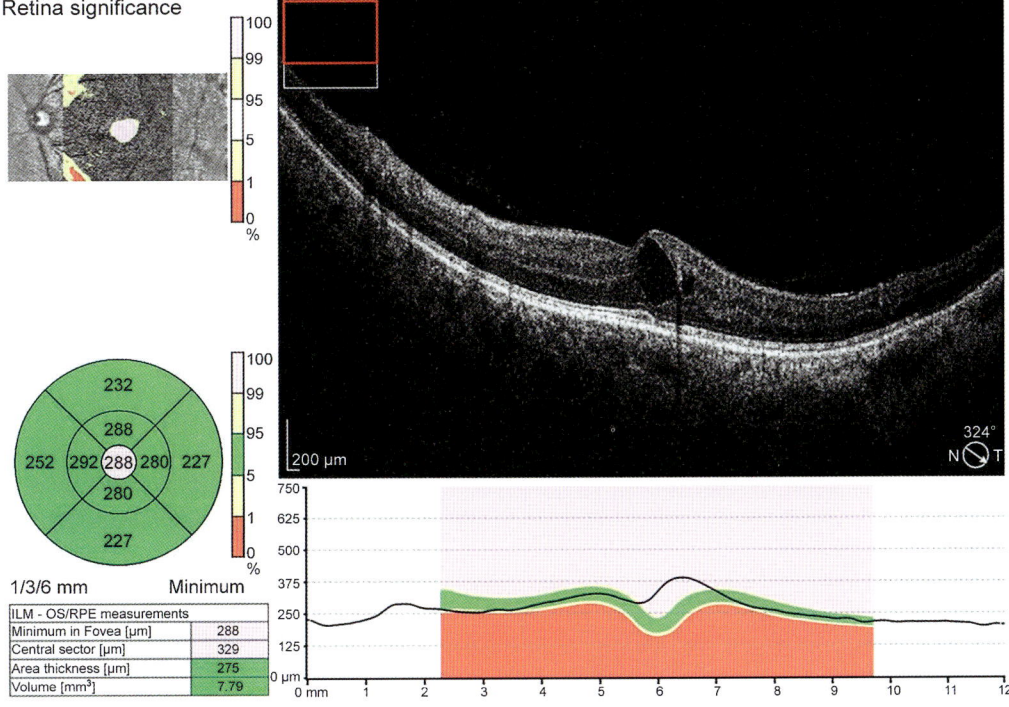

Fig. 4: Spectral-domain optical coherence tomography (SD-OCT) image of left eye showing center-involved diabetic macular edema (CI-DME) sparing the central 1 mm ETDRS circle.

TABLE 1: OCT-based DME classification systems.

Authors	Year	OCT type	Classification
Otani et al.	1999	TD-OCT	*Tomographic fluid distribution:* Type 1 = Sponge-like retinal swelling Type 2 = Cystoid macular edema Type 3 = Serous retinal detachment
Koleva Georgieva et al.	2008	SD-OCT	*Macular thickness and retinal morphology:* Type 1 = Early, CMT > normal + 2 SD Type 2 = Simple Type 3 = Cystoid *Type 3A, mild:* Cystoid spaces with horizontal diameter < 300 μm *Type 3B, intermediate:* Cystoid spaces with horizontal diameter 300–599 μm *Type 3C, severe:* Cystoid spaces with horizontal diameter ≥600 μm, or large confluent cavities like retinoschisis
Bolz et al.	2014	SD-OCT and fundus fluorescein angiography (FFA)	S = Subretinal fluid A = Area of retinal thickening V = Vitreoretinal abnormalities E = Etiology of leakage (focal, nonfocal, ischemic, and atrophic)
Parodi et al.	2016	SD-OCT	• Vasogenic = DME with vascular dilation • Nonvasogenic = DME without vascular dilation • Tractional • Mixed

(DME: diabetic macular edema; SD-OCT: spectral-domain optical coherence tomography; TD-OCT: time-domain OCT)

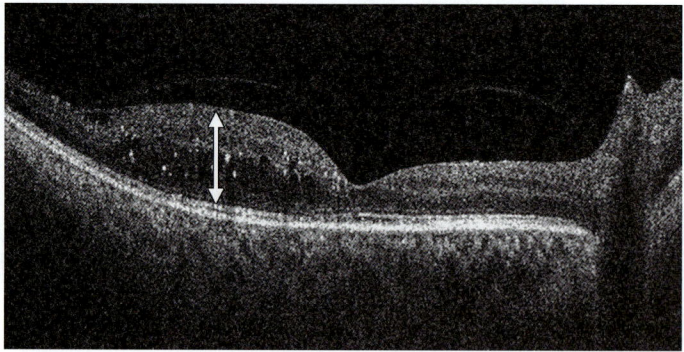

Fig. 5: Spectral-domain optical coherence tomography (SD-OCT) image of the right eye showing multiple cystic spaces along with retinal thickening (spongiform macular edema).

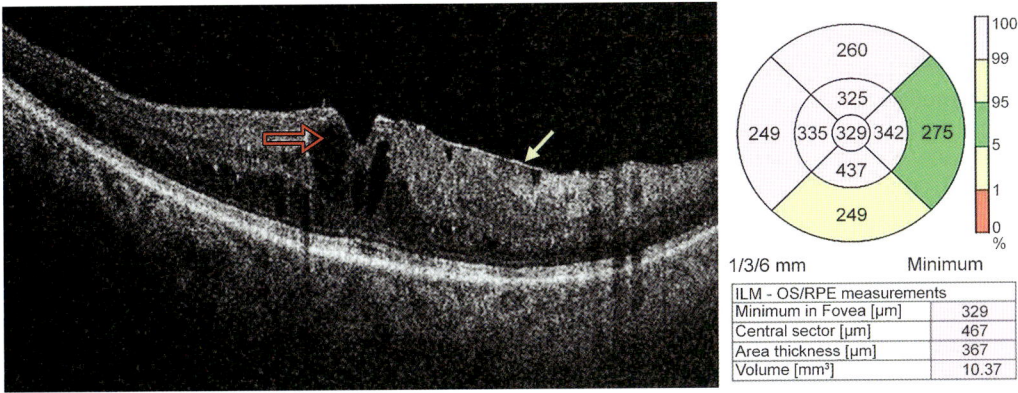

Fig. 6: Spectral-domain optical coherence tomography (SD-OCT) image of the right eye showing center-involved diabetic macular edema (CI-DME) with large oval cystic spaces (red hollow arrow) involving the central 1 mm ETDRS circle. Patchy epiretinal membrane (yellow solid arrow) is also noted.

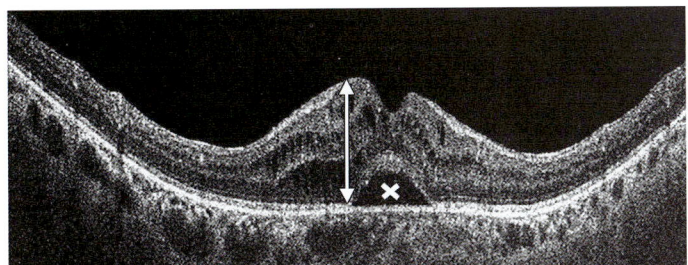

Fig. 7: SD-OCT image of the left eye showing multiple cystic spaces along with retinal thickening, suggesting CI-DME and SRF in the foveal region. (CI-DME: center-involved diabetic macular edema; SD-OCT: spectral-domain optical coherence tomography; SRF: subretinal fluid)

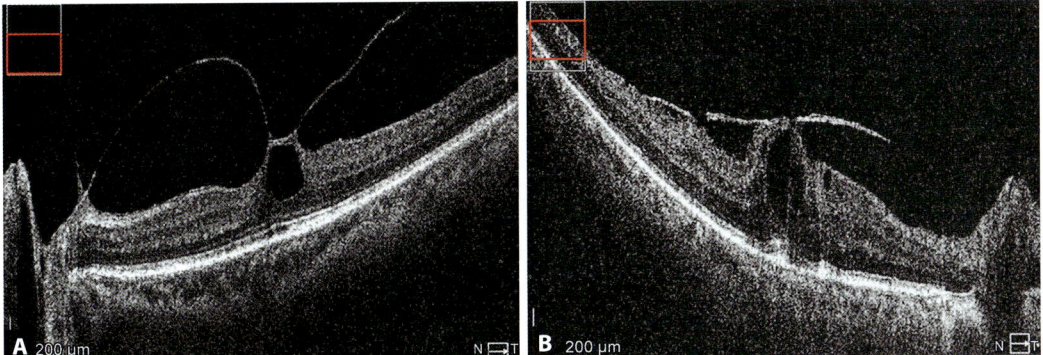

Figs. 8A and B: (A) Spectral-domain optical coherence tomography (SD-OCT) image of left eye showing focal vitreomacular traction with intraretinal large cystic edema and (B) SD-OCT image of right eye showing cystoid macular edema with taut posterior hyloid.

TABLE 2: Retinal OCT biomarkers.

Biomarkers	Prognosis	Retinal layers involved	Description
1. Hyperreflective dots (HRDs) **(Fig. 9)**	—	Inner retinal layers	• Inflammatory biomarker • *Composition:* Subclinical lipoprotein deposits/activated microglial cells/degenerated photoreceptors • <30 µm size • No back shadowing
2. Pearl necklace sign **(Figs. 10A and B)**	Poor (if subfoveal location)	Inner retinal layers	• Hyperreflective dots arranged in a contiguous ring along the inner wall of cystoid spaces • Precursor to HEs • Following intravitreal treatment, clinically noticeable HEs occur in the same location once the edema resolves
3. Hard exudates (HEs)	Poor (if subfoveal plaque or cholesterol crystal formation)	Outer plexiform layer	• Lipoproteinaceous (albumin and fibrin) deposits • Associated with abnormal lipid profile • >30 µm size • Back shadowing is present
4. Disorganization of retinal inner layers (DRILs) **(Fig. 11)**	Poor	Ganglion cell layer—inner plexiform layer complex, inner nuclear layer, and outer plexiform layer	• Inability to distinguish between the inner retinal layers at the central 1 mm retinal zone • Disorganization of >50% or >500 µm of this area is considered significant. • Signifies macular capillary nonperfusion • Can also be associated with outer retinal layers disruption
5. Intracystic hyperreflective material (ICHRM) **(Fig. 12)**	Poor	Outer plexiform layer	• Clumps of hyperreflective material within the intraretinal cystic space without back shadowing • Transudation of proteins, fibrin, macrophages, fluid, lipids, and/or heme from the intravascular space to the extravascular space • Complete ICHRM filling within the retinal cyst is suggestive of a prolonged course of edema and a poor response to treatment
6. Bridging retinal processes **(Fig. 13)**	Good	Between the cystic cavities	• Represent residual neural elements connecting outer and inner retina • Believed to be composed of Muller cells and bipolar cells

Contd...

Contd...

Biomarkers	Prognosis	Retinal layers involved	Description
7. Photoreceptor outer segment (PROS)	Good	Ellipsoid zone (EZ) and RPE	• Length between the photoreceptor inner and outer segment junction and the RPE[4] • Outer segments are more critical than inner segments since they act as opsin reservoirs
8. External limiting layer (ELM) and ellipsoid zone integrity **(Fig. 14)**	Good	ELM and EZ	• Directly related to the vitality of photoreceptors • Long-standing DME associated with disruption of these layers
9. Subretinal fluid (SRF) **(Figs. 15A and B)**	Good		• Protective role • Assists in preserving and healing the photoreceptor layers • Baseline SRF correlates with a rapid recovery of DME following intravitreal injections[5]

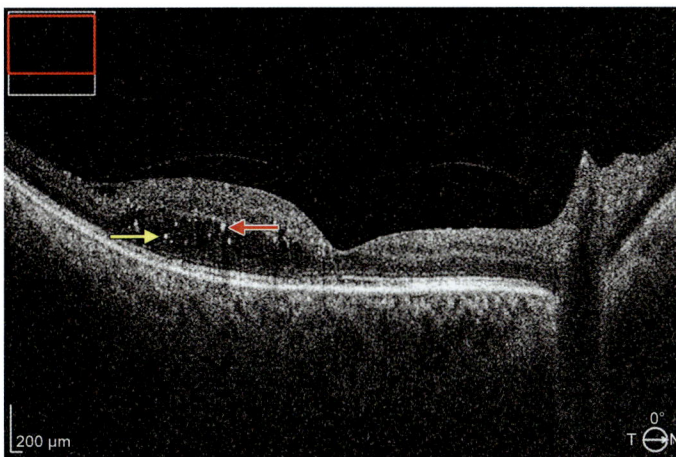

Fig. 9: Spectral-domain optical coherence tomography (SD-OCT) image of the right eye showing hyperreflective dots and spots without backshadowing (yellow arrow) and hard exudates with backshadowing (red arrow).

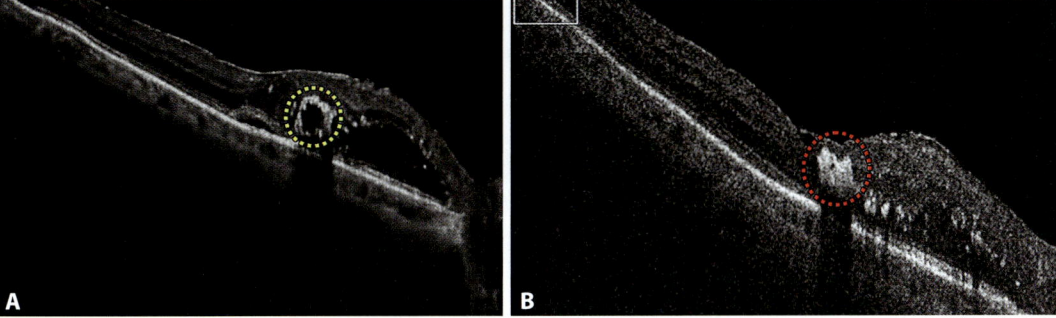

Figs. 10A and B: (A) SD-OCT image of right eye showing DME with juxtafoveal pearl necklace sign and (B) SD-OCT image of right eye at 1 month following intravitreal aflibercept injection showing clumps of hard exudates forming hard exudate plaque (dotted red circle) at the previous location of the pearl necklace sign. (DME: diabetic macular edema; SD-OCT: spectral-domain optical coherence tomography)

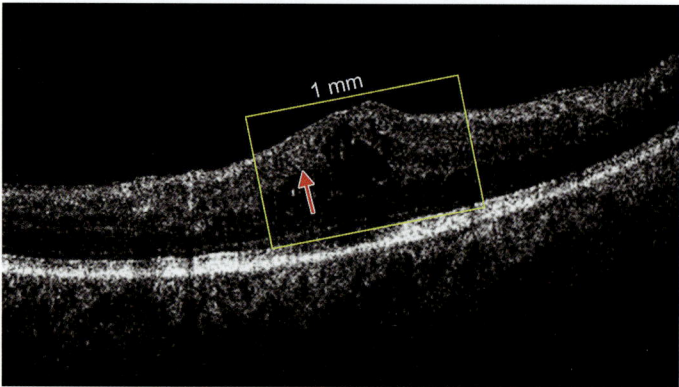

Fig. 11: Spectral-domain optical coherence tomography (SD-OCT) image of right eye showing disorganization of retinal inner layer (DRIL) in the central 1 mm zone centered around fovea, inner retinal layers cannot be distinguished (red arrow) unlike the other half of the central 1 mm zone.

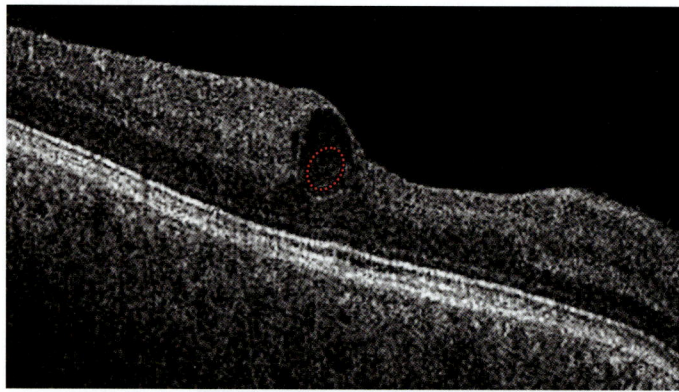

Fig. 12: Spectral-domain optical coherence tomography (SD-OCT) image of right eye showing partial filled intracystic hyperreflective material (ICHRM).

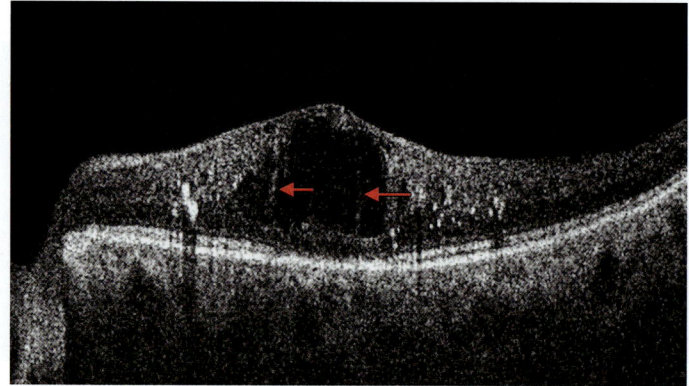

Fig. 13: Spectral-domain optical coherence tomography (SD-OCT) large cystic space, hyperreflective dots (HDRs) with backshadowing, and retinal thickening.

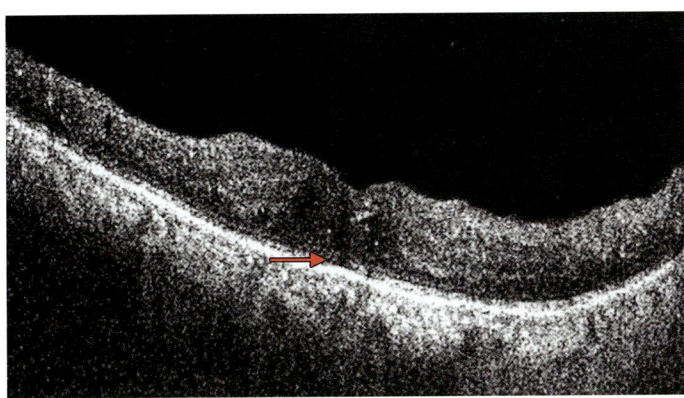

Fig. 14: SD-OCT image of the left eye showing CI-DME with subfoveal ellipsoid zone and external limiting membrane disruption, also with alteration in the inner retinal layer. (CI-DME: center-involved diabetic macular edema; SD-OCT: spectral-domain optical coherence tomography)

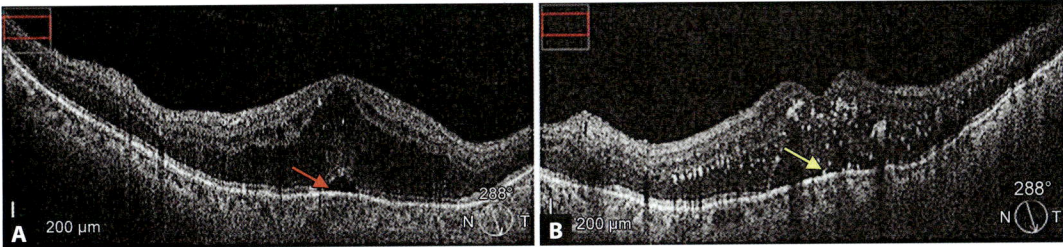

Figs. 15A and B: (A) SD-OCT image of left eye showing CI-DME with subfoveal NSD with SRF (red arrow) and (B) Image of the left eye at 1 month following intravitreal dexamethasone implant injection showing resolving subfoveal NSD. (CI-DME: center-involved diabetic macular edema; NSD: neurosensory detachment; SD-OCT: spectral-domain optical coherence tomography; SRF: subretinal fluid)

integrity of inner retinal layers (bipolar and ganglion cells/axons) and the photoreceptor and RPE layers. Patients can have poor visual acuity despite resolution of CST following intravitreal injections or a good visual acuity despite an increased CST. Hence, CST assessment alone cannot accurately prognosticate the final visual outcomes.

With the introduction of OCT angiography (OCTA), it has now become possible to calculate the automated central macular fluid volume (CMFV) using the deep-learning algorithm.[6] The standard CST assessment, while informative, frequently fails to capture the entire level of fluid collection in the macula. CST only considers the thickness of a single location, which may not correctly indicate the overall disease condition or therapy response. In contrast, CMFV gives a thorough assessment of fluid distribution, providing a more holistic perspective of the pathological alterations occurring in the retina. Studies have found that changes in CMFV correspond more strongly with visual outcomes than CST. Reduction in CMFV after treatment has been related to increased visual acuity, implying that monitoring CFMV might optimize patient management strategies.[7]

Retinal OCT biomarkers are often the focus of the majority of OCT biomarker studies in DME. Due to the dynamic nature of choroid, several confounding factors

TABLE 3: Choroidal OCT biomarkers.

Biomarkers	Prognosis	Description
1. Hyperreflective choroidal foci	Poor	• Sign of migration of HRD into the choroid • Inflammatory biomarker • Associated with increasing severity of DR (seen more in proliferative cases versus nonproliferative DR) • Associated with higher CT[8]
2. Subfoveal choroidal thickness (CT)		• CT increases with increasing severity of DME[9] • It also correlates with the severity of microangiopathy within the retina (greater with diffuse DME than focal) • Among diffuse DME, CT is found to be greater in CME than spongiform edema • Vary with systemic disorders—hypertension, renal failure, fluctuating blood glucose levels, or history of previous treatment with intravitreal injections/laser
3. Choroidal vascularity index		• Ratio of choroidal luminal area to total choroidal area[10] • *Better biomarker* than CT since it is unaltered by the abovementioned confounding variables • Associated with increasing severity of DR (seen more in proliferative cases versus nonproliferative DR) • *Earliest biomarker* to be affected (predictor of occurrence of a DR or DME)

(CME: cystoid macular edema; CT: computed tomography; DME: diabetic macular edema; DR: diabetic retinopathy; HRD: hyperreflective dots)

may alter the choroidal thickness (CT) like the presence of other systemic disorders—hypertension, renal failure, fluctuating blood glucose levels, or history of previous treatment with intravitreal injections/laser. However, CT with other choroidal biomarkers may still act as a potential biomarker in establishing visual prognosis in concordance with retinal OCT biomarkers. **Table 3** summarizes some important choroidal OCT biomarkers.

In conclusion, the comprehensive assessment of both retinal and choroidal OCT biomarkers plays a pivotal role in diagnosing, monitoring, and predicting the visual prognosis of DME. These biomarkers, combined with advanced OCT technologies such as swept-source OCT and OCT angiography, enhance our ability to personalize treatment plans, optimize patient outcomes, and guide clinical decisions. By leveraging these insights, ophthalmologists can ensure more accurate predictions regarding disease progression and tailor therapies that preserve vision, especially in the presence of complex DME subtypes.

REFERENCES

1. Zheng F, Deng X, Zhang Q, He J, Ye P, Liu S, et al. Advances in swept-source optical coherence tomography and optical coherence tomography angiography. Adv Ophthalmol Pract Res. 2022;3(2):67-79.
2. Diabetic Eye Care - International Council of Ophthalmology.
3. Panozzo G, Cicinelli MV, Augustin AJ, Battaglia Parodi M, Cunha-Vaz J, Guarnaccia G, et al. An optical coherence tomography-based grading of diabetic maculopathy proposed by an international expert panel: The European School for Advanced Studies in Ophthalmology classification. Eur J Ophthalmol. 2020;30(1):8-18.

4. Forooghian F, Stetson PF, Meyer SA, Chew EY, Wong WT, Cukras C, et al. Relationship between photoreceptor outer segment length and visual acuity in diabetic macular edema. Retina. 2010;30(1):63-70.
5. Park J, Felfeli T, Kherani IZ, Altomare F, Chow DR, Wong DT. Prevalence and clinical implications of subretinal fluid in retinal diseases: a real-world cohort study. BMJ Open Ophthalmol. 2023;21:8(1):e001214.
6. Tsuboi K, You QS, Guo Y, Wang J, Flaxel CJ, Bailey ST, et al. Automated Macular Fluid Volume as a Treatment Indicator for Diabetic Macular Edema. J Vitreoretin Dis. 2023;7(3):226-31.
7. You QS, Tsuboi K, Guo Y, Wang J, Flaxel CJ, Bailey ST, et al. Comparison of Central Macular Fluid Volume With Central Subfield Thickness in Patients With Diabetic Macular Edema Using Optical Coherence Tomography Angiography. JAMA Ophthalmol. 2021;139(7):734.
8. Saurabh K, Roy R, Herekar S, Mistry S, Choudhari S. Validation of choroidal hyperreflective foci in diabetic macular edema through a retrospective pilot study. Indian J Ophthalmol. 2021;69(11):3203.
9. Amjad R, Lee CA, Farooqi HMU, Khan H, Paeng DG. Choroidal Thickness in Different Patterns of Diabetic Macular Edema. J Clin Med. 2022;11(20):6169.
10. Agrawal R, Gupta P, Tan KA, Cheung CMG, Wong TY, Cheng CY. Choroidal vascularity index as a measure of vascular status of the choroid: Measurements in healthy eyes from a population-based study. Sci Rep. 2016;6:21090.

CHAPTER 28

Ocular Ultrasonography in Retinal Disorders

Mousumi Banerjee

INTRODUCTION

Ocular ultrasonography (USG) is a painless, noninvasive, safe, rapid, cost-effective, rapidly evolving real-time diagnostic tool for precise diagnosis of ocular lesion. Henry Mundt and William Hughes described the use of one-dimensional acoustic display in which echoes are represented as vertical spikes from a baseline (A-scan) in 1956 for the first time. Baum and Greenwood (1958) codeveloped two-dimensional B scan USG in 1958 with the help of a water bath as a coupling agent between globe and probe.[1] Bronston and workers introduced the first handheld contact B scan without the need for a water bath.[2] Standardization of A-scan combined with contact B scan led to the development of Standardized Echography by Ossoinig, leading to highly accurate detection and differentiation of oculo-orbital disorders.[3]

PRINCIPLE OF ULTRASOUND (FLOWCHART 1)

With increase in frequency of USG, wavelength of USG decreases which determines the depth of tissue penetration and resolution. Wavelength of USG is directly proportional to the depth of tissue penetration and inversely proportional to resolution.

Thus, ocular USGs are of higher frequency (10 MHz) as it needs less tissue penetration and higher resolution. Recently, a high-frequency 20 MHz contact probe has been introduced.[4] 20 MHz USG has superior resolution and can detect details at the posterior pole and in the orbit, orbital fat imaging and differentiating lesions in the orbit, extraocular muscles, and optic nerve. However, 10 MHz has superior sensitivity and a closer focal distance, thus, better appreciates low intensity weakly reflective particles like detection of posterior

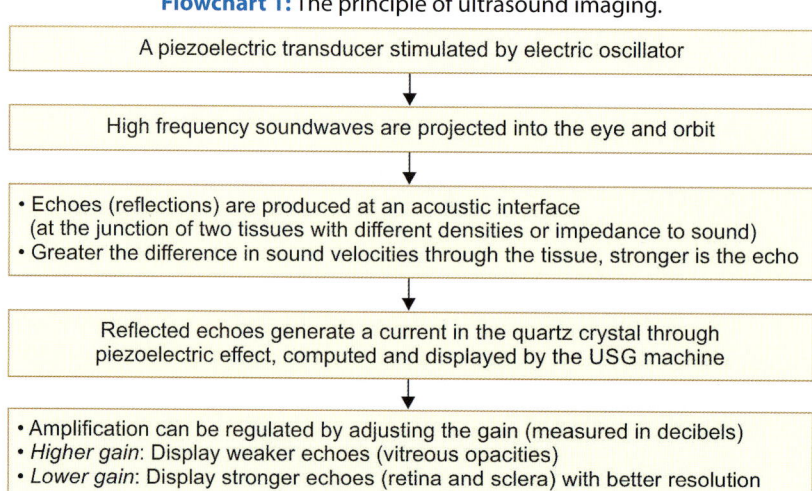

Flowchart 1: The principle of ultrasound imaging.

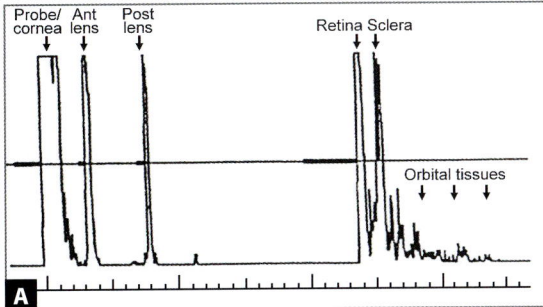
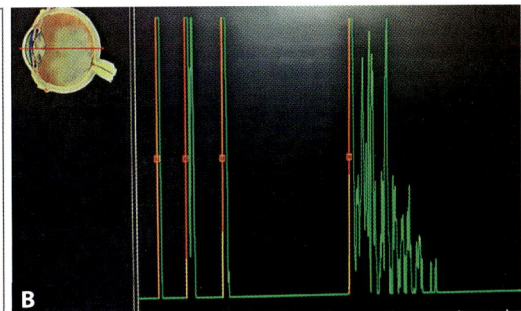

Figs. 1A and B: First spike: Probe interface meets the cornea. Second and third spike: Anterior and posterior lens surface respectively followed by flat line representing vitreous. Fourth and fifth spike: Retinal and sclera spike respectively followed by progressively reducing spikes representing orbital fat.

vitreous detachment (PVD), vitreous hemorrhage, and subtle vitreous change such as inflammatory cells, etc.[4]

TYPES OF OCULAR ULTRASONOGRAPHY SCANS

There are two main types of display modes currently used in ophthalmic practice: (1) Amplitude (A-scan) and (2) brightness (B-scan). C-scan has been described in literature to demonstrate the normal orbital fat and optic nerve, together with selected pathological conditions in the orbit. The C-scan facility permits imaging of the orbital contents in the coronal plane.[5]

A-Scan

A single sound beam is sent from the transducer and the returning echoes are converted into a series of spikes with height proportional to the strength of the echo. An ideal A-scan comprises five spikes followed by series of progressively reducing spike heights representing orbital fat **(Figs. 1A and B)**.

A-scan probe is a small pencil-sized probe with no mark emitting parallel and nonfocused ultrasound beam **(Fig. 2)**. The probe can be directly placed over the globe after instillation of topical anesthetics.

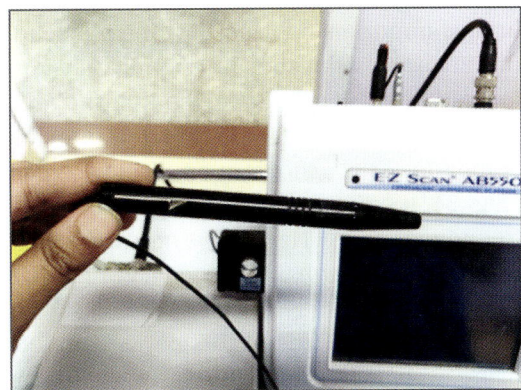

Fig. 2: Standardized A-scan probe of 8 MHz emitting parallel sound beam of 5 mm width at the highest decibel gain and 0.5 mm at the lowest.

B-Scan

Two-dimensional B scan can be performed either directly on the surface of the anesthetized eye using a protective cap or through the eyelids using a coupling jelly (transpalpebral approach). A gray-scale image representing the reflectivity of the structures is displayed on the screen. Low reflectivity is denoted by black whereas high reflectivity is depicted by white. Gain of the machine needs to be increased while visualizing low-reflective structures. Earlier USG machines used to have low gain, whereas recent machines have a maximum gain of 100 dB.

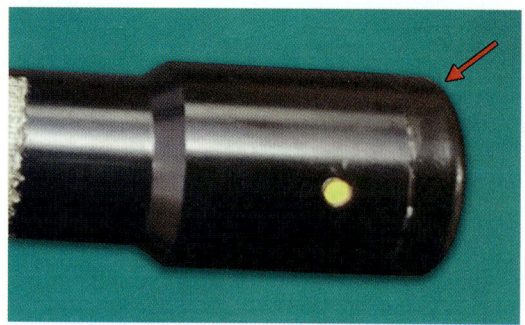

Fig. 3: B-scan probe with a mark (red arrow) for beam orientation.

Orientation of the B-scan probe is of utmost importance for performing a B scan. B-scan probe is thicker with a mark at the top indicating beam orientation so that the area toward which the mark is directed appears at the top of the echogram on display screen **(Fig. 3)**. It emits focused sound beams at a frequency of 10 MHz. *Recent machines emit focused sound beams at a frequency of 12 MHz and 20 MHz.*

Based on the axis of the globe, which is being evaluated, three scan descriptions are used—(1) axial scan, (2) transverse scan, and (3) longitudinal scan **(Table 1)**.

SPECIAL EXAMINATION TECHNIQUES

There are three special examination techniques used together to derive an echographic diagnosis.
1. *Topographic echography:* Performed using B-scan probe. It helps in documenting shape, extent, location, and dimension of the mass lesion.
2. *Kinetic echography:* Determines the mobility and vascularity of the lesion. Example: Posterior vitreous detachment (PVD) has moderate—marked after movements, retinal detachment (RD) has moderate—none after movements based on the duration of detachment, while choroidal detachment (CD) has mild—none after movements.
3. *Quantitative echography:* Performed using A-scan probe. It consists of reflectivity, internal composition, and sound absorption.

INDICATIONS FOR OCULAR SONOGRAPHY

- Evaluation of details of intraocular structures obscured by opacities, e.g., corneal opacity, hyphema, dense cataract, vitreous hemorrhage, and retinoblastoma.
- Differentiation of solid and cystic masses
- Biometry (determination of axial length of the eyeball)
- Documentation of posteriorly dislocated crystalline lens, intraocular lens, intraocular foreign body, and ocular cysticercosis
- Choroidal lesions (melanoma and hemangioma), metastasis, macular lesions (e.g., osteoma by characteristic calcification)
- Detection of T sign in posterior scleritis
- Differentiating RD from PVD.
- Optic disc cupping, increased optic nerve sheath diameter in papilledema, calcification at optic nerve head in optic disc drusen.

DESCRIPTION OF OCULAR SONOGRAPHY IN VARIOUS VITREO-RETINAL CONDITIONS

Retinal Detachment (Videos 1 and 4)

Retinal detachment has moderate-to-high reflectivity in view of the higher thickness and multiple layers of neurosensory retina and is tethered posteriorly to both margins of optic disc and anteriorly to ora serrata with limited after movements which sometimes appear like whip-lash movement **(Figs. 4A and B)**.

TABLE 1: Ultrasound biomicroscopy (UBM) scan orientations: Axial scan, transverse scan, and longitudinal scan.

Axial scan

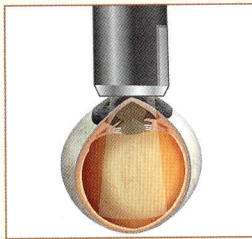

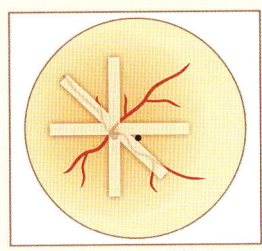

The patient fixates in the primary gaze and the probe is placed on the globe and directed axially.

Depending on the clock hour location of the mark, three sections obtained: (1) Axial–horizontal, (2) axial–vertical, and (3) axial–oblique.

Demonstrates optic nerve head and posterior pole.

Transverse scan

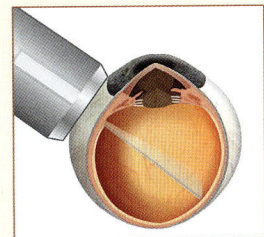
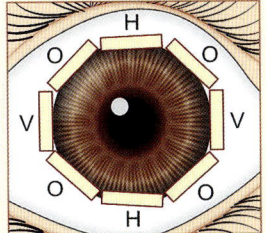
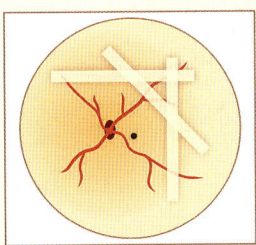

The mark on the probe is kept parallel to the limbus.

Depending on the clock hour location of the mark, three sections obtained: (1) Horizontal-transverse, (2) vertical-transverse, and (3) oblique-transverse.

Optic nerve head is not visualized. It depicts the lateral extent of a lesion.

Longitudinal scan

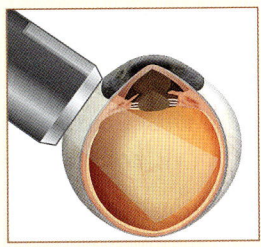
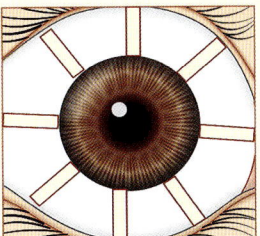
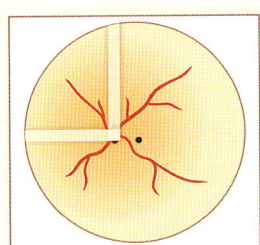

The mark on the probe is kept perpendicular to the limbus.

Depending on the clock hour location of the mark, three sections obtained: (1) Horizontal-longitudinal, (2) vertical-longitudinal, and (3) oblique-longitudinal.

Optic nerve head is visualized at the bottom of the scan. Demonstrates the antero-posterior extent of the lesion.

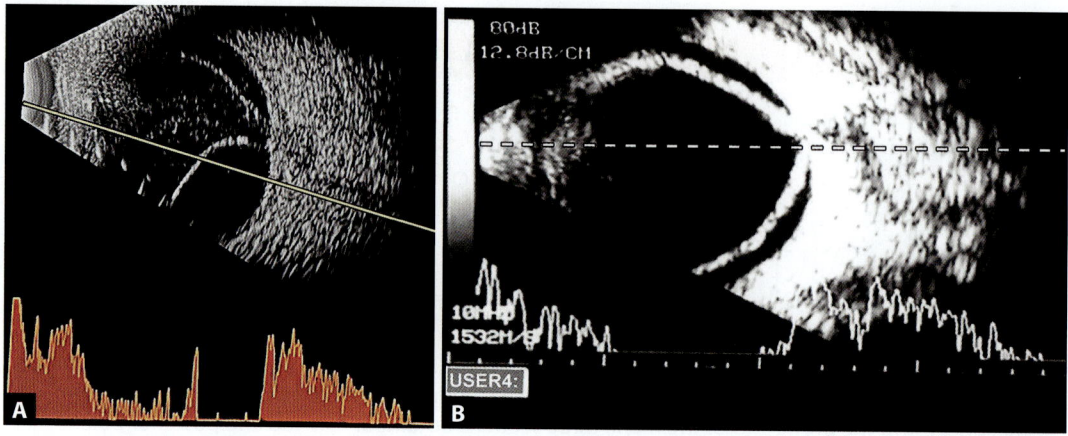

Figs. 4A and B: Ultrasound biomicroscopy (UBM) images showing retinal detachment.

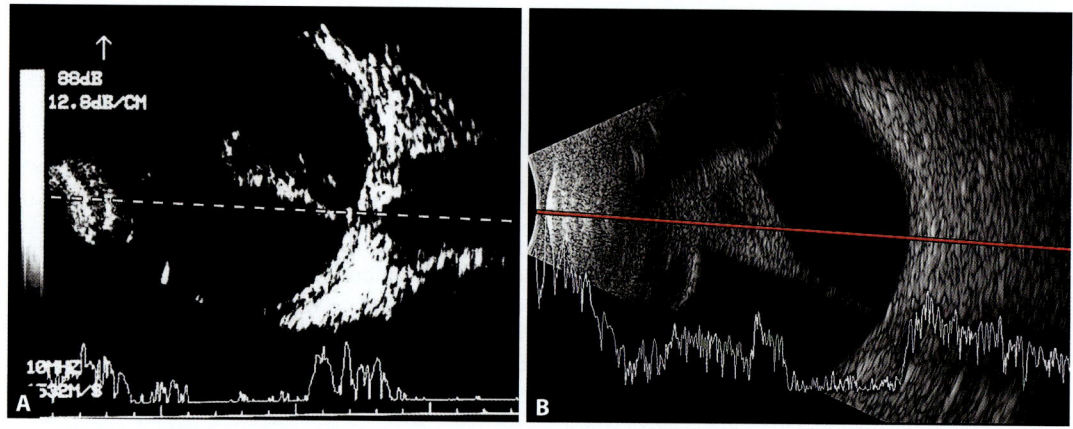

Figs. 5A and B: Ultrasound biomicroscopy (UBM) images of closed funnel retinal detachment.

Closed Funnel Retinal Detachment

Thick membrane is attached on both sides of the optic nerve with no after movements and a closed funnel configuration is noted **(Figs. 5A and B)**.

Giant Retinal Tear (Video 2)

A thick membrane is attached to the optic nerve with curled-up posterior flap of giant retinal tear rolled inward. A-scan depicts high amplitude spike corresponding to the rolled-up edge of the giant retinal tear **(Fig. 6)**.

Vitreous Hemorrhage with Posterior Vitreous Detachment (Video 3)

B-scan depicts bright dot-like echoes in the vitreous cavity corresponding to low-medium reflectivity spikes along the A-scan vector. A thin membrane with pinpoint attachment to the optic disc is noted having low-to-moderate reflectivity and good after movements. Dot-like echoes are also noted posterior to the membrane (subhyaloid hemorrhage) **(Fig. 7)**.

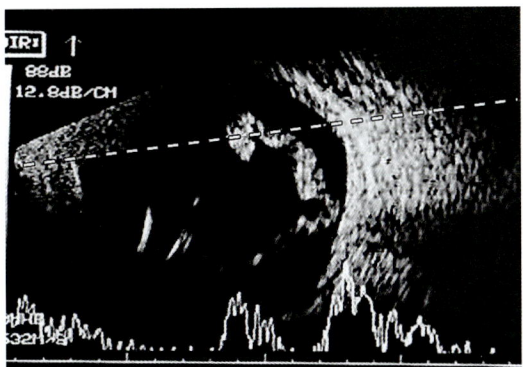

Fig. 6: Ultrasound biomicroscopy (UBM) image of a giant retinal tear, showing a thick membrane attached to the optic nerve with a curled posterior flap.

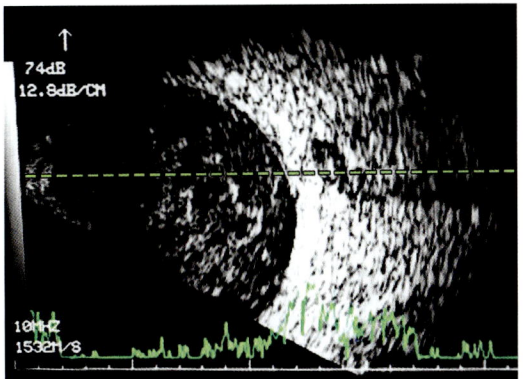

Fig. 8: Ultrasound biomicroscopy (UBM) image of endophthalmitis, showing dot-like echoes and pseudomembrane-like structures in the vitreous cavity, corresponding to mild–moderate amplitude spikes on the A-scan.

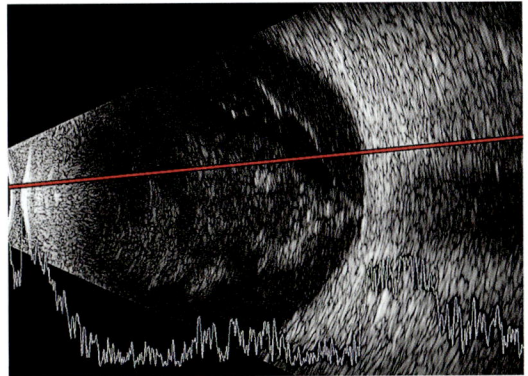

Fig. 7: Ultrasound biomicroscopy (UBM) image illustrating vitreous hemorrhage with posterior vitreous detachment.

Endophthalmitis

Multiple dot-like and pseudomembrane like echoes noted in the vitreous cavity corresponding to mild–moderate amplitude spikes on A-scan suggestive of endophthalmitis **(Fig. 8)**.

Choroidal Detachment

Left image **(Fig. 9A)***:* A dome-shaped elevation with limited after-movement with dot-like echoes and apposed membranes on USG suggestive of kissing choroidals in hemorrhagic CD.

Right image **(Fig. 9B)***:* A dome-shaped echolucent elevation (serous CD) with no retinal apposition seen after drainage of the kissing choroidals.

Fundal Coloboma

Excavation of the ocular coats (white arrow) with a moderate amplitude spike corresponding with the detached intercalary membrane (red arrowhead) overlying the colobomatous area **(Fig. 10)**.

Optic Nerve Head Drusen

Anechoic on B-scan with localized hyperechoic focus at the optic nerve head corresponding to high reflectivity on A-scan vector **(Fig. 11)**.

Optic Nerve Head Cupping

A depression or bean pot-like configuration is noted at optic nerve head (red arrow) suggestive of glaucomatous optic nerve head cupping **(Fig. 12)**.

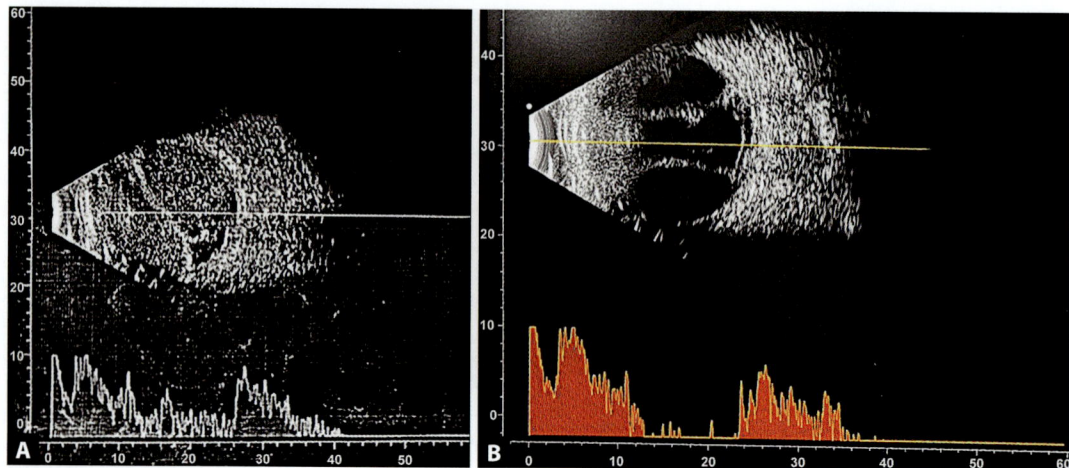

Figs. 9A and B: Ultrasound biomicroscopy (UBM) image of (A) Choroidal detachment—a dome-shaped elevation with limited after-movement and dot-like echoes, along with apposed membranes, indicating hemorrhagic choroidal detachment and kissing choroidals. (B) Serous choroidal detachment—a dome-shaped echolucent elevation with no retinal apposition seen after drainage of the kissing choroidals.

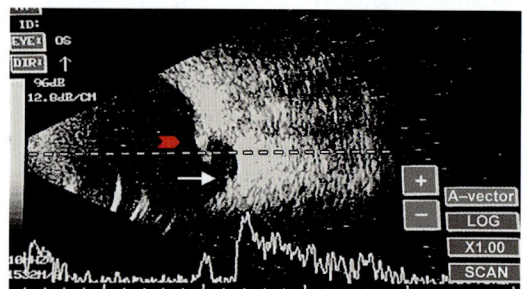

Fig. 10: Ultrasound biomicroscopy (UBM) image showing fundal coloboma, depicting ocular coat excavation (white arrow) and a moderate amplitude spike corresponding to the detached intercalary membrane (red arrowhead) overlying the colobomatous area.

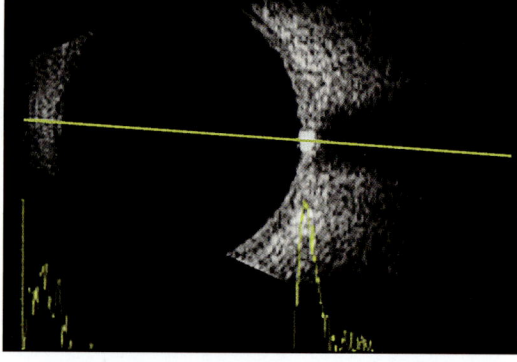

Fig. 11: Ultrasound biomicroscopy (UBM) image showing optic nerve head drusen, which appears anechoic on B-scan with a localized hyperechoic focus at the optic nerve head, corresponding to high reflectivity on A-scan.

Asteroid Hyalosis

Medium-to-high amplitude spikes noted in the vitreous cavity, localized to the core of the vitreous body with clear lucid interval noted in retrovitreal/preretinal space (red arrow) **(Fig. 13)**.

T-sign in Posterior Scleritis

A hypoechoic space in the subtenon space and around the optic nerve head giving the appearance of the letter "T". It indicates accumulation of fluid in the subtenon space **(Fig. 14)**.

Ocular Ultrasonography in Retinal Disorders

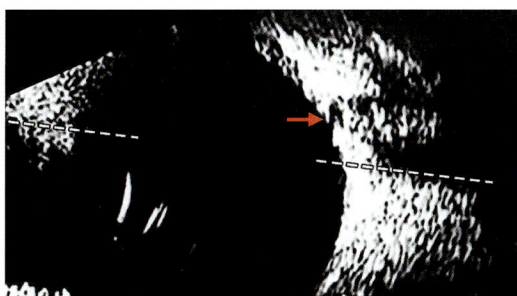

Fig. 12: Ultrasound biomicroscopy (UBM) image of optic nerve head cupping, demonstrating a depression or bean pot-like configuration at the optic nerve head (red arrow), suggestive of glaucomatous cupping.

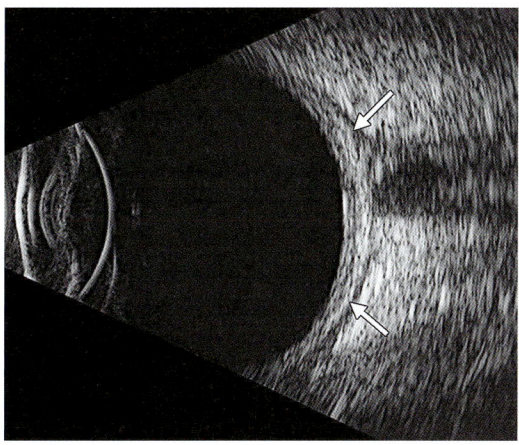

Fig. 14: Ultrasound biomicroscopy (UBM) image of T-sign in posterior scleritis, showing a hypoechoic space around the optic nerve head and in the subtenon space, forming the appearance of the letter "T", indicating fluid accumulation in the subtenon space.

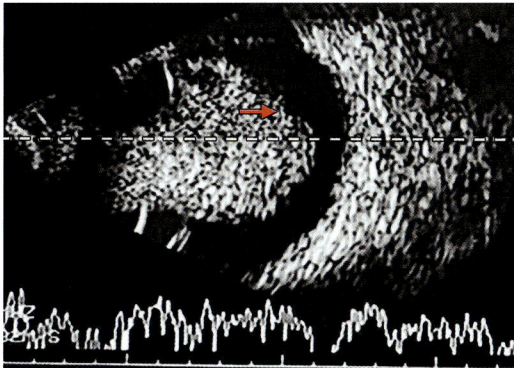

Fig. 13: Ultrasound biomicroscopy (UBM) image of asteroid hyalosis, showing medium-to-high amplitude spikes in the vitreous cavity, localized to the core of the vitreous body with a clear lucid interval in the retrovitreal/preretinal space (red arrow).

REFERENCES

1. Baun G, Greenwood I. The application of ultrasonic locating techniques to ophthalmology. Arch ophthalmol. 1958; 60(2):263-79.
2. Ossoinig KC, Cennamo G, Byrne SF. Echographic differential diagnosis of optic nerve lesions. In: Thijssen JM, Verbeek AM (Eds). Ultrasonography in Ophthalmology, Dordrecht/Boston/Lancaster: Dr. W. Junk Publishers; 1981. p. 327.
3. Ossoinig KC. Standardized echography: Basic principles, clinical applications, and results. Int Ophthalmol Clin. 1979;19(1):127-210.
4. Hewick SA, Fairhead AC, Culy JC, Atta HR. A comparison of 10 MHz and 20 MHz ultrasound probes in imaging the eye and orbit. Br J Ophthalmol. 2004;88(4):551-5.
5. Restori M, Wright JE. C-scan ultrasonography in orbital diagnosis. Br J Ophthalmol. 1977; 61(12):735-40.

VIDEO LEGENDS

Video 1: Retinal detachment.
Video 2 Giant retinal tear.
Video 3: Vitreous hemorrhage.
Video 4: Tractional retinal detachment.

Vitrectomy

N Shastikaa, Prasanna Venkatesh Ramesh, Shruthy Vaishali Ramesh, Anugraha Balamurugan, Ashik Azad, Navaneeth Krishna MP, Ajanya K Aradhya

INTRODUCTION

- Vitrectomy is a surgical procedure involving the partial or complete removal of the vitreous humor, and it is rarely performed as an isolated procedure.
- *Indications:*
    - For posterior segment diseases like:
        - Rhegmatogenous retinal detachment with proliferative vitreoretinopathy (PVR)
        - Giant retinal tears
        - Tractional retinal detachment
        - Epiretinal membranes
        - Macular holes
        - Long-standing vitreous hemorrhage
        - Endophthalmitis
        - Retained foreign body
    - Anterior segment indications include:
        - Along with cataract surgeries for subluxated cataract, pediatric cataract, etc.
        - Persistent primary hyperplastic vitreous
        - Pupillary block
        - Malignant glaucoma

Procedure

- *Vitrectomy* uses an operating microscope with a contact or noncontact viewing system for a magnified and binocular image.
- It involves a closed-system approach with three ports placed 3–4 mm behind the surgical limbus **(Fig. 1)**.
- One port infuses balanced salt solution to maintain intraocular pressure, with epinephrine added to reduce bleeding and cause mydriasis.
- The other two ports allow access to the vitreous cavity with tools like a fiber-optic endoilluminator and various instruments for manipulating, dissecting, or removing intraocular tissues, fluids, and objects.
- Instruments required:
    - Vitreous cutter
    - Intraocular forceps
    - Micro-pick forceps
    - Intraocular scissors
    - Endolaser probe
    - Extrusion cannula
    - Fragmatome
- Retinal tamponade can be achieved by using air, sulfur hexafluoride (SF6), perfluoropropane (C3F8), or silicone oil as a vitreous substitute.

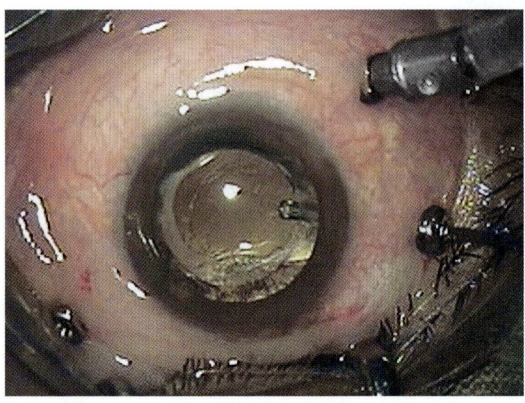

Fig. 1: Three port 23-gauge vitrectomy.

Possible complications include:
- Endophthalmitis
- Cataract
- Hypotony
- Iatrogenic phototoxicity

INTRAVITREAL INJECTION

This being one of the most common ophthalmic procedures performed involves administering drugs directly into the vitreous using a fine needle.

Uses
- *Antiangiogenic drugs:* Antivascular endothelial growth factor (VEGF) and antivascular endothelial growth factor receptor (VEGFr) agents such as aflibercept, ranibizumab, bevacizumab, faricimab, and brolucizumab.
  - *Contraindications:* Stroke, cardiac arrest, uncontrolled hypertension, and anticoagulants.
  - *Adverse effects:* Subconjunctival hemorrhage and increased intraocular pressure (IOP).
- Steroid preparations
- Antimicrobials

COMMON INDICATIONS
- Age-related macular degeneration
- Diabetic retinopathy
- Macular edema from venous occlusive disease
- Endophthalmitis

Procedure
- Performed under strict aseptic conditions with topical or subconjunctival anesthesia.
- *Site of injection:* 3–4 mm posterior to the limbus (4 mm for phakic, 3.5 mm for pseudophakic, and 3 mm for aphakic).
- *Direction of needle:* Toward the midvitreous.
- The ocular surface is rinsed with sterile saline, and optic nerve perfusion is confirmed.

Complications
- Endophthalmitis
- Raised IOP
- Severe corneal endothelial toxicity (with dexamethasone)

SCLERAL BUCKLING

By externally indenting the sclera, scleral buckling closes retinal breaks. Transscleral cryopexy is used to create a permanent bond between the retina and the retinal pigment epithelium at the break sites. The key step is identifying all retinal breaks and any additional vitreoretinal pathology.

Techniques
- Segmental buckles
- Encircling episcleral buckles
- Radial placement
- Intrascleral techniques

These methods are chosen based on the number and location of retinal breaks, eye size, patient's age, presence of posterior vitreous detachment (PVD), and other vitreoretinal findings.

Complications
- Induced myopia
- Anterior ocular ischemia
- Diplopia
- Extraocular muscle disinsertion
- Ptosis
- Orbital cellulitis
- Subretinal hemorrhage from drainage
- Retinal incarceration at the drainage site

LASER PHOTOCOAGULATION

This procedure involves using lasers to heat target tissue above 65°C, causing protein denaturation. Lasers such as argon, krypton, diode (810 nm), and frequency-doubled neodymium-doped yttrium aluminum garnet (Nd:YAG) are commonly used. The effectiveness depends on light transmission through ocular media and pigment absorption in the target tissue. The laser wavelength is chosen based on the target's absorption characteristics.

Modes of Light Delivery
- *Transpupillary:* Using a slit lamp or indirect ophthalmoscope.
- *Endophotocoagulation:* During vitrectomy.
- *Transscleral:* Using a contact probe.

Procedure
- May require topical, peribulbar, or retrobulbar anesthesia.
- Negative-power planoconcave lenses and high-plus-power lenses can be used for slit-lamp delivery.
- *Macular:* Focal laser photocoagulation is useful for certain macular edema types, extrafoveal choroidal neovascularization, and focal retinal pigment epithelium abnormalities.
- *Peripheral retinal photocoagulation:*
  - *Focal:* Targets specific leakage areas in the retina, treating lesions like retinal arterial microaneurysms and macroaneurysms.
  - *Grid:* Laser applied in a grid pattern over edematous retina.
  - *Barrage:* Argon laser treats retinal tears or holes to prevent detachment.
  - *Panretinal photocoagulation (PRP):* Laser applied to peripheral retina in a scattered pattern, sparing the central macula, reducing retinal oxygen demand, and causing abnormal blood vessels to shrink.

Complications
- Excess energy or misdirected light can cause corneal and iris burns, leading to corneal opacities, iritis, and iris atrophy.
- Optic neuropathy.
- Chorioretinal issues like foveal burns, Bruch membrane ruptures, retinal or choroidal lesions, and exudative detachment.

CONCLUSION

In the management of retinal diseases, vitrectomy serves as a cornerstone for mainly treating conditions like retinal detachment and macular hole.

Scleral buckling, though less commonly performed now with the advent of vitrectomy, it remains as a valuable option for treating retinal breaks without PVD. Additionally, laser photoagulation techniques like panretinal photocoagulation and focal laser treatments continue to play a critical role in stabilizing conditions like diabetic retinopathy and retinal vein occlusions where as anti-VEGF are used for treating macular edema. These procedures are performed with careful consideration of potential complications such as raised intraocular pressure, endophthalmitis, and retinal toxicity, ensuring the best outcomes for patients with retinal disorders. The integration of these procedures is crucial in preserving vision and improving quality of life in patients with retinal diseases.

Vogt–Koyanagi–Harada Disease

Sameeksha Agrawal, Ankit Agrawal

A multisystemic disorder is characterized by:
- Granulomatous panuveitis affecting both anterior and posterior segments.
- Exudative retinal detachments due to choroidal inflammation.
- Associated neurologic (e.g., meningismus and headache) and cutaneous manifestations (e.g., vitiligo and poliosis).
- Poliosis + vitiligo + ocular inflammation → *Vogt* in 1906.
- Primary posterior uveitis + exudative retinal detachments (RDs) + cerebrospinal fluid (CSF) pleocytosis, prodromal phase of malaise and meningeal irritation→ *Harada* in 1926.
- Bilateral anterior uveitis + skin and hair depigmentation → *Koyanagi* in 1929.

PATHOGENESIS

Flowchart 1 showing the pathogenesis of Vogt–Koyanagi–Harada (VKH) disease.

CLASSIFICATION

Flowchart 2 showing the revised diagnostic criteria proposed by the first international workshop on Vogt–Koyanagi–Harada disease.

STAGES

1. Prodromal stage
2. Uveitic stage

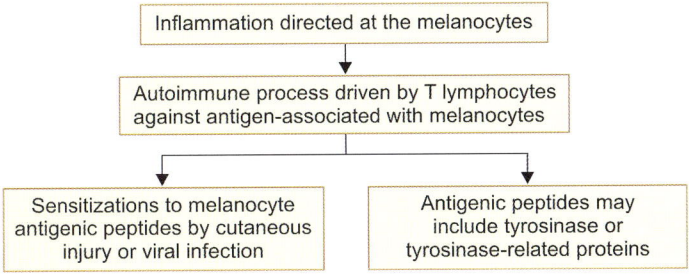

Flowchart 1: The pathogenesis of Vogt–Koyanagi–Harada disease.

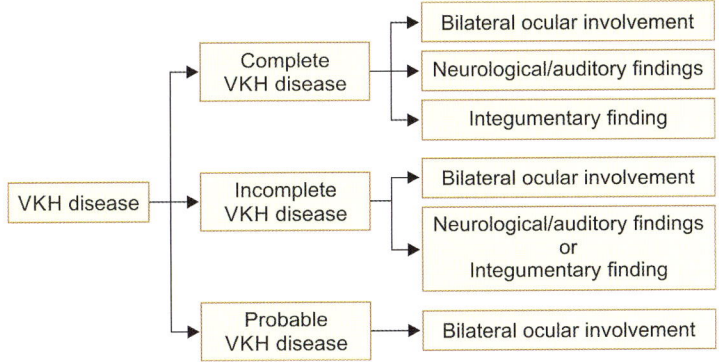

Flowchart 2: The revised diagnostic criteria proposed by the first international workshop on Vogt–Koyanagi–Harada (VKH) disease.

3. Chronic (Convalescent) stage
4. Chronic recurrent stage

Prodromal Stage
- May last for a few days
- Headaches, nausea, dizziness, fever, orbital pain, and meningismus
- Light sensitivity and tearing may occur 1–2 days following the above symptoms.
- Rarely neurological signs such as cranial nerve palsies and optic neuritis
- Cerebrospinal fluid pleocytosis

Uveitic Stage
- Presents with blurring of vision in both eyes.
- One eye may be affected first followed a few days later by the second eye.
- Thickening of the posterior choroid with elevation of the peripapillary retinochoroidal layer.
- Multiple serous retinal detachments
- Hyperemia and edema of the optic nerve head
- The inflammation eventually becomes diffuse, extending into the anterior segment and revealing the presence of flares and cells in the anterior chamber.
- Less commonly—mutton-fat keratic precipitates (KPs), small nodules on the iris surface and pupillary margin. The inflammatory infiltrate in the ciliary body and choroid may cause forward displacement of the lens iris diaphragm, leading to acute angle-closure glaucoma or annular choroidal detachment.

Chronic Stage
- Occurs several weeks after the acute uveitic stage.
- Characterized by development of vitiligo, poliosis, and depigmentation of the choroid.
- Perilimbal vitiligo, also known as "Sugiura's sign" may develop at this stage (Japanese patients)
- Choroidal depigmentation occurs a few months after the uveitic phase.
- Characteristic pale disc with a bright red-orange choroid known as *"sunset-glow fundus".*
- The juxtapapillary area may show marked depigmentation.
- In Hispanics, the sunset-glow fundus may show foci of retinal pigment epithelium (RPE) changes in the form of hyperpigmentation or hypopigmentation.
- Small, yellow, and well-circumscribed areas of chorioretinal atrophy may appear mainly in the inferior mid-periphery of the fundus.

Chronic Recurrent Stage
- The juxtapapillary area may show marked depigmentation.
- Smoldering panuveitis with acute episodic exacerbations of granulomatous anterior uveitis.
- The anterior uveitis may be resistant to local and systemic corticosteroid therapy.
- Iris nodules may be seen during this phase and these appear as round, whitish, well-circumscribed nodules on a background of atrophic iris stroma.
- Visually debilitating complication—subretinal neovascular membranes
- Other features may include:
  - Posterior subcapsular cataract
  - Glaucoma (angle-closure or open-angle)
  - Posterior synechiae

INVESTIGATIONS

Mainly a clinical diagnosis when the patient presents with ocular and extraocular manifestations.

TABLE 1: Clinical diagnostic procedure, when the patient presents without extraocular manifestations.		
Imaging modality	*Acute*	*Chronic*
Fluorescein angiography	• Delayed choroidal filling • Choroidal hyperfluorescence • Numerous punctate hyperfluorescent dots at level of RPE—enlarge and stain the surrounding SRF • Optic disc hyperfluorescence	Moth-eaten appearance, with multiple hyperfluorescent RPE window defects without progressive staining
Indocyanine green angiography	• Diffuse delayed choroidal perfusion • Segmental hypercyanescence and hypocyanescence	Multiple hypocyanescent spots
Optical coherence tomography	• Subretinal fluid with septae • Presence of fibrin in subretinal space • Increased choroidal thickness • Choroidal undulation and excavation	RPE changes
Fundus autofluorescence	Diffuse hyperautofluorescence with areas of blockage due to subretinal fluid	RPE changes, atrophic nummular scars—Decreased FAF
Ultrasonography	Diffuse, low-to-medium reflective thickening of the choroid posteriorly	

(FAF: fundus autofluorescence; RPE: retinal pigment epithelium; SRF: subretinal fluid)

When the disease presents without extraocular changes **(Table 1)**:
- Optical coherence tomography (OCT)
- Fluorescein angiography
- Indocyanine green (ICG) angiography
- Ultrasonography
- Lumbar puncture

DIFFERENTIAL DIAGNOSIS

- Sympathetic ophthalmia
- Uveal effusion syndrome
- Posterior scleritis
- Acute posterior multifocal placoid pigment epitheliopathy
- Central serous chorioretinopathy
- Primary intraocular B-cell lymphoma
- Sarcoidosis

TREATMENT

- Steroids—Early and aggressive use of systemic corticosteroids followed by slow tapering over 3–6 months is the treatment of choice to suppress the intraocular inflammation and to prevent the development of complications related to the ocular inflammation.
- Immunosuppressive agents
- Patients with inflammatory cell infiltration in the anterior chamber require topical corticosteroids and cycloplegics to reduce ciliary spasm and prevent posterior synechiae formation.

COMPLICATIONS

The complications of chronic recurrent Vogt–Koyanagi–Harada disease include:
- Cataract
- Glaucoma
- Choroidal neovascularization
- Subretinal fibrosis
- Optic atrophy

CHAPTER 31

Optic Neuritis

Sameer Chaudhary, Deepika Beeraka

INTRODUCTION

Optic neuritis (ON) encompasses a group of conditions characterized by inflammation of the optic nerve. It is the most common cause of optic nerve dysfunction in young adults and an important cause of visual dysfunction.[1] That said, it is also often associated with several systemic conditions that are known to cause significant morbidity. This makes it imperative to be familiar with ON and its various systemic associations. As a large proportion of cases of ON is associated with demyelinating disorders, this chapter mainly focuses on them.

Much of the knowledge about ON was established by the optic neuritis treatment trial (ONTT), a multicenter collaborative clinical trial that included 457 patients with acute optic neuritis and randomized them to either one of the three treatment groups: oral prednisolone alone (1 mg/kg/day for 14 days), intravenous methylprednisolone (IVMP) (1 g/day for 3 days) followed by oral prednisolone for 11 days, or placebo. The patients were followed up for 15 years.[2]

Case (Video 1)

ETIOLOGY

The causes of ON are protean **(Table 1)**. Despite the numerous entities that can present with ON, most of the cases are due to demyelinating lesions, which are either idiopathic (isolated) or associated with systemic demyelinating disorders. The most commonly associated demyelinating disorder is multiple sclerosis (MS), followed by neuromyelitis optica spectrum disorder (NMOSD) and myelin oligodendrocyte antibody disease (MOGAD).[3,4] Approximately 20% of the patients with MS present with ON as the foremost demyelinating episode, and half of the MS patients develop ON during the disease.[5]

TABLE 1: Different etiologies of optic neuritis.

Demyelinating	Infectious	Other inflammatory/autoimmune causes
• Idiopathic • MS • NMOSD • MOGAD	Viral: • VZV • HIV Bacterial: • TB • Syphilis • Borrelia • Bartonella • Toxoplasma	• Sarcoidosis • Granulomatous polyangiitis • SLE • Sjögren syndrome • CRMP-IgG mediated • Autoimmune GFAP astrocytopathy

(CRMP: collapsin response mediator protein; GFAP: glial fibrillary acidic protein; HIV: human immunodeficiency virus; MOGAD: myelin oligodendrocyte antibody disease; MS: multiple sclerosis; NMOSD: neuromyelitis optica spectrum disorder; SLE: systemic lupus erythematosus; TB: tuberculosis; VZV: varicella zoster virus)

TABLE 2: Comparison of the demographic profile of MS, NMOSD, and MOGAD.

Patient's profile	MS	NMOSD	MOGAD
Age	20–50 years (32 years)	40 years	Biphasic 5–10 years, 20–45 years (20–35 years)
Gender	F:M = 3:1	F:M = 7:1–9:1	No clear sex predilection
Course	Relapsing Progressive	Relapsing	Monophasic or relapsing

(MOGAD: myelin oligodendrocyte antibody disease; MS: multiple sclerosis; NMOSD: neuromyelitis optica spectrum disorder)

TABLE 3: Features of typical and atypical optic neuritis.

Characteristics	Typical optic neuritis	Atypical optic neuritis
Age	20–50 years	<12 or >50 years
Gender	Female predominant	No clear sex predilection
Onset	Acute or subacute	Gradual
Laterality	Unilateral	Bilateral
Presenting visual acuity	Better than 6/60	Worse than 6/60
Pain	Present, worsens on extraocular movements (90%)	Absent
RAPD	Present	May or may not be present
Fundus	Two-thirds of cases normal	Severe disc swelling, macular exudates, optic disc or retinal hemorrhages
Course	Stablizes over 2 weeks	Progresses beyond 2 weeks, recurrent disease course
Response to steroids	Excellent	Can be refractory
Prognosis	Excellent	Poor

DEMOGRAPHICS

Although the most common etiology of ON remains demyelination and MS remains the most common association, in India, more atypical presentations and a relatively suboptimal prognosis have been reported as compared to the western part of the world.

For acute demyelinating ON, there is a predilection for the female gender, and it more commonly affects the age group of 20–50 years **(Table 2)**.

CLINICAL FEATURES

Based on the clinical presentation, ON has been broadly classified as typical and atypical **(Table 3)**. The classical set of complaints is painful (90%), acute or subacute, unilateral loss of vision **(Fig. 1)**.

- The axons of the papillomacular bundle are predominantly affected, and most of the clinical features result from it. As these fibers project from the macula, their affliction grossly impairs central visual

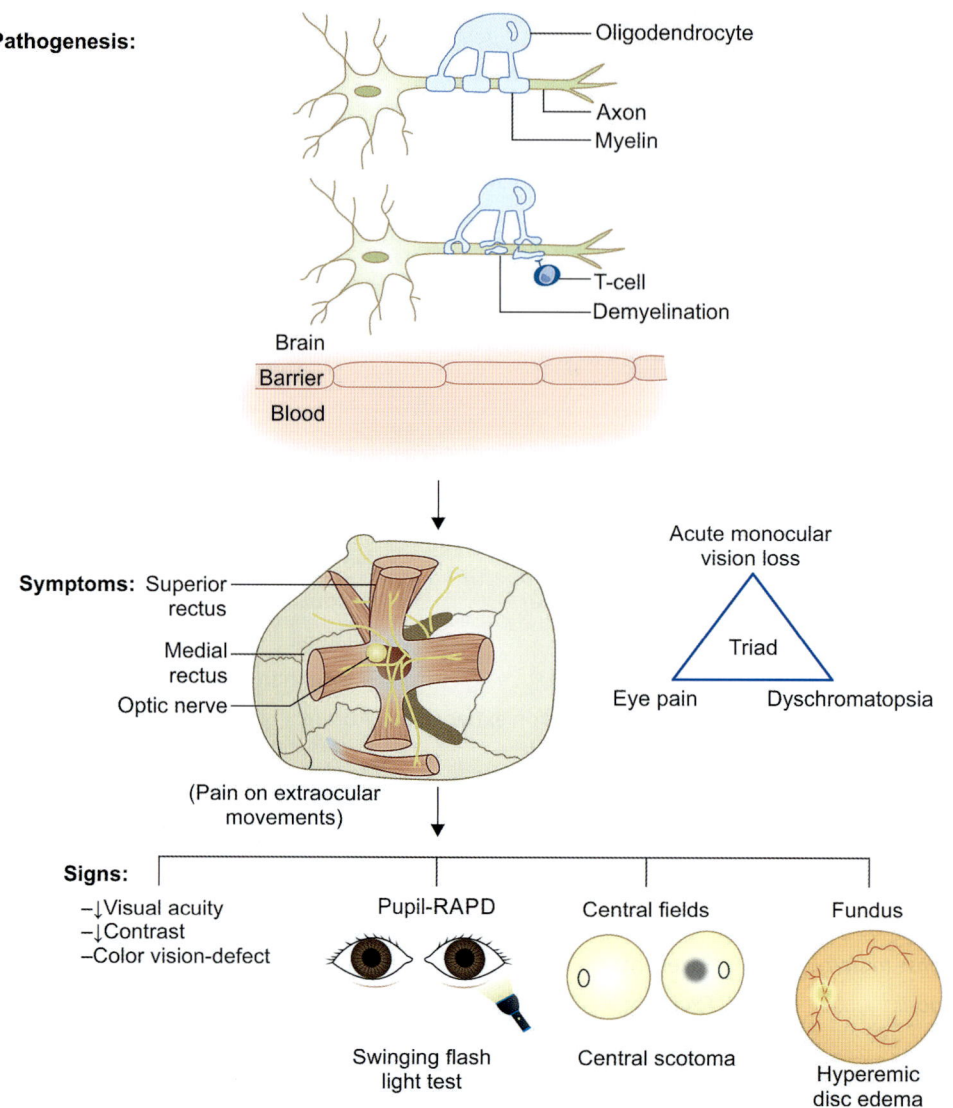

Fig. 1: Illustration depicting the pathogenesis and clinical features of demyelinating optic neuritis. The top section shows immune infiltration, which consists predominantly of CD8 + T cells, which destroy the oligodendrocytes and result in demyelination of the optic nerve. The middle section (left) depicts *Whitnall's hypothesis*, which states that the pain worsens during ocular movements due to the traction at the origin of the superior and medial rectus at the optic nerve sheath. The middle section (right) and bottom section show the other classical clinical features.

acuity (90%) and color vision and most commonly results in a central scotoma. Although central scotoma is present in almost half of the patients (48%), other field defects such as paracentral scotoma (Fig. 2), centro-cecal scotoma and peripheral field defects can also be present.

- When the ON is unilateral, as in typical ON, it almost always presents with a relative afferent pupillary defect.

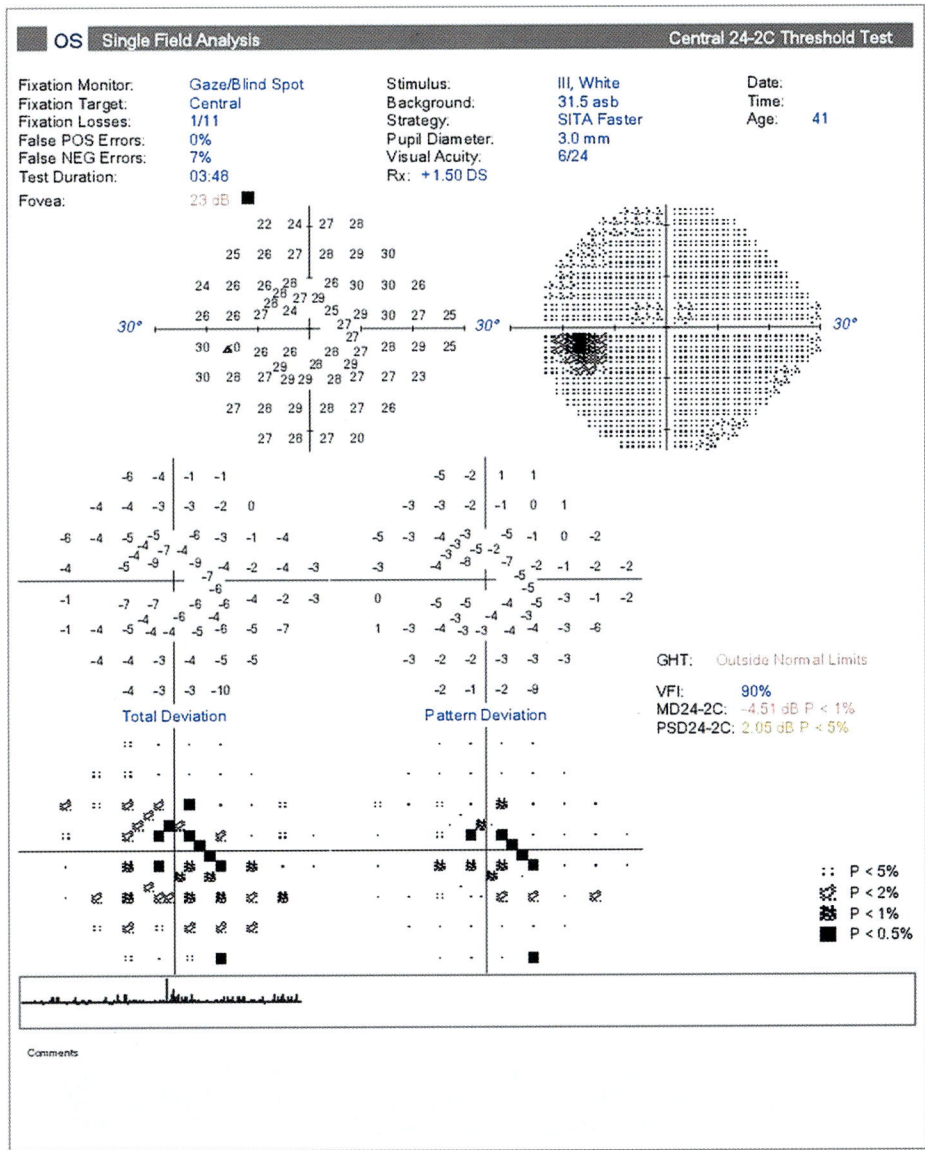

Fig. 2: Automated perimetry of the left eye done using Humphreys Field Analyzer in a 41-year-old female patient with optic neuritis showing a paracentral scotoma with mild generalized depression of the field. The foveal threshold is reduced, and the pattern standard deviation plot shows a paracentral scotoma. The mean deviation value is suggestive of generalized depression.

- The pain typically worsens on extraocular movements. According to *Whitnall's hypothesis,* this is due to traction on the origins of the medial and superior rectus on the optic nerve sheath **(Fig. 1)**.
- Fundus examination can either be normal or show optic disc swelling **(Fig. 3)**. The presence of perineuritis and neuroretinitis can suggest MOGAD, sarcoidosis, and infectious etiologies.

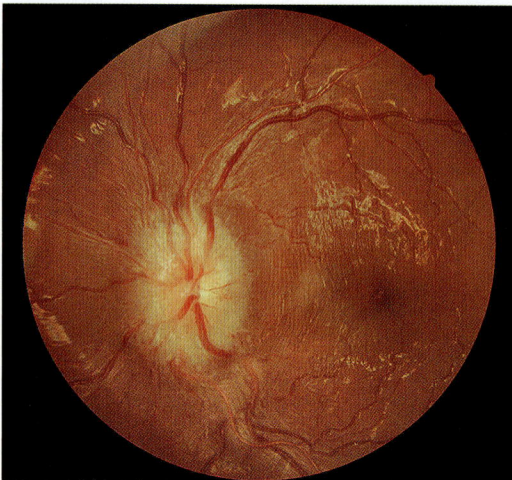

Fig. 3: Fundus photo of left eye with acute demyelinating optic neuritis presenting as papillitis. The image shows significant disc swelling with chorioretinal folds temporal to it.

SYSTEMIC PHENOMENON

- *Uhthoff's phenomenon:* Transient worsening of neurological function due to increase in body temperature. This might cause transient obscuration of vision as well following exercise or hot bath.
- *Pulfrich phenomenon:* Due to a delay in signal conduction in one of the optic pathways due to demyelination, there is a discrepancy in visual perception between the two eyes. This results in an illusion where two-dimensional objections are perceived as three-dimensional.
- *Lhermitte's phenomenon:* Electric shock-like sensation in the neck and back when the former is flexed.
- *Multiple sclerosis hug:* A tight band-like sensation around the upper body seen in association with thoracic cord lesions.
- *Area postrema syndrome:* Specific of NMOSD, this is characterized by intractable hiccups and vomiting due to the involvement of area postrema in dorsal medulla.

DIAGNOSIS

The diagnosis of ON is essentially clinical. However, imaging is often required to confirm the diagnosis and rule out central nervous system (CNS) demyelinating lesions. When the presentation is atypical, other ancillary investigations might be ordered.[3,6]

IMAGING

Magnetic resonance imaging (MRI) remains the imaging of choice. The following MRI imaging protocols are usually preferred:

- Short T1 inversion recovery (STIR) images are used to visualize optic nerves and spinal cord demyelinating lesions. STIR inverts the magnetization of hydrogen atoms from fat (present in orbit and around the spinal cord) and suppresses their signal.
- Fluid-attenuated inversion recovery (FLAIR) images for visualization of demyelinating lesions in the brain. FLAIR inverts the magnetization of water molecules from cerebrospinal fluid (CSF) and allows the visualization of periventricular demyelinating lesions in MS.
- Gadolinium enhancement
- 1–3 mm thin sections of optic nerve

When evaluating the MRI of a patient with suspected ON, the following points should be considered:

- Location of lesions along the optic nerve
- Location of lesions in the brain and spinal cord
- Length of the lesions along the optic nerve and spinal cord
- Presence of perineural and orbital enhancement

The presence of contrast enhancement of the optic nerve is highly specific (94%) for ON and helps to differentiate it from

Optic Neuritis

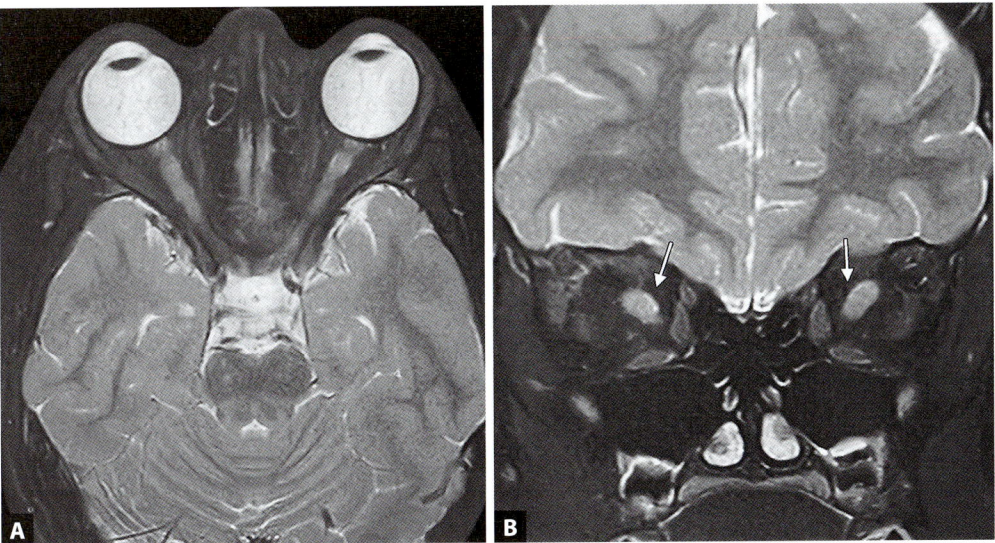

Figs. 4A and B: T2-weighted (T2W) MRI axial and coronal section, showing thickening and enhancement of both optic nerves suggestive of bilateral optic neuritis.

noninflammatory optic neuropathies **(Figs. 4A and B)**. **Table 4 and Figure 5** compare the MRI features of the three demyelinating syndromes.

ANCILLARY INVESTIGATIONS

- *Serum antibodies:* Both AQP4-immunoglobulin G (IgG) and MOG-IgG have significant diagnostic value for NMOSD and MOGAD, respectively. Cell-based assays have been recommended over indirect immunofluorescence antibody assay and enzyme-linked immunosorbent assays (ELISAs). As testing them remains costly and is not widely available in the Indian subcontinent, they should be investigated when the presentation is atypical and significant clinical suspicion is present. Both AQP4-IgG and MOG IgG have >95% specificity and a sensitivity between 75 and 80%. The latter means that a negative serology does not rule out the disease.[7]
- Cerebrospinal fluid analysis:
  - *Pleocytosis:* It is frequently seen in MOGAD-ON and NMOSD-ON. Whereas for MS, it is variable and is rarely very high.
  - *Oligoclonal bands:* These are bands of immunoglobulins present in CSF and indicate inflammation of the CNS **(Fig. 6)**. These have 95% sensitivity and 87% specificity for MS.
  - *Protein:* It might be elevated in MOGAD-ON and NMOSD-ON.
- *Visual evoked potentials (VEPs):* Increased latency with preserved wave morphology is indicative of a demyelinating process. The sensitivity of VEP is around 85% **(Fig. 11)**.

TREATMENT

The standard of treatment remains high-dose corticosteroids, as established by the ONTT. This involves the administration of 1 g IVMP for 3 days, followed by oral prednisolone 1 mg/kg/day for 11 days and weekly tapering.

TABLE 4: Comparison of MRI features of MS, NMOSD, and MOGAD.

Feature	MS	NMOSD	MOGAD
Location of lesions along optic nerve	• Unilateral **(Fig. 7)** • Anterior optic nerve predominantly	• Bilateral • Affects posterior segments, chiasma, and optic tract more commonly **(Figs. 8 and 9A)**	• Bilateral • Can affect all segments, anterior more common
Length of the lesion (Most useful parameter)	Focal	Longitudinally extensive (≥50% of the prechiasmal length)	Longitudinally extensive
Perineural and orbital enhancement	Rarely found	Rarely found	Majority of MOGAD patients (Can also be present in sarcoidosis and infectious causes)

Brain	• Well-defined lesions involving the periventricular, juxtacortical, and infratentorial white matter
	• Perpendicular periventricular lesions—"Dawson's fingers" **(Figs. 9B and 10A)**
		• Periventricular lesions involving:
		  – Thalamus and hypothalamus
		  – Cerebellar and dorsal brainstem lesions
		  – Corpus callosum **(Fig. 10B)**
		• Area postrema
		• Subcortical cerebral white matter
			• Deep gray matter lesions
			• Multiple ill-defined lesions in supratentorial and infratentorial white matter
			• Ill-defined lesions involving medulla, pons, or middle cerebellar peduncle

Spinal cord	Lesions <1 vertebral segments, involving peripheral regions of the cord—nodular enlargement of the cord	More frequently involves the lower cord (conus) and the central gray matter—"H" sign	LETM (≥3 contiguous vertebral segments)

(LETM: longitudinally extensive transverse myelitis; MOGAD: myelin oligodendrocyte antibody disease; MS: multiple sclerosis; NMOSD: neuromyelitis optica spectrum disorder)

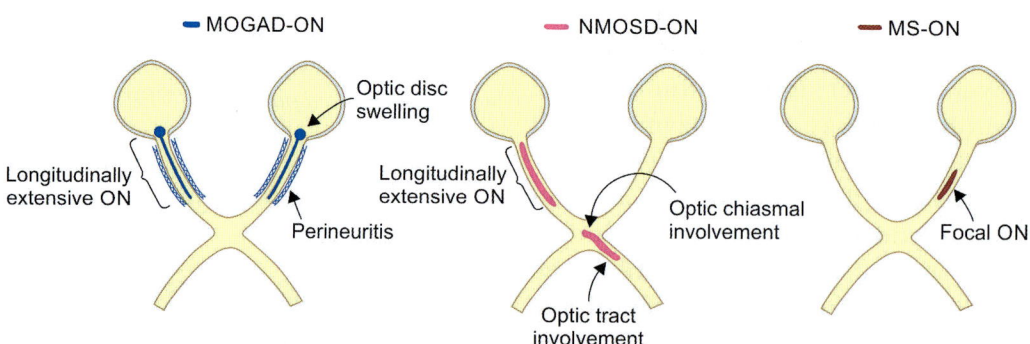

Fig. 5: Illustration comparing the MRI features of MOGAD-ON, NMOSD-ON, and MS-ON. (Left) MOGAD-ON shows bilateral longitudinally extensive ON with perineuritis and optic disc swelling. (Middle) NMOSD-ON shows longitudinally extensive ON with optic chiasmal and optic tract involvement. (Left) MS-ON shows focal ON. (MOGAD: myelin oligodendrocyte antibody disease; MS: multiple sclerosis; NMOSD: neuromyelitis optica spectrum disorder; ON: optic neuritis)

Optic Neuritis

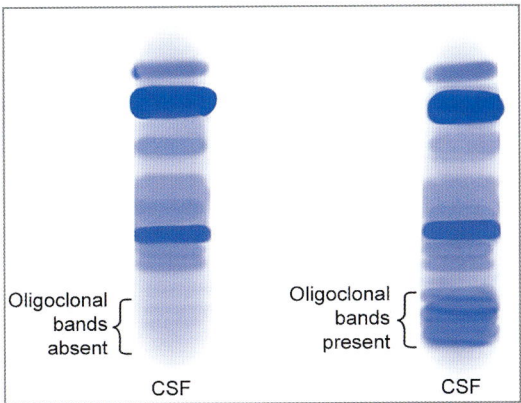

Fig. 6: Illustration depicting the result of cerebrospinal fluid (CSF) analysis for oligoclonal bands using immunofixation electrophoresis. The result on the left is normal, and the one on the right is abnormal.

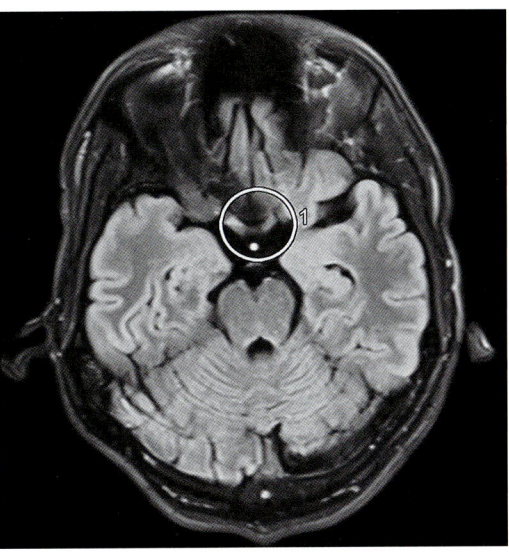

Fig. 8: FLAIR MRI axial section. Hyperintense lesions seen in the optic chiasma, suggestive of NMOSD related optic neuritis.

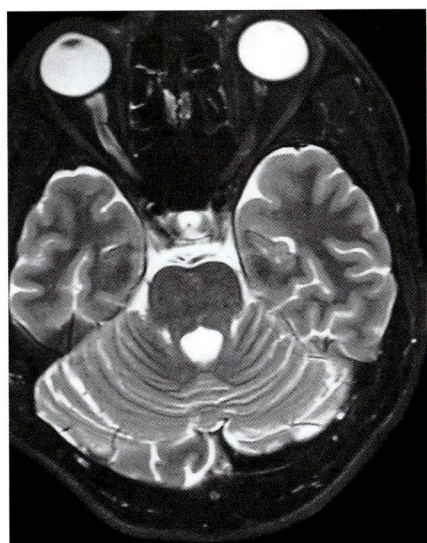

Fig. 7: T2W MRI axial section showing thickening and enhancement of right optic nerve suggestive of right sided optic neuritis in a case of multiple sclerosis.

Although the end visual outcome does not differ significantly when compared to placebo, it accelerates visual recovery and delays conversion to MS. Oral steroids should not be used alone as they have been shown to double the risk of recurrence.

In steroid-refractory cases, which is relatively common in NMOSD, immunotherapy should be started in the form of plasma exchange or intravenous immunoglobulin. Long-term immunosuppression might be required to prevent relapses. Azathioprine is the first-line steroid-sparing agent, and other alternatives include mycophenolate mofetil and methotrexate. Rituximab is a monoclonal antibody against CD20 and is widely used.

COURSE AND PROGNOSIS

Acute demyelinating ON usually stabilizes over 2 weeks, followed by a phase of rapid improvement and a phase of gradual improvement. More than 90% of the patients improve within 5 weeks of onset. Overall, the prognosis is excellent with more than two-thirds of the patients achieving the best corrected visual acuity of 6/6.

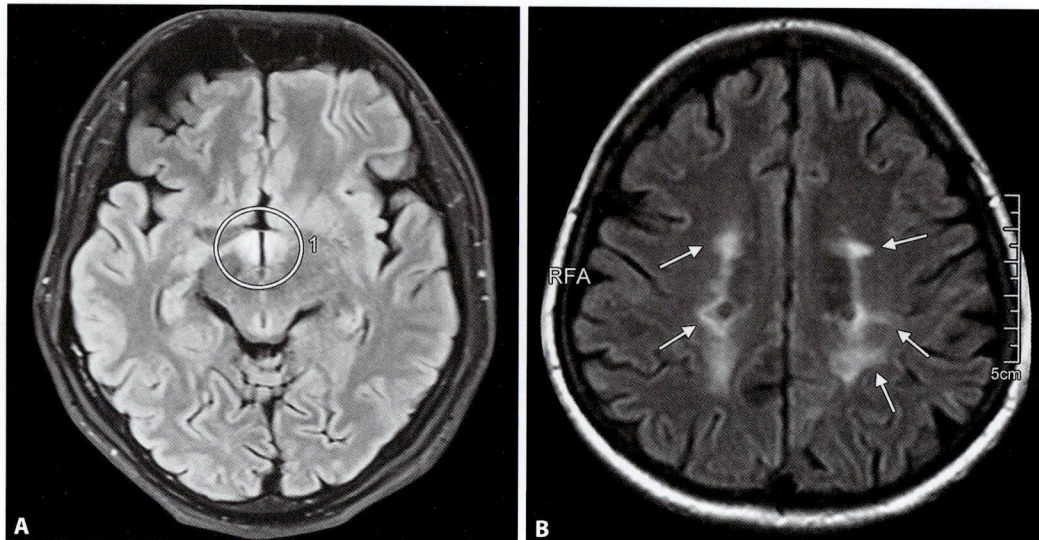

Figs. 9A and B: (A) FLAIR MRI axial section. Hyperintense lesions seen in the pre-chiasmal optic nerve bilaterally, suggestive of NMOSD related optic neuritis; (B) FLAIR MRI axial section. Hyperintense periventricular lesions seen oriented perpendicularly in multiple sclerosis, suggestive of "Dawson's fingers".

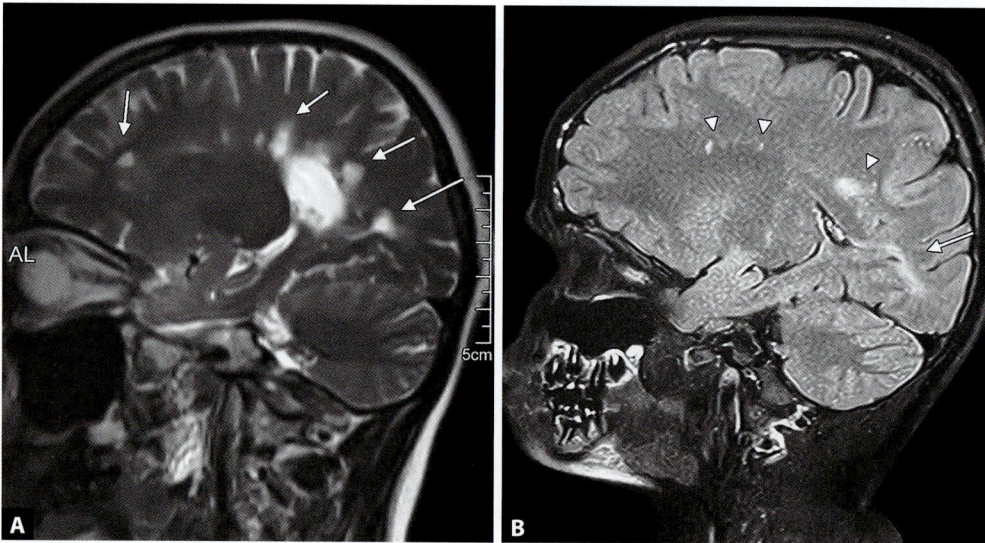

Figs. 10A and B: (A) T2W MRI sagittal section. Hyperintense periventricular lesions seen oriented perpendicularly in multiple sclerosis, suggestive of "Dawson's fingers"; (B) FLAIR MRI sagittal section. The image depicts hyperintense periventricular lesions involving the corpus callosum in a patient with neuromyleitic optica spectrum disorder.

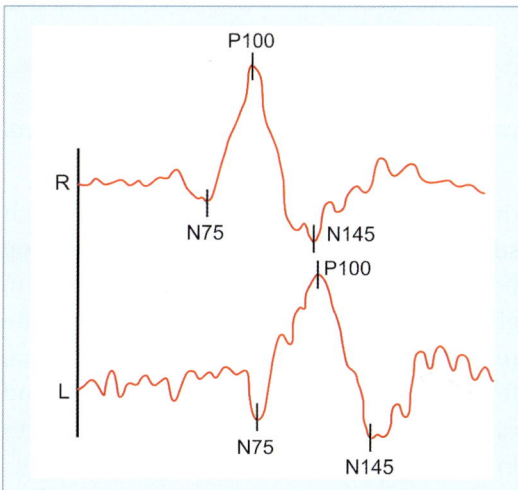

Fig. 11: Illustration depicting visual evoked potential (VEP) of the right optic pathway (top section), which is normal and the left optic pathway (bottom section), which is affected by optic neuritis. Between the two eyes, the amplitude is almost similar. However, the latency is significantly increased in the left optic pathway.

VIDEO LEGEND

Video 1: Animation showing a case scenario of a typical case of optic neuritis—its presentation, clinical features, and management.

REFERENCES

1. Bennett JL. Optic Neuritis. Continuum (Minneap Minn). 2019;25(5):1236-64.
2. Beck RW, Cleary PA, Anderson MM Jr, Keltner JL, Shults WT, Kaufman DI, et al. A randomized, controlled trial of corticosteroids in the treatment of acute optic neuritis. The Optic Neuritis Study Group. N Engl J Med. 1992;326(9):581-8.
3. Winter A, Chwalisz B. MRI Characteristics of NMO, MOG and MS Related Optic Neuritis. Semin Ophthalmol. 2020;35(7-8):333-42.
4. Jeyakumar N, Lerch M, Dale RC, Ramanathan S. MOG antibody-associated optic neuritis. Eye (Lond). 2024;38(12):2289-301.
5. Greco G, Colombo E, Gastaldi M, Ahmad L, Tavazzi E, Bergamaschi R, et al. Beyond Myelin Oligodendrocyte Glycoprotein and Aquaporin-4 Antibodies: Alternative Causes of Optic Neuritis. Int J Mol Sci. 2023;24(21):15986.
6. Phuljhele S, Kedar S, Saxena R. Approach to optic neuritis: An update. Indian J Ophthalmol. 2021;69(9):2266-76.
7. Al-Ani A, Chen JJ, Costello F. Myelin oligodendrocyte glycoprotein antibody-associated disease (MOGAD): current understanding and challenges. J Neurol. 2023;270(8):4132-50.

Thyroid Eye Disease

Ankita Aishwarya Agrawal, Rachna Agrawal, Ankit Agrawal

INTRODUCTION

Thyroid eye disease (TED) or Graves' ophthalmopathy (GO) or thyroid-associated ophthalmopathy (TAO) is an autoimmune inflammatory disease affecting the orbit and periorbital tissues associated with thyroid dysfunction. This is the most common cause of both unilateral and bilateral proptosis in adults. The quality of life is significantly affected in these patients due to its effects on vision, protrusion of eyeball, and recurrence, necessitating an understanding of its clinical presentation, pathogenesis, and management options.

EPIDEMIOLOGY

Approximately 25–50% of Graves' disease (GD) cases develop TED.[1] Globally, the prevalence of TED is 86.2% for hyperthyroidism, 10.36% for hypothyroidism, and 7.9% for euthyroidism.[2] The overall incidence of pediatric TED is 0.79–6.5 per 100,000 children.[3] Both age groups show a female predominance. Both active and passive smoking are known risk factors.

PATHOPHYSIOLOGY

The management of TED remains highly challenging due to its complex pathogenesis targeting the thyroid gland and the tissues around the eyes. In Graves' disease, the immune system produces antibodies against the thyrotropin receptor [thyroid-stimulating hormone receptor (TSH-R)], which is expressed not only in the thyroid but also in the orbital tissues. The disease process involves the activation of orbital fibroblasts which stimulate the inflammatory cascade affecting both B and T cells leading to inflammation, glycosaminoglycan deposition, and tissue remodeling.[4] Various risk factors are genetics, female sex, advanced age, smoking, and radioactive iodine therapy.[5] The key features include:

- *Orbital inflammation:* Immune cells infiltrate the orbital tissues, causing swelling.
- *Glycosaminoglycan accumulation:* Increased production of these molecules leads to tissue expansion and impaired venous drainage leading to chemosis, proptosis, and optic neuropathy.
- *Fibrosis:* Chronic inflammation results in the fibrosis of orbital tissues, contributing to restricted eye movement.

PHASES OF THYROID EYE DISEASE

Historically, Rundle's curve has described TED as biphasic disease:[6]
- *Active/Inflammatory phase:* This phase typically lasts 6–18 months, characterized by inflammation and progressive symptoms.
- *Inactive/Chronic phase:* Following the resolution of inflammation, residual fibrosis and structural changes may persist.

CLINICAL PRESENTATION

Symptoms

The patient complains of foreign body sensation, sensitivity to light, bulging of the eyes, retraction of eyelid, double vision, and blurred vision.

Signs[7]

Lid Signs

- *Dalrymple's sign:* Eyelid retraction (most common).
- *Joffroy sign:* Absent crease in the forehead on upgaze.
- *Stellwag sign:* Incomplete and frequent blinking.
- *Von Graefe sign:* Retarded descent of upper lid in downgaze.
- *Kocher sign:* Staring and frightened appearance of eyes.
- *Gifford sign:* Difficulty while everting the upper eyelid.
- *Boston sign:* Jerky movements of eyelids in downgaze.
- *Enroth sign:* Lower eyelid edema.
- *Griffith sign:* Lid lag on upgaze.
- *Vigouroux sign:* Eyelid fullness.

Muscle Signs

- *Mobius sign:* Not able to converge eyes.
- *Ballet sign:* One or more extraocular muscle restriction.
- *Jendrassik sign:* Limitation of abduction and rotation of the eye.

Globe Signs

- *Wilders sign:* Twitching of eyeball on adduction or abduction.
- *Mean sign:* Increased scleral show on upgaze (globe lag).
- *Goldzeiher sign:* Deep temporal bulbar conjunctiva congestion.

Pupillary Signs

- *Cowen sign:* Extensive hippus of consensual pupillary light reflex.
- *Knies sign:* Uneven pupillary dilatation in dim light.

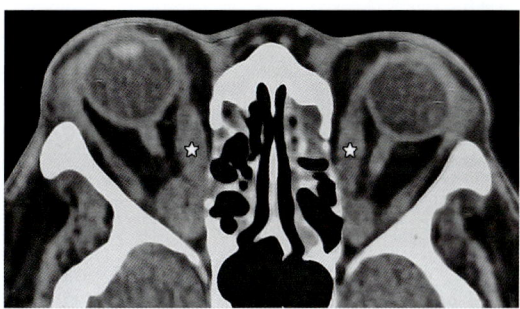

Fig. 1: Axial CT scan of the orbit showing bilateral enlargement of the medial rectus muscle bellies with tendon sparing, characteristic of thyroid eye disease (TED).

Investigations

It is mainly a clinical diagnosis. However, thyroid hormone levels and anti-thyroid antibodies can help us to aid in diagnosis.

Imaging

Computed tomography (CT) scan: CT scan typically shows an enlarged muscle belly with sparing of tendons **(Fig. 1)**. CT scan helps in calculating Barett's muscle index for dysthyroid optic neuropathy. It also helps in planning orbital decompression surgeries.

Magnetic resonance imaging (MRI): It helps to correlate clinical activity status.

DIFFERENTIAL DIAGNOSIS

- Nonspecific orbital inflammatory disorders (NSOID)
- Caroticocavernous fistula
- Orbital myositis (OM)
- Immunoglobulin G 4 (IgG4) disease

MANAGEMENT

The management of TED depends on the activity and grading of the disease. Various scoring systems have been used, such as "NO SPECS" and the VISA scoring system. However, the currently used systems are the "clinical activity score (CAS)" and the

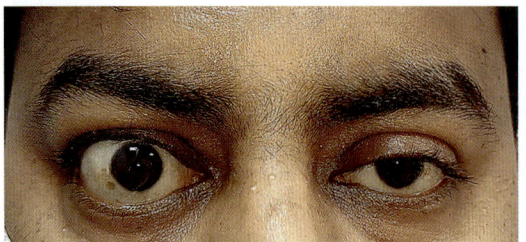
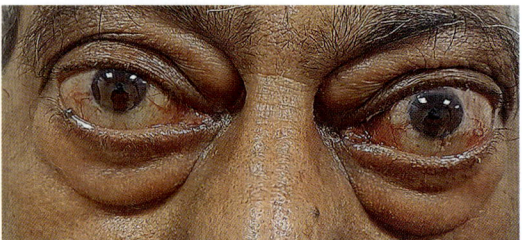

Fig. 2: Clinical photograph of a 32-year-old male with mild thyroid eye disease (TED) and hyperthyroidism, demonstrating right eyelid retraction and 2 mm of proptosis.

Fig. 3: Clinical photograph of a 55-year-old male with moderate thyroid eye disease (TED) and hypothyroidism showing bilateral 4 mm proptosis, periocular edema, pain on extraocular movements, and conjunctival and caruncular congestion.

European Group of Graves' Orbitopathy (EUGOGO) classification.[8] CAS includes spontaneous orbital pain, pain on eye movement, eyelid erythema, conjunctival redness, chemosis, swelling of the eyelids, and inflammation of the caruncle or plica. The score ranges from 0 to 7 initially and from 0 to 10 during follow-up, with a score of ≥3/7 or ≥4/10 indicating active disease that requires intervention.[9]

MILD DISEASE (FIG. 2)

- Eyelid retraction <2 mm
- Proptosis <3 mm
- Transient or no diplopia

Treatment

- *Lifestyle modification:* Cessation of smoking.
- Tablet selenium 100 μg twice daily for 6 months
- Lubricants

MODERATE-TO-SEVERE DISEASE (FIG. 3)

- Eyelid retraction >2 mm
- Proptosis >3 mm
- Constant or inconstant diplopia in functional gaze
- No imminent
- Threat to sight

Treatment

- *Oral steroids:* They have suboptimal response and higher recurrence rate. Not recommended.
- *Intravenous methyl prednisolone (IVMP):* The EUGOGO recommended dose is 500 mg once weekly for 6 weeks, followed by 250 mg once weekly for the next 6 weeks.
- *Immunomodulators:* These are steroid sparing agents.
- *Biologicals:* Newer and promising modality of treatment. Drugs used are rituximab, etanercept, tocilizumab, and teprotumumab. Teprotumumab is the first and only Food and Drug Administration (FDA)-approved biological for TED and has shown a decrease in proptosis.[10]
- Radiotherapy

VERY SEVERE OR SIGHT THREATENING DISEASE (FIG. 4)

- Imminent threat to sight
- Dysthyroid optic neuropathy
- Corneal exposure leading to corneal breakdown

Treatment

- *High-dose IVMP:* 500–1,000 mg/day for 3 days, followed by 500–1,000 mg weekly for six cycles.

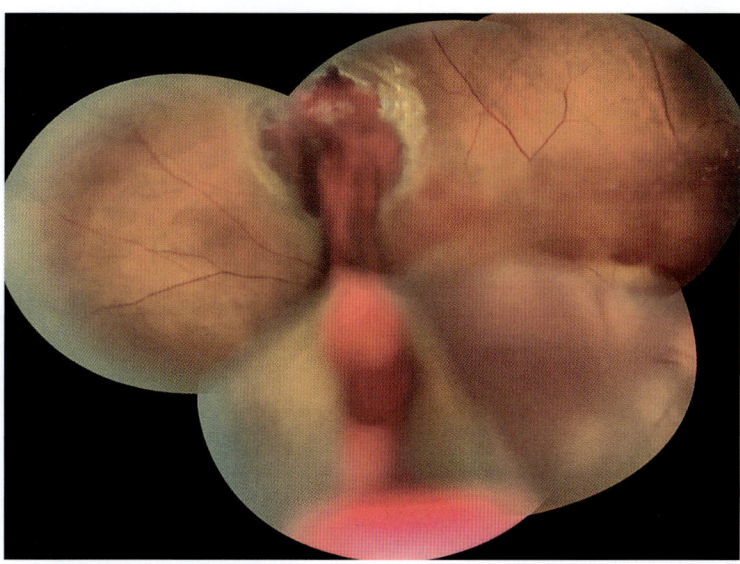

Fig. 1: The fundus photograph showing a large retinal hole, superotemporal to the superior vascular arcade, oozing fresh blood in the vitreous cavity, like a waterfall.

performing a cosmetic procedure. Her best corrected visual acuity (BCVA) in the right eye was 1/60. On fundus examination, there was a large retinal hole, superotemporal to the superior vascular arcade, oozing fresh blood in the vitreous cavity, like a waterfall **(Fig. 1)**. The size of the retinal hole was approximately 4 disc diameters.

A "barrage laser" (double frequency Nd:YAG laser—532 nm) was done around the retinal hole to prevent the development of retinal detachment **(Fig. 2)**. The large "retinal hole" was successfully barraged.

The vitreous hemorrhage gradually absorbed leading to complete recovery of the vision of the patient. Her final BCVA was 6/6 **(Fig. 3)**.

Long-term complications include "choroidal neovascularization" at the site of injury and long-term follow-up of the patient is required to keep a check for the same.

Laser injury during the cosmetic procedure in a dermatologist is very rare with very few prior case reports.[2]

Q-switched Nd:YAG laser has a wavelength of 1,064 nm. It is used to treat nevus of Ota and Hori, or to remove tattoo. It penetrates into the deeper regions of the skin and destroys deep-seated dermal melanocytes by selective photothermolysis.[3]

CASE OF SUBINTERNAL LIMITING MEMBRANE BLEED FOLLOWING INJURY BY LASER LIGHT

A 20-year-old male had exposure to laser light while dancing on the DJ Floor during a party. Laser used for decorative lighting had caused him a subinternal limiting membrane (sub-ILM) bleed **(Figs. 4 and 5)**. His BCVA was CF@1 m at presentation, but it improved to 6/6 in 1 month with only observation.

Many such cases have been reported during festive season where people get exposed to strong laser light which is used for decorative purposes.

Another common presentation of laser-induced ocular injury is damage to photoreceptors at fovea which is called as

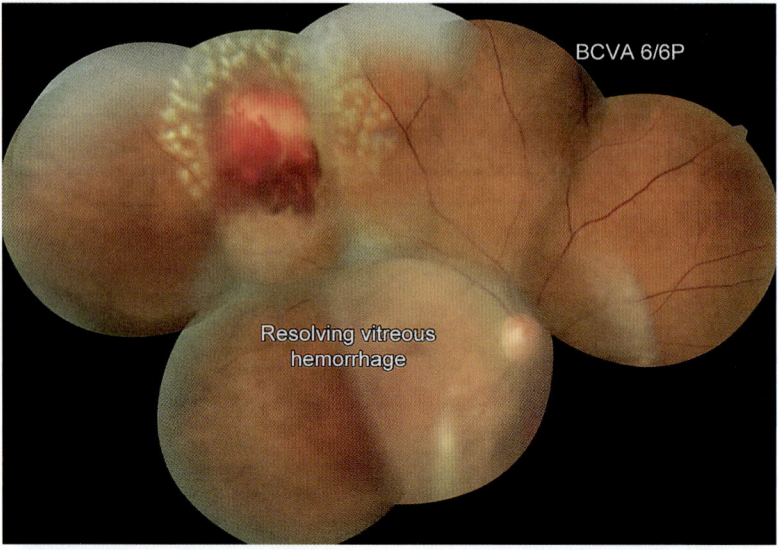

Fig. 2: The fundus photograph showing a "barrage laser" was done around the retinal hole.

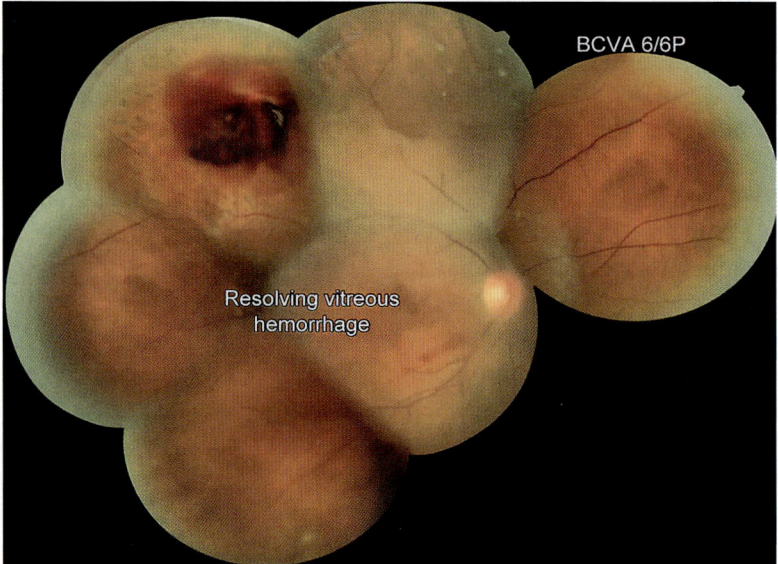

Fig. 3: The fundus photograph showing resolving vitreous hemorrhage.

"Photic Maculopathy" **(Fig. 6)**. Such patients usually have irreversible loss of vision of varying degrees and optical coherence tomography (OCT) of macula reveals disruption of inner segment–outer segment (IS–OS) junction at fovea **(Fig. 7)**.

Complications

- Chorioretinal scarring
- Choroidal neovascular membrane (CNVM)
- Macular cysts

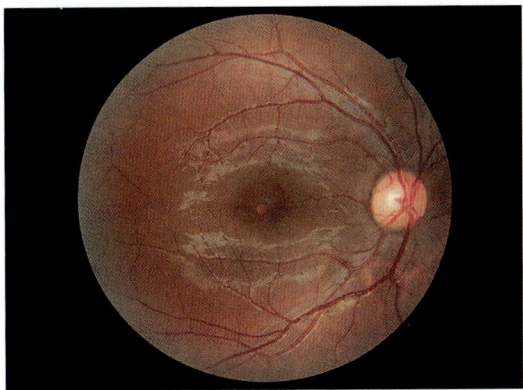

Fig. 4: The fundus photograph showing subinternal limiting membrane (ILM) bleed.

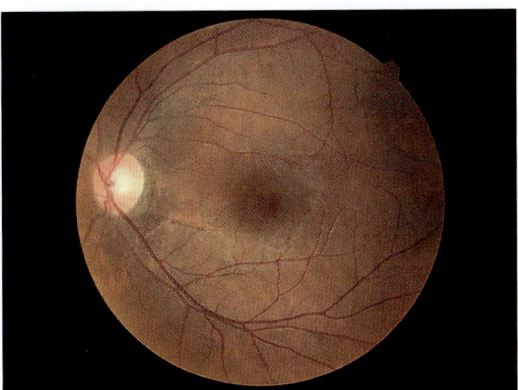

Fig. 6: The fundus image showing "photic maculopathy".

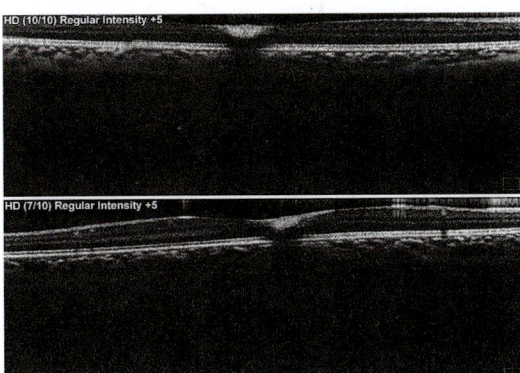

Fig. 5: The optical coherence tomography (OCT) image showing hyperreflective spots on fovea, suggestive of subinternal limiting membrane (ILM) bleed.

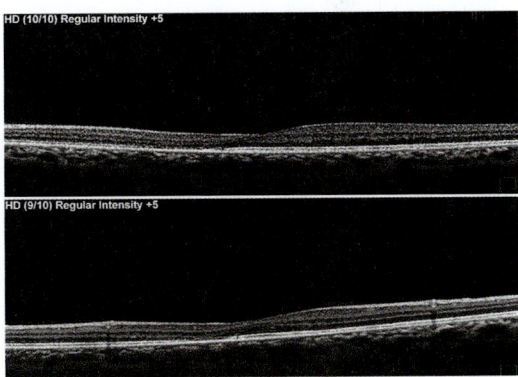

Fig. 7: The optical coherence tomography (OCT) image showing disruption of inner segment–outer segment (IS–OS) junction at fovea, suggestive of photic retinopathy.

- Epiretinal membrane (ERM) and macular pucker
- Full-thickness macular hole (FTMH) (Some FTMHs may close spontaneously, but most cases require surgical repair)

Prevention

- *Laser safety eyewear*
- *Strict safety requirements for use of lasers during public events.*
- *All laser users should be registered with the authorities before a show.*
- *Accountability in case mishaps occur.*

The most effective means to prevent laser-induced ocular injuries is to avoid unprotected exposure and to use "protective safety wear" while using them. Caution must be exercised to avoid ocular injuries and catastrophic visual sequelae.

VIDEO LEGEND

Video 1: Large retinal hole following injury by Q-Switched Nd:YAG laser.

REFERENCES

1. Shah RP, Dabre ZG, Sengupta S. An outbreak of subhyaloid hemorrhage after accidental laser exposure during an Indian festival. Indian J Ophthalmol. 2023;72:S144-7.
2. Lee YH, Kim YC. Foveal choroidal neovascularization secondary to accidental laser exposure in a dermatologist: A case report. Medicine (Baltimore). 2019;98(18):e15429.
3. Kim YJ, Whang KU, Choi WB, Kim HJ, Hwang JY, Lee JH, et al. Efficacy and safety of 1,064 nm Q-switched Nd:YAG laser treatment for removing melanocytic nevi. Ann Dermatol. 2012;24(2):162-7.

Index

Page numbers followed by *b* refer to box, *f* refer to figure, *fc* refer to flowchart, and *t* refer to table.

A

Accommodation 27
    diopters of 37
    near point of 35, 39
    stimulus for 38
    test for 33
Accommodative esotropia 38, 39*f*
    classification of 39*fc*
Acoustic shock waves 11
Active force generation test 46
Adjacent ocular sites 114
Aflibercept 141
Alagille syndrome 71
Allergic 55, 56
Allergy testing 55
Altered plasma fibrinogen levels 127
Amblyopia 39, 48
    classification 49*fc*
    management of 49*fc*
    therapy 86
Amplitude 161
Amplitude spike 166*f*
    mild-moderate 165*f*
Amyloidosis 115
Angle-closure glaucoma
    secondary 107, 108
Angle, neovascularization of 107*f*
Angle recession glaucoma 104
Aniridia 71
Annular fibrovascular proliferation 135*f*
Anomalous collagen 71
Anomalous head posture 35*f*
Anterior chamber cells, minimal 106*f*
Anterior segment barriers, clinical significance 20
Anti-blocking suction tip 13, 13*f*
Anti-inflammatory agents 55, 56
Antioxidant systems 4
Anti-vascular endothelial growth factor 140
Aqueous humor dynamics 21
Aqueous humor formation 20, 21*f*
Argentinian flag sign
    management 101
Artificial intelligence 73
Artificial tears 54
A-scan biometry 84*f*
Asteroid hyalosis 114, 115*f*, 166, 167*f*
Astigmatic neutral zone 15*f*
Astigmatism 31
Aurora borealis 117*f*
Automated perimetry 177*f*
Autosomal dominant pattern 74

B

Bagolini-striated glass 39
Ballet sign 185
Barrage laser 189, 190
Beam orientation 162*f*
Bergmeister papilla 113, 113*f*
Bevacizumab 141
Binocular vision 24
    concept of 35
Binocularity
    and stereopsis, tests for 37*t*
    test for 37
Birmingham Eye Trauma Terminology system 58
Blepharitis 56
Blood aqueous barrier 20
Blood pressure 109*f*
Blunt trauma 79*f*
Boston sign 185
Brolucizumab 141
Brown's syndrome 47, 48
    mild 48
    moderate 48
    severe 48
Brunescent cataract grade 15
Bull's eye 75*f*

C

Capillary occlusion 126
Capsular polish 98
Capsule 2
Capsulorhexis 15, 16, 76, 84, 94, 174
    mastering art of 88
Caruncular
    chemosis 187*f*
    congestion 186*f*
Cataract 5
    acquired 79
    based on maturity of 6
    bilateral 83
        congenital 79*f*
    cerulean 81*f*
    classification of 6
    congenital 40*f*, 71, 79
    coralliform 81, 82*f*
    developmental 79
    formation, pathophysiology of 5
    lamellar 79*f*, 80
    leaking hypermature 106*f*
    lens opacities classification system 6
    mature 101
    membranous 82*f*
    nuclear 80, 80*f*
    posterior polar 18, 74, 74*f*, 81*f*
        classification of 75
    posterior subcapsular 80, 80*f*, 81*f*
    rosette 79*f*
    surgery 77*fc*
    symptomatology of 5
    syndromic 79
    total intumescent 108*f*
    traumatic 67, 68*f*
        oblique with
        unilateral 84
    with phacoemulsification, management of 7
Cavitation energy 11
Center-involved diabetic macular edema 149, 153*f*, 157*f*
Central safe zone 12, 12*f*
Central subfield thickness 150
Cerebrospinal fluid analysis 179, 181*f*
Charleaux oil droplet reflex 72
Chop
    horizontal 17
    vertical 17

Chopping 97
Chorioretinal
　folds temporal 178f
　scarring 190
Choroidal
　detachment 165
　lesions 162
　neovascular membrane 190
　neovascularization 189
　thickness 158
Ciliary body
　band, widening of 104f
　cysts 107
　　multiple 107f
　epithelium of 20
Ciliary congestion, minimal 106f
Closed funnel retinal detachment 164, 164f
Closed-globe
　injury, classification 59b
　trauma, injury zones in 59b, 60f
CM-T flex intraocular lens 103
Collapsin response mediator protein 174
Color vision 24
　reduced 136
　theories of 24
Compliance 13
Computed tomography 158
Concomitant esotropia, acute 40
　classification 40t
　management of 40t
　pathogenesis 40t
Conjunctivitis 54, 55
Consecutive esotropia 40
Contact lens, placement of bandage 63f
Continuous curvilinear capsulorhexis 12, 16f, 90, 95f, 96f, 96
　with forceps 90
　physics of 89
　technique of 88
Convergence
　near point of 39
　types of 41fc
Core vitrectomy 142
Cornea 70f
Corneal biomechanics 72
Corneal collagen crosslinking 73
Corneal decompensation, left eye 187f
Corneal hydrops, acute 72
Corneal injuries 58

Corneal laceration 63f
　management protocols 58
Corneal optical coherence tomography 72
Corneal peripheral tear 68f
Corneal protrusion 72f
Corneal staining
Corneal suturing 62f
　principles 61
Corneal tear 68f
　scarring 69f
　with iris prolapse 68f
Corneal topography 72
Corneal transparency 23f
Corneal visualization Scheimpflug technology 109
Corneoscleral laceration 65
Corneoscleral tear 68f
Cortex 3
　cleaving hydrodissection 16
　management 18
　wash 98, 98f
Cortical matter removal 77
Corticosteroids 56
Cover test 33, 35
Cowen sign 185
Creating limbal groove 94f
Crystallins 4
　proteins, synthesis of 2
Curled posterior flap 165f
Curvilinear laceration 66f
Cyanoacrylate glue
Cyclic esotropia 40
Cyclosporine A 56
Cystic
　changes, minimal 150f
　spaces, right eye multiple 152f
Cystitome 90, 95
Cystoid macular edema 150, 158
Cystotome 88
　versus forceps, technique 89
Cytoskeletal proteins 4

D

Dalrymple's sign 185
Dawson's fingers 182f
Decoding secondary glaucomas 104
Delamination 142
Demyelinating optic neuritis, acute
　clinical features of 176f
Descemet's membrane 72
Dexamethasone 141

Diabetes 128
　type of 128
　eye disease 125
Diabetic eye disease, advanced 135f
Diabetic macular edema 149, 150f, 151f, 152, 153f, 158
　classification of 137b, 149
　location of 149
Diabetic maculopathy 137
Diabetic retinopathy 125, 131f, 136, 140t, 150f, 158
　clinical diagnosis of 128
　clinical stages of 129
　early treatment 136
　ETDRS classification of 136
　management of 138
　mild 150f
　pathogenesis of 125, 125fc
　pathological changes in 126
　rheological changes in 127
　stage of 136, 140
　strategies to treat 139
　surgery for 142
　symptoms of 135
Dilated and tortuous episcleral vessels 105f
Diplopia 32, 169
Direct chopping techniques, types of 96
Disc damage 104f, 105f, 107f
Disc, neovascularization of 136
Dissociated vertical deviation 43, 43f
　management of 43fc
Divide and conquer 16
Domain optical coherence tomography 156f
Dot-like echoes 165f
Double vision and distortions 6
Down syndrome 71, 79
Dry eye disease 54
　chronic severe 54f
Dual-linear foot pedal 8f
　control of 7
Duane's retraction syndrome 44
　management of 47fc
Duke and Elder's classification 75
Dyslipidemia 128

E

Edinger-Westphal nucleus 27f
Edwin Land's theoretical model 24

Ehlers-Danlos syndrome 71
Electrical potential changes 23
Elliptical 10
Embryonal nucleus 3
Emulsified oil particle deposits in angle 105*f*
Emulsified silicone oil in situ 105*f*
Encircling episcleral buckles 169
Endolaser 142
    probe 168
Endophotocoagulation 170
Endophthalmitis 62, 165, 165*f*, 168, 169
    and suture-related infection 86
Endothelial dysfunction 126
Energy delivery, linear mode methods 10*t*
Enroth sign 185
Epicanthal fold 38*f*
Epinuclear material layer 77*f*
Epinucleus 3
Epinucleus management 15, 18
Epinucleus removal 77
    layer-by-layer technique 77
Epiretinal membrane 168, 191
Epithelial cells, migration of 2
Epithelium 3
Esodeviation 35
Esotropia 49
    causes of consecutive 40*t*
Exodeviation 41
    classification of 42*t*
Exotropia 49
    classification 41
Extracellular vesicles 73
Extraocular
    manifestations 173*t*
    movements 35, 186*f*
    muscle
        actions of 34*t*
        disinsertion 169
Extrusion cannula 168
Exudative retinal detachments 171
Eye and vision, physiology of 20
Eye
    irritation 57
    rubbing 71
    sclera's structure 20
Eyeball 20
Eyelid disorders 54
Eyelids 59
    fullness 185
    jerky movements of 185
    retraction 186

F

Faricimab 141
Fat Müller sign 145
Fetal nucleus 3
Fibrosis 184
Fibrous tissue 135
Fibrovascular proliferation 135
Fine keratic precipitates 106*f*
Fleischer's ring 71, 72*f*
Floaters 11, 135
Fluidics 7, 11
    components of 11
    terminologies in 12
Focal laser 141
Focal maculopathy 137
Focal vitreomacular traction 153*f*
Followability, area of
    highest 12
    poor 12
Followability, zones of 12
Foot pedal 7, 8*f*
    controlling machine with 7
    dual-linear control of 7
    excursion, total 10
Forced duction test 46
Forceps 91
    capsulorhexis, safe and effective 90*t*
    in focus 89
    only technique 91
    right 91
    tactile feedback with 91
    transitioning to 89
Foreign body
    retained 168
    type of 58
Foveal burns 188
Fracturing 16
Fuch's corneal dystrophy 71
Fundal coloboma 165, 166*f*
Fundus autofluorescence 173
Fundus fluorescein angiography 137
Fusional vergences, tests for 33

G

Galactosemia 79, 80*f*
Gas 143
Genetic predisposition 128
Ghost cell glaucoma 106
Giant papillary conjunctivitis 56
Giant retinal tear 164, 165*f*, 168
Gifford sign 185

Glaucoma 110*f*
    dynamics 109
    in iridocorneal endothelial syndrome 108
    monitor for 86
    secondary 86
        angle-closure 107
        to raised episcleral venous pressure 105
Glial fibrillary acidic protein 174
Glutathione peroxidase 4
Glycation end products, advanced 125
Glycolytic enzymes 4
Glycosaminoglycan accumulation 184
Golden ring formation 76*f*
Goldmann applanation tonometer 109, 110*f*
    clinical tips 110*f*
Goldzeiher sign 185
Granulomatous panuveitis 171
Grasping 91
Griffith sign 185
Grip 90

H

Handheld laser pointers 188
Hard exudates 127, 131
Head tilt test 46
Heavy eye syndrome, management of 48*fc*
Heminuclei 97*f*
Hereditary vitreoretinopathies 114
Hering opponent theory 24
Hering's law of equal innervation 34
Hirschberg pupillary
    light reflex 36*f*
    reflex test 35
Hormones 71
Horopter, concept of 32
Human immunodeficiency virus 174
Hyaloid traction, posterior 150
Hydrocannula, direction of 95*f*
Hydrodelineation 16, 76*f*
    technique 16*f*
Hydro procedure 15, 16, 76, 95
Hygiene 56
Hyperburst mode 11
Hypercoagulability 127
Hyperintense lesions 181*f*, 182*f*

Hyperpigmented trabecular meshwork 104*f*
Hyperreflective dots 158
Hyperreflective spots, fovea
Hypertension 46, 128
Hyperthyroidism 186*f*
Hypothyroidism 186*f*

I

Incision, triplanar 94
Infantile esotropia 38
Infectious 174
Inferior oblique
    antero-nasal transposition 46
    over-action 43
    paresis 48
    total anterior positioning 43, 46
Inflammation, severe anterior chamber 86
Intense pulse light therapy system 55, 56
Interferometry 55
Intermittent divergent squint 41*f*, 41
    calhounz staging of 42*t*
    management of 42*fc*, 42
Internal limiting membrane 145*f*, 146, 147*f*
International Dry Eye Workshop 54
Intracorneal ring segment 73
Intracystic hyperreflective material 156*f*
Intraocular lens SICSM oblique 66*f*
Intraocular forceps 168
Intraocular foreign body 58
Intraocular lens 103
    foldable 18
    implantation 78
        of foldable 18*f*
    insertion 99
        techniques 85
    secondary 76
    symmetrical 99*f*
Intraocular pressure 20, 21, 22*fc*, 109*f*, 110, 110*f*
    insights into 109
    measure 109*fc*
Intraocular scissors 168
Intraretinal hemorrhage 188

Intraretinal microvascular abnormalities 127, 132, 136
Intrascleral techniques 169
Intravitreal
    anti-VEGF agents, types of 141*t*
    dexamethasone implant injection 157*f*
    injection 140, 169
    steroid injections, types of 141*t*
    triamcinolone acetonide 116*f*
Inverse horseshoe technique 77
Iridocorneal endothelial syndrome 71
Iris
    colour of 68*f*
    multiple 107
    neovascularization of 107*f*
    sphincter tears 104*f*
Ischemic maculopathy 137

J

Jendrassik sign 185
Joffroy sign 185
Juvenile open-angle glaucoma 105

K

Kelman phaco tip 9*f*, 10
Keratoconus 70, 71
    advanced 72*f*
    management 73
Keratoplasty 73
Kinetic echography 162
Kissing choroidals 166*f*
    drainage of 165
Knies sign 185
Kocher sign 185
Krimsky test 35
Krukenberg spindles 104*f*

L

Laceration 63, 63*f*
    full-thickness 62
    partial thickness 62
Lambda technique 76
Laser
    induced ocular injury 188
    light 188
        wavelengths 188

    photocoagulation 170
    treatment, types of 141*t*
Laws governing extraocular movements 34
Lens
    anatomy of 2
    biochemistry 4
    embryology and growth 2
    epithelial cells, proliferation of 2
    equator 2
    growth 2
    induced glaucoma 106, 110*fc*
    physiology 4
    pit formation 2
    placode formation 2
    vesicle formation 2
Lenticonus
    anterior 82*f*
    posterior 82*f*
Lesser vacuum 97
Leukostasis 127
Lhermitte's phenomenon 178
Lid signs 185
Lifestyle modification 55, 186
Light
    delivery, modes of 170
    sensitivity and glare 6
Limbus, anatomy of 1
Linear 10
Linear laceration 65*f*
    repair with intraocular lens 68
    with traumatic cataract 65*f*
Looping 127

M

Mackool phaco tip 9*f*
Macular cysts 190
Macular edema 127
    clinically significant 137
Macular hole 168, 188
Magnetic resonance angiography 46, 185
Magnetostrictive 9
Malignant glaucoma 107
Marfan's syndrome 71, 79, 80*f*, 85*f*
Matrix metalloproteinase-9 test 55
Mean sign 185
Meibomian gland expression 56
Membrane dissection 142
Membrane proteins 4
Metabolic enzymes 4

Microaneurysms 126
 multiple 150*f*
Microphthalmia 75
Micro-pick forceps 168
Micropulse phaco 13
Microtropia 38, 39
 management of 39
Microvascular damage 126
Mittendorf dot 113
Mobius sign 185
Monocular elevation deficiency
  46*f*, 48
 management of 48*fc*
Motion, vertical 8*f*
Mucin secretagogues 55
Munson's sign 71, 72*f*
Muscle signs 185
Myelin oligodendrocyte antibody
  disease 174, 175,
  180, 180*f*
Myopic strabismus fixus 47, 49*f*

N

Nasal regressive pterygium 57*f*
Needle puncture 91
Neodymium-doped yttrium
  aluminum garnet
  76, 188
Neovascular glaucoma 107, 135
Nerve palsy 44, 45*f*
 management of 44, 45*fc*,
  46*fc*, 47*fc*
Neurofibromatosis 71
Neuromyelitis optica spectrum
  disorder 174, 175, 180,
  180*f*, 182*f*
Neurosensory detachment 157*f*
Night vision problems 136
Noncomitant squint 43
Noncontact tonometer 109
Non-Hodgkin's diffuse 117
Nonproliferative diabetic
  retinopathy 129, 136
 mild 131*f*
 moderate 131*f*
Nuclear fragment, removal of 18
Nucleotomy
 standard techniques of 96
 techniques 76
Nucleus 3
 and cortical removal 76
 grade of 10
 management 15, 16

O

Obesity 128
Oblique laceration 66*f*
Oblique overaction, primary
  superior 48
Ocular
 coat excavation 166*f*
 disorders 71
 ischemia, anterior 169
 motility, grading of 36*f*
 perfusion pressure 110*f*
 response analyzer 109
 sonography 162
 surface disease 54
 surface disorders 54
  clinical manifestations 54
  diagnosis 54
  management 54
 surface staining 54
 trauma 58
  classification of 58, 58*fc*
 ultrasonography 160
 types of 161
Oil droplet cataract 80*f*
Oligoclonal bands 179
Oozing fresh blood 189*f*
Open-angle glaucoma,
  secondary 104
Open-globe injury
  classification 59*b*
Open-globe trauma, zones of
  injury in 59*b*, 60*f*
Ophthalmic viscosurgical device
  14, 14*t*, 90
 actions of 14
 advantages of dispersive 14
 disadvantages of
  cohesive 14
  dispersive 14
 use of 14
Optic capture 85
 posterior 85*f*
Optic chiasmal 180*f*
Optic disc 23
 cupping 162
 swelling 180*f*
Optic nerve 165*f*
 head
  cupping 165, 167*f*
  drusen 165, 166*f*
 right 181*f*
Optic neuritis 174, 180*f*, 183*f*
 atypical 175, 175*t*
 bilateral 179*f*

 clinical features 175
 course and prognosis 181
 demographics 175
 diagnosis 178
 etiology 174, 174*t*
 imaging 178
 systemic phenomenon 178
 treatment 179
 typical 175, 175*t*
Optic pathway
 left 183*f*
 right 183*f*
Optical coherence tomography
  15*f*, 113*f*, 137, 137*b*,
  145, 145*f*, 146, 147*f*,
  149*b*, 191*f*
 angiograph 137
 based DME classification
  systems 152*t*
 biomarkers 149
 structural 149
 time-domain 152
 type 152
Orbit
 cellulitis 169
 fat 161*f*
 inflammation 184
 rim 59
Osmotic stress 5
Osteogenesis imperfecta 71
Oval cystic spaces, large 153*f*
Oxidative stress 5, 71
Ozurdex 141

P

Panretinal photocoagulation
  141, 170
Par focalization 93
Paracentral scotoma 177*f*
Paralytic squint 43
 clinical characters of 44
 phases of 44
Parfocalization 94*f*
Pediatric cataract 79
 evaluation of 82
 surgery, complications of 86
 types of 79
Pellucid marginal degeneration
  71
Pentose phosphate pathway
  enzymes 4
Perfluorohexyloctane eye drop 55
Periocular edema 186*f*
Peripheral cortex 3

Peripheral retinal
  holes 188
    photocoagulation 170
Peripheral unsafe zone 12*f*
Peristaltic machine 13
Peristaltic pump 11, 11*f*
Persistent fetal vasculature 75, 113
Persistent hyperplastic primary vitreous cataract 83*f*
Persistent tunica vasculosa lentis remnants 113
Persistent vitreous hemorrhage 135*f*
Phaco chop 17
  technique 76
Phaco console 7
Phaco foot pedal, features of 8*t*
Phaco handpiece 9
Phaco power 8*f*
  delivery 10
Phaco, journey of 7
Phaco tip 9, 12, 13
  in the nucleus 97*f*
  movements, types of 10
Phacodynamics 7
Phacoemulsification 8*f*, 76, 93
  complications of 18
  instrument 16
  machine, components of 7, 8*f*
  partial-occlusion 13
  tips and tricks in 93
  venting mechanism in 13*f*
Phacolytic glaucoma 106
Phacomorphic glaucoma 108
Phosphokinase c 125
Photic maculopathy 188, 190, 191*f*
Photic retinopathy 191*f*
Photochemical alterations 23
Photorefractive keratectomy 73
Phototoxicity, iatrogenic 169
Piezoelectric 9
Pigment dispersion glaucoma 104
Placido disc 72
Platelet dysfunction 127
Pleocytosis 179
Polar cataract, anterior 75, 80, 81*f*
Polycystic ovarian disease 71
Polyol pathway activation 125
Posner–Schlossman syndrome 106
Postcorneal tear OPK 69*f*
Posterior capsular polish 99*f*

Posterior capsular rupture 18
  managing 77*fc*
Posterior capsule
  management 84
  opacification 3
    risk of 3, 84
Posterior capsulorhexis 85*f*
Power delivered, amount of 10
Power
  delivery, effects of 11
  thumb rule for 10
Prepapillary vascular loops 113
Preretinal hemorrhages 146*t*
Prism bar cover tests 33
Prism diopters 42, 43
Proliferative diabetic retinopathy 132, 136
Proptosis 186, 186*f*
Protein 179
  aggregation 5
Pseudoesotropia 35, 38*f*
Pseudoexfoliation
  deposits 104*f*
  glaucoma 104
Pseudomembrane-like structures 165*f*
Pterygium 56
Ptosis 169
Pulfrich phenomenon 178
Pumps, outflow 11
Punctate lens opacities 81, 81*f*
Pupillary
  pathway and reflex 27
  reflex 27*f*
  signs 185

Q

Qualitative tests 54
Quality of life 54
Quantitative echography 162
Quantitative tests 54
Quattro pump 11

R

Radial placement 169
Randot stereoacuity 38*f*
Ranibizumab 141
Rectus
  inferior 43
  lateral 43, 46
  medial 43, 46
  superior 43
Rectus muscle, medial 185*f*

Refraction
  focuses 30
  fundamental principles of 30
  part 30, 31
Refractive
  correction 86
  errors, types of 31
Retina 23
Retinal
  detachment 86, 162, 164
    risk of 135
  disorders 160
  edema 131
  hemorrhages 126, 131, 132*f*
  hole 189, 190
    large 188, 189*f*
  layers 154, 155
  lesions 129*f*
  microvasculature 125
  optical coherence tomography biomarkers 154*t*
  pigment epithelium 173, 188
  tamponade 168
  tear 115*f*
  thickening 153*f*
Retinopathy of prematurity 35, 118
Retinopathy, pathogenesis of 125
Retrofixated iris-claw intraocular lens postimplantation 85*f*
Retroillumination 79*f*, 81*f*, 82*f*
Rhegmatogenous retinal detachment 168
Rigid gas 69
Rizzuti's sign 71, 72*f*

S

Schirmer test 54
  strip 55*f*
Schlemm's
  canal, blood in 105*f*
  classification 75
Scleral
  buckling 169
  incision 15*f*
  lenses 55
Sclerosis, multiple 174, 175, 178, 180, 180*f*, 181*f*
Sculpting 16
Segment structures, anterior and posterior 20*f*
Segmental buckles 169
Segmentation 142

Sensory
  adaptation tests 33
  esotropia 40
    in left eye 40f
  exotropia 42
Serous retinal detachment 150
Serum antibodies 179
Shallow anterior chamber 86
Sherrington's law 34
Sidekicks 7
Silicon oil 143
  induced glaucoma 105
Singh's classification 75
Slit-lamp
  image 70f, 72f, 115f
  microscope 54f
Small incision cataract surgery 7
Smart tips 13
Special examination techniques 162
Spectral-domain optical coherence tomography 151f, 152, 152f, 153f, 155f, 156f, 157f
  left eye 157f
Spongiform macular edema 152f
Squint
  correction of 39f
  evaluation of 33
  restrictive 46f
  surgeries 52f
Stelate laceration 67f
Stellwag sign 185
Stereopsis 24
  concept of 35
  test for 37
Stereopsisbucket handle orientation 26f
Steroid-induced glaucoma 105
Stickler syndrome 114
Stop and chop 18, 96
Strabismus 34
  basic concepts 32
  basics of 34
  classification and management of 43fc
  fixus, etiologies of 47
  large angle of 38
  pattern 42
  sensory evaluation of 35
  surgeries 52
Stroke length 8
Subhyaloid hemorrhage 146
Sub-internal limiting membrane 144

bleed 189, 191f
hemorrhage 144, 144f, 146, 146t, 147f, 148f
  diagnostic criteria 144
  etiopathogenesis 144
  management 146
Subretinal fluid 153f, 157f, 173
Subtenon block 61
Sulphur hexafluoride 143
Superior oblique
  overaction 43
  tendon, shortening of 48
Superior vascular arcade 189f
Superotemporal lens subluxation 80f
Supranuclear cortex 3
Surge 12
  surgeon's control of 14
Sutural cataract 82f
Suture 3
  knot burial 64f
  material 61
  removal 67
Suturing techniques 64, 85
Systemic disorders 71
Systemic lupus erythematosus 174
Systemic phenomenon 178

T

T2W MRI axial section 181f
Tamponade 142
  agents, types of 143
Tan hyphema 106
Tarsal conjunctiva 56
Tear
  film break-up time test 54
  osmolarity test 55
Terrien marginal degeneration 71
Thyroid eye disease 184, 185f
  differential diagnosis 185
  epidemiology 184
  management 185
  mild 186f
  pathophysiology 184
  phases of 184
  sight-threatening 187f
Tilt and chop 17
Tissue
  loss 65
  prevent prolapse of 62
Toothpaste-like material 56f
Topographic echography 162
Torsional 10

Trabecular outflow 22f
Tractional retinal detachment 135, 136
Transpupillary 170
Transscleral cryopexy 169
Triamcinolone acetonide 141
Trivarate tear 67f
  repair 67f
True exotropia 41
True versus pseudoesotropia 35, 41
T-sign posterior scleritis 166
Tuberculosis 174
Tubings, compliance of 13

U

Uhthoff's phenomenon 178
Ultrasonic power 7
Ultrasound
  biomicroscopy 107f, 163t, 165f-167f
  power active 8f
  principle of 160, 160fc
Ultraviolet radiation 71
Uncover test 35
Uveal effusion 108
Uveitic stage 172

V

Vacuum 11
  tubings, high 13
Varicella zoster virus 174
Vasavada classification 75
Vascular lesions 129f
Venous beading 127
  and dilatation 132
Venting 13
Venturi pump 11, 12f
Vernal keratoconjunctivitis 71
Vigouroux sign 185
Visco wash 99
Viscodissection 77
Vision
  basic physiology of 23
  blurred 135
  grades of binocular 35
  loss, sudden painless 136
  threatening diabetic retinopathy 125
Visual acuity 35, 59
  changes in 6
Visual axis opacification 84, 86
Visual evoked potential 179, 183f

Visual field defect 104*f*, 105*f*, 107*f*
Visual pathway 25, 26*f*
Visual recovery 102
Vitrectomy 168
   three port 23-gauge 168*f*
Vitreoretinal
   conditions 162
   lymphoma 117*f*
      primary 117
Vitreous
   anatomy of 113
   cavity 116*f*, 165*f*
   cutter 168
   cyst 116, 116*f*
   degeneration 114, 114*f*
   detachment, posterior 164, 165*f*, 169
   disorders of 113
   hemorrhage 114, 135, 135*f*, 161, 164, 188, 190*f*
      fundus image of 115*f*
      in proliferative diabetic retinopathy 115*f*

Vitritis 116, 116*f*
Vogt–Koyanagi–Harada disease 171, 171*fc*
   classification 171
   complications 173
   differential diagnosis 173
   investigations 172
   pathogenesis of 171, 171*fc*
   treatment 173
Von Graefe sign 185

W

Wagner syndrome 114
Wald's visual cycle 24, 24*fc*
Wald's visual pathway 23
Wedge shaped 81
   cataract 82*f*
   fragmentation 16
Whitnall's hypothesis 176*f*, 177
Wilders sign 185
Worth four dot test 37*f*

Wound
   construction 15, 94
   hydrating 99
   leak 86
   triplanar 15*f*, 4

X

XNIT technique 103
   for scleral fixation of intraocular lens 103

Y

Yoke muscles 34
Young-Helmholtz trichromatic theory 24

Z

Zepto-assisted technique 84
Zonular stress 18